H. Bender, H. Palmedo,
H.-J. Biersack and P. E. Valk
(Editors)

**Atlas of Clinical PET in Oncology
PET versus CT and MRI**

Springer-Verlag
Berlin Heidelberg GmbH

H. Bender, H. Palmedo,
H.-J. Biersack and P. E. Valk (Editors)

Atlas of Clinical PET in Oncology

PET versus CT and MRI

With 157 Figures in 471 Separate Illustrations

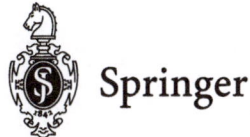 Springer

Hans Bender, MD, ass. Prof.
Holger Palmedo, MD, ass. Prof.
Hans-Jürgen Biersack, MD, Prof. and Chairman

Department of Nuclear Medicine
University of Bonn
Sigmund-Freud-Str. 25
53105 Bonn, Germany

Peter E. Valk, MD

Northern California PET Imaging Center
3195 Folsom Blvd.
Sacramento, CA 95816-5233, USA

ISBN 978-3-642-64093-3   ISBN 978-3-642-59706-0 (eBok)
DOI 10.1007/978-3-642-59706-0

Library of Congress Cataloging-in-Publication Data
Atlas of the Clinical PET in oncology: PET versus CT, MRI /
H. Bender ... [et al.]. p.; cm. Includes bibliographical refer-
ences and index.   .1.   Cancer–   Tomo-
graphy–Atlases. 2. Tomography, Emission–Atlases. 3. Cancer-
Magnetic resonance imaging–Atlases. I. Title: PET versus CT,
MRI. II. Bender, H. (Hans), 1957– . [DNLM: 1. Neoplasms–dia-
gnosis–Atlases. 2. Magnetic Resonance Imaging– Atlases]. 3.
Tomography, Emission-Computed–Atlases. 4. Tomography, X-
Ray Computed–Atlases. QZ 17 A88065 2000] RC270.3.T65 A87
2000 616.99'40757–dc21 99-059592

Springer-Verlag is a company in the
BertelsmannSpringer publishing group.
© Springer-Verlag Berlin Heidelberg 2000
Originally published by Springer-Verlag
Berlin Heidelberg New York in 2000
Softcover reprint of the hardcover 1st edition 2000

Typesetting: Data conversion by B. Wieland, Heidelberg

SPIN: 10693805   21/3135 – 5 4 3 2 1 0
Printed on acid-free paper

Preface

During the past decade positron emission tomography (PET) has been introduced into the clinical management of patients suffering from different malignant tumor entities, such as head and neck cancer, malignant melanoma, colorectal and lung cancer, breast cancer and lymphoma. It has been proven that PET significantly changes the therapeutic strategy in many patients and, additionally, can achieve reduction of costs by improving the staging. Besides the option of whole-body staging, PET offers the unique possibility of monitoring tumor vitality after chemotherapy at a very early time, giving the clinician valuable information for further therapeutic decisions.

The authors of this atlas have accrued great experience in the field of clinical PET. They have undergone a long and intensive phase of autodidactic training in different techniques and pitfalls of PET. High sensitivity and acceptable specificity can be achieved with fluorine-18 deoxyglucose and PET if the nuclear medicine specialist refers to a standardized scheme categorizing the results into malignancy-typical, suspicious and unspecific areas of glucose metabolism.

It is the goal of this atlas to help nuclear medicine specialists and radiologists to overcome the learning phase and typical diagnostic problems of PET. In the editors' experience it is necessary in this context to correlate PET images with CT, MRI and histopathology, not only in order to achieve the best available information about the patient but also to learn about the advantages and limitations of PET.

The book was also written with the intention to present the results of PET as a modern functional imaging technique to the general practitioner, oncologist and oncological surgeon, the source of referrals to the specialist.

The applications of PET will, we firmly believe, become broader with the development of new radiopharmaceuticals aiming to improve diagnosis and staging in oncological patients.

H. PALMEDO
for the editors
Spring 2000

Contents

List of Authors

Abdulaziz Al-Sugair, MD
Department of Radiology
Division of Nuclear Medicine
Box 3949, Duke University Medical Center
Durham, NC 27710, USA

Elma Abella-Columna, MD
Northern California PET Imaging Center
3195 Folsom Boulevard
Sacramento, CA 95816-5233, USA

Peter Albers, MD, ass. Prof
Department of Nuclear Medicine
University of Bonn
Sigmund-Freud-Str. 25
53105 Bonn, Germany

Hans Bender, MD, ass. Prof
Department of Nuclear Medicine
University of Bonn
Sigmund-Freud-Str. 25
53105 Bonn, Germany

Hans-Jürgen Biersack, MD, Prof. and Chairman
Department of Nuclear Medicine
University of Bonn
Sigmund-Freud-Str. 25
53105 Bonn, Germany

Uwe Cremerius, MD
Department of Nuclear Medicine
University of Aachen
Pauwelsstr. 1
52057 Aachen, Germany

R. Edward Coleman, MD
Department of Radiology
Division of Nuclear Medicine
Box 3949, Duke University Medical Center
Durham, NC 27710, USA

Christoph G. Diederichs, MD
Department of Nuclear Medicine
University of Ulm
Robert-Koch-Str. 8
89081 Ulm, Germany

Frank Grünwald, MD, Prof. and Chairman
Department of Nuclear Medicine
University of Frankfurt
Theodor-Stern-Kai 7
60590 Frankfurt, Germany

Rosalie J. Hagge, MD
Department of Radiology
Division of Nuclear Medicine
Box 3949, Duke University Medical Center
Durham, NC 27710, USA

Hartwig Newiger, MD
Siemens AG
Medical Engineering, Nuclear Medicine
Henkestr. 127
91052 Erlangen, Germany

Holger Palmedo, MD, ass. Prof.
Department of Nuclear Medicine
University of Bonn
Sigmund-Freud-Str. 25
53105 Bonn, Germany

Hans-Joachim Straehler-Pohl, MD
Department of Otorhinolaryngology
University of Bonn
Sigmund-Freud-Str. 25
53105 Bonn, Germany

Jörn H. Risse, MD
Department of Nuclear Medicine
University of Bonn
Sigmund-Freud-Str. 25
53105 Bonn, Germany

Peter E. Valk, MD
Northern California PET Imaging Center
3195 Folsom Boulevard
Sacramento, CA 95816-5233, USA

Terry Z. Wong, MD, Prof.
Department of Radiology
Division of Nuclear Medicine
Box 3949, Duke University Medical Center
Durham, NC 27710, USA

Introduction

H.-J. Biersack

Because of managed health care and other economic changes in this area, it is no longer possible to consider numerous different imaging procedures for the solution of a particular problem. In the economic arena of health care, many modalities, such as computed tomography (CT), magnetic resonance imaging (MRI), sonography and nuclear medicine procedures, are becoming competitive rather than complementary. The time has come for nuclear medicine to be promoted for the functional, physiologic, and biochemical capabilities of its radionuclide procedures and to make clear that it is distinctly different in diagnostic capability from the mainly morphologic radiological procedures.

In these "troubled waters" a new clinical – and expensive – imaging procedure has arrived, namely positron emission tomography (PET). While the indications for its use in neurological and myocardial diseases – at least so far – have been limited, malignant tumors are the target for this promising technology. Again, its advantage over radiological procedures such as MRI and CT is its capability to differentiate between viable and dead tumor tissue. MRI and CT can only detect enlarged lymph nodes (above 1 cm) and not whether tumor remnants are alive or dead. On the other hand, normal-sized lymph nodes are considered normal although they may be invaded by tumor tissue. After radiation or chemotherapy, a tumor remnant may be present. Viable tissue can only be detected by 3-month follow-up with CT and MRI. Another advantage of PET is its ability to look at the entire body and not only at restricted areas. Clinical studies during the past 10 years have shown that PET is more sensitive than CT and MRI in many tumors. However, in many cases the combination with radiological procedures is necessary, for example in head and neck tumors. It may be speculated that PET should be the first study on a malignant tumor when metastatic spread is suspected. MRI and CT may then be restricted to those body areas which present with sites of physiologically increased glucose metabolism e. g. brain. Thus, a combination of metabolic and morphologic procedures will certainly enhance tumor detection and change the therapeutic strategy. In this case, newer and expensive imaging procedures may reduce overall expenditure by reducing the cost of therapy. Another field for the combined use of PET and CT/MRI will be monitoring of the response to therapy. As mentioned above, radiological procedures require a follow-up period of 1–3 months, but PET may immediately predict the outcome as glucose metabolism is reduced as early as 3 days after therapy. PET studies can be restricted to radiology-proven tumor sites. These remarks make it evident that an atlas including PET, CT, MRI, and histology data is desirable to combine metabolic and morphologic imaging. The chapters in this volume on distinct tumor entities present an overview of these data, which will not only assist the training of our colleagues from radiology and nuclear medicine, but will also help to convince our partners in oncology. At the turn of the millennium, PET needs to fulfill its promise in one of the most threatening diseases facing mankind: cancer.

Principles of Positron Emission Tomography

H. Newiger

The existence of positrons was predicted by P. A. M. Dirac in the year 1927. The first positrons were observed by C. Anderson 5 years later. Shortly after these physical experiments, the use of positron emitters for medical imaging was discussed. An initial technical prototype of a PET scanner was described by H. O. Anger, who used two gamma cameras operating in coincidence mode. But due to physical and engineering challenges it took some time before commercial systems started to expand the availability of PET in the late 1980s. Today in more than 300 centers worldwide PET is in clinical use and demonstrates the additional sensitivity and specificity this method is able to contribute to diagnostic procedures in oncology.

The most commonly used positron emitter is ^{18}F. This isotope of fluorine has a half-life of 110 min and can therefore easily be distributed from its site of production to the hospital for clinical use. In addition fluorine can replace an OH group in many biologically relevant molecules, for example in ^{18}F-FDG, which is the "working horse" of clinical PET today. It is described in Sect. 2.1.

The ideal physical properties of the positrons allow the design of sophisticated positron emission tomographs. Its intrinsic technology will be described in Sect. 2.2.

2.1 F-18 Fluorodeoxyglucose (FDG)

Today, the most commonly used PET tracer is 2-[^{18}F]-2-deoxy-D-glucose (FDG). Its biochemical properties together with ^{18}F's half-life of 110 min allow an effective use in clinical PET.

2.1.1 Production of FDG

^{18}F$^-$, produced by a cyclotron, is used for the synthesis of FDG. Today, commercial modules (Fig. 1) are available, which allow the fully automated production of FDG. The synthesis is based on the method described by Hamacher et al. (1986). When the FDG has successfully passed the necessary quality control it can be distributed to the PET center, ready for patient use.

2.1.2 Biochemical Characteristics of Glucose and FDG

As FDG has a very similar metabolism to glucose, FDG can be used to determine the glucose metabolism in vivo. Cells with glucose consumption will also accumulate FDG.

In the body glucose is needed mainly by the nervous system and the erythrocytes, but other organs and cells also consume glucose. This is especially true for fast growing tumors.

Whereas glucose is metabolized completely into water and CO_2, the metabolism of FDG stops after the first step (Fig. 2), which is the phosphorization. The 2-FDG-6-phosphate is trapped in the cell. FDG imaging therefore allows the detection of cells metabolizing glucose with a high contrast.

2.1.3 The Tracer FDG

Approximately 50% of the injected FDG is not metabolized. It is extracted by the kidneys and then accumulates in the bladder. Another 20% is found in the brain. The rest is accumulated by other organs and cells. Especially

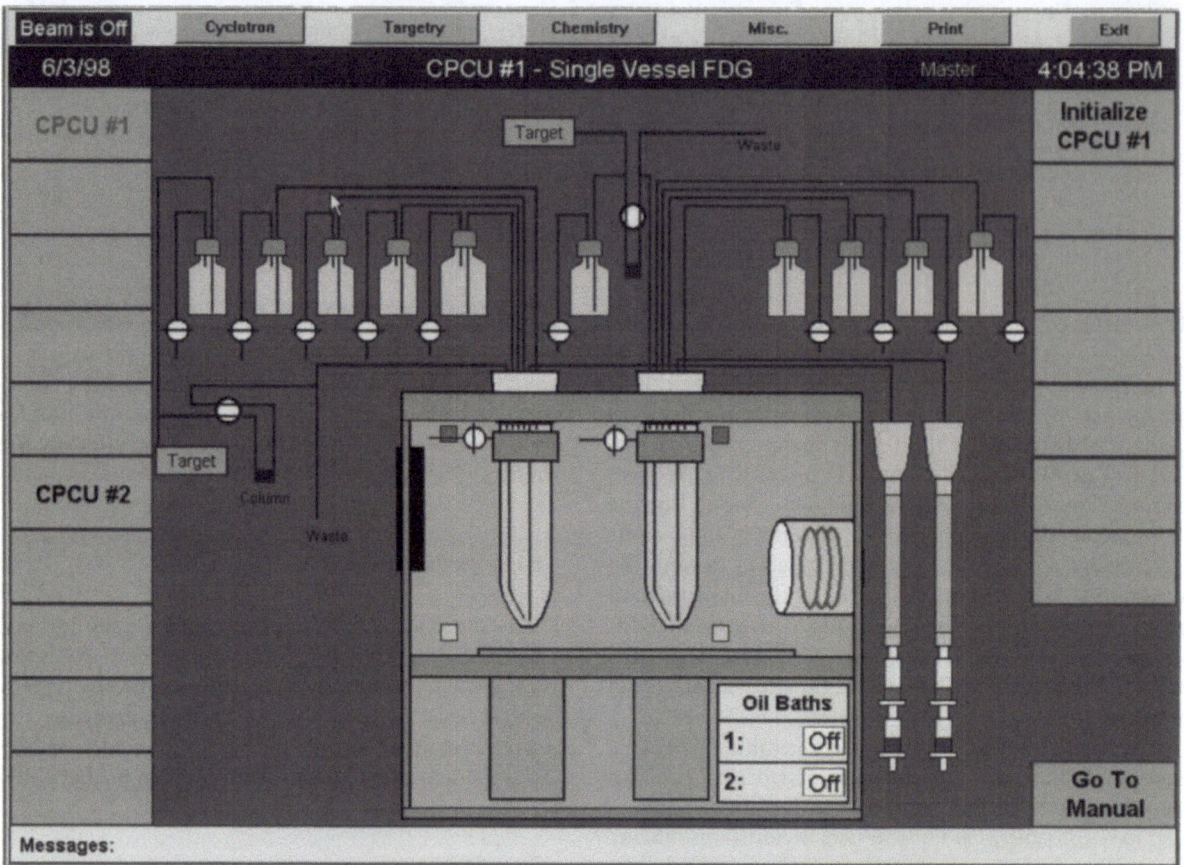

Figure 1 ▲

Synthesis module for FDG. Display of the monitor controlling the cyclotron and the chemical synthesizer for production of FDG

Figure 2 ▼

Metabolism of glucose and FDG. Comparison of the metabolic pathway of glucose and FDG

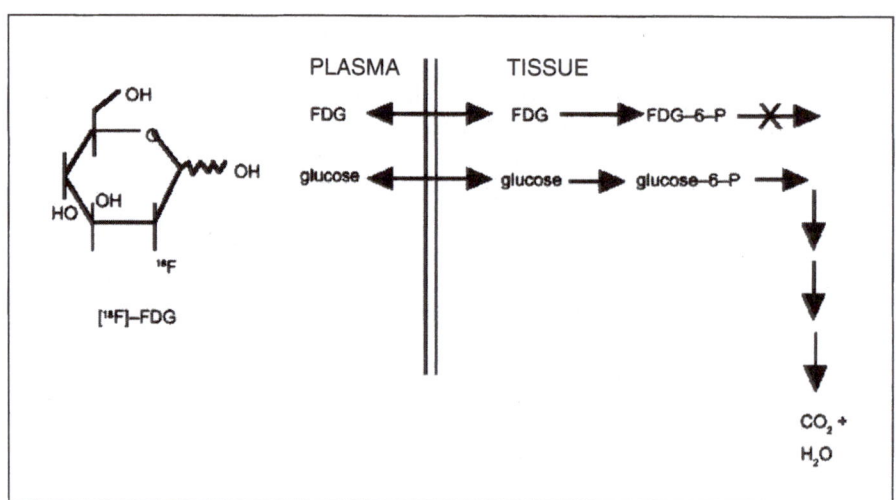

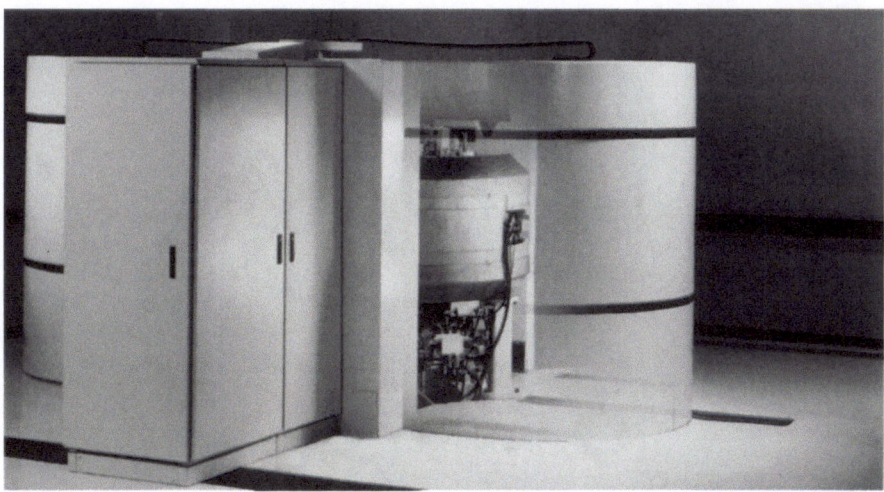

cancer cells have the tendency for a high metabolic rate of glucose (Warburg 1931).

This phenomenon is the basis of clinical PET in oncology: tumors and metastasis often have a high metabolic rate of glucose and accumulate FDG. With high contrast these lesions can be visualized and quantified by PET.

Figure 3

Compact cyclotron for the production of positron emitters (CTI RDS 111). Computer aided graphic of the CTI's cyclotron RDS 111: the actual cyclotron is overlaid by the self shielding of the cyclotron

2.2 Principles of Measurement

2.2.1 Production of Positron Emitters

Positrons are elementary particles like electrons. Their physical properties are the same. The only difference is their positive charge (compared to the negative charge of the electrons). In positron emitters the number of protons is high compared to the number of neutrons. As a consequence these atomic nuclei are unstable. Their half-life is so short that positron emitters cannot be found in nature. They have to be produced using, for example, a cyclotron (Fig. 3).

In a cyclotron, for example, charged particles like protons or deuterons are accelerated. When their energy is high enough, they are extracted and directed to a target. Such a target could be, for example, $H_2^{18}O$. In a nuclear reaction the ^{18}O of this water will be converted into the positron emitter ^{18}F.

Other clinically used positron emitters which can be produced with a cyclotron like the RDS 111 are ^{11}C, ^{13}N, and ^{15}O.

In a chemical synthesis, biological tracers are labeled with these positron emitting isotopes, ready for clinical use.

2.2.2 ß⁺-Decay and Detection of Positrons

When a positron emitter is decaying a proton of the nucleus is converted into a neutron, a neutrino and a positron. The neutron stays in the nucleus of the nuclide, but the neutrino and the positron are emitted. Due to its physical properties there is nearly no interaction of the neutrino with surrounding material. It just disappears.

As the physical properties of the positron are basically the same as for an electron, the positron reacts with matter next to the positron emitter. Scatter processes slow it down. When it nearly comes to a halt, the positron captures an electron. For a very short moment in time they form a structure called a positronium. However, since they act as material and antimaterial, in a process called annihilation the two masses are converted into two gamma rays traveling in exactly the opposite direction. Due to the law of conservation of energy, the energy of these two quanta is 511 keV each. Detecting the two quanta with two opposing detectors "at the same time" (coincidence) results in information on the position of the positron emitter (Fig. 4). To allow the detection of annihilations which are not exactly in the center between two detectors, a coincidence timing window is used. If the two detectors register an event within 12 ns, this is counted as a coincidence.

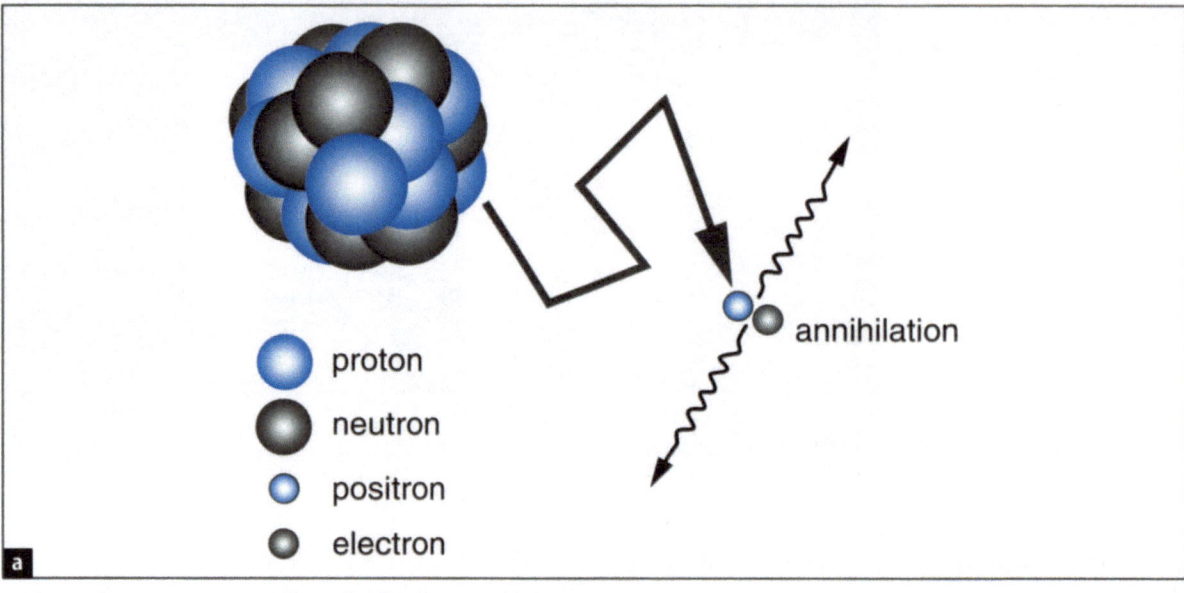

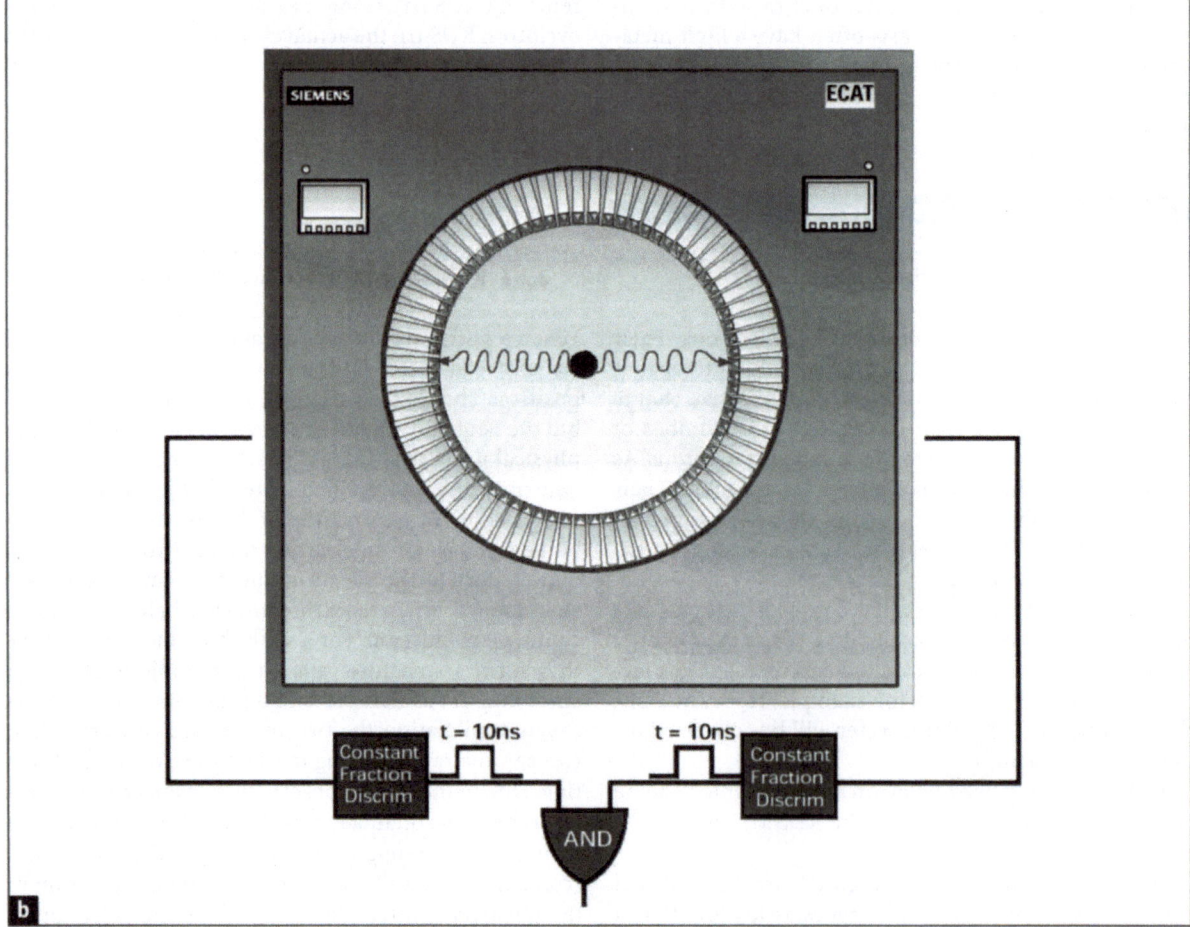

Figure 4 a, b

Schematics of β⁺-decay and detection of positrons. The principle of positron decay and detection of the gamma rays generated by the annihilation of the positron is shown

Table 1. Characteristics of positron emitters used. [a] From Derenzo (1979) except the values marked with [b], which are estimates.

Isotope	Half-life (min)	Maximum energy (MeV)	FWHM[a] (mm)	FWTM[a] (mm)
F-18	109.7	0.635	0.22	1.09
C-11	20.4	0.96	0.28	1.86
N-13	9.96	1.19	0.60[b]	2.8[b]
O-15	2.07	1.72	1.1[b]	5.3[b]
Ga-68	68.3	1.90	1.35	5.92
Rb-82	1.25	3.35	2.6	13.2

As the two gamma quanta with an energy of 511 keV originate from the annihilation process, the point of annihilation is between the two detectors detecting the two quanta. The positron emitter may be somewhat off this line, depending on the distance the positron has traveled from the point of emission to the point of annihilation. The length of this path depends on the intrinsic kinetic energy of the positron, which relates to the physical properties of the positron emitter itself (see Table 1). This effect will limit the theoretical resolution of a PET scanner. A similar effect is that the remaining angular momentum of the positron and/or electron causes a deviation in the opposite direction of the two gamma rays. Both effects limit the intrinsic resolution of a clinical positron emission tomograph to 2–3 mm.

2.2.3 Detectors for PET

Due to the high energy of 511 keV the detectors for PET have to be designed carefully. Historically NaI(Tl) was the first PET detector. But the physical properties of this material are not ideal for the detection of positrons. Therefore, today nearly all scanners are equipped with BGO scintillators (bismuth germanate). BGO offers both a high density for effective stopping of the gamma quanta and easy handling and manufacture.

The breakthrough in detectors for clinical PET was the introduction of the block detector. With this detector a high resolution can be achieved within an image plane together with a small spacing of adjacent image planes. In a typical clinical PET scanner, such a block detector (Fig. 5) combines an array of 8 × 8 individual crystals. Four photomultiplier tubes (PMT) convert the scintillations into electrical signals.

Using adjacent rings of such block detectors, axial FOVs of 15–16 cm can easily be achieved. If for large organs or for whole body scans, more extended axial field of views are needed, the patient bed will translate axially. Using this method whole body scans up to a total length of 195 cm can be performed.

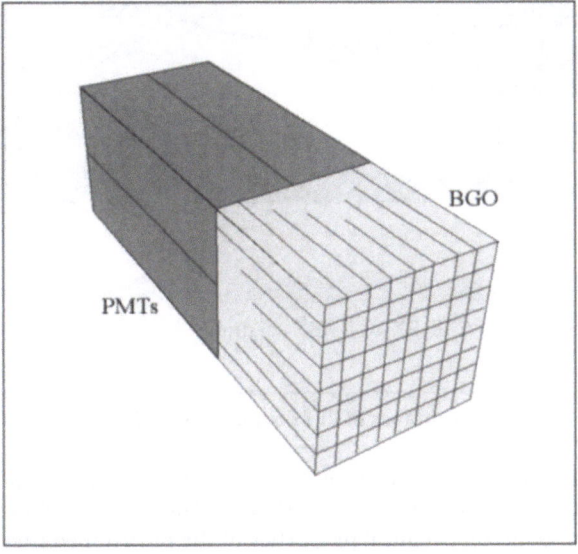

Figure 5

Schematics of a block detector for PET. The block detector of ECAT scanners combining 64 individual BGO (bismuth germanate) detectors with 4 PMTs (photomultiplier tubes) is shown

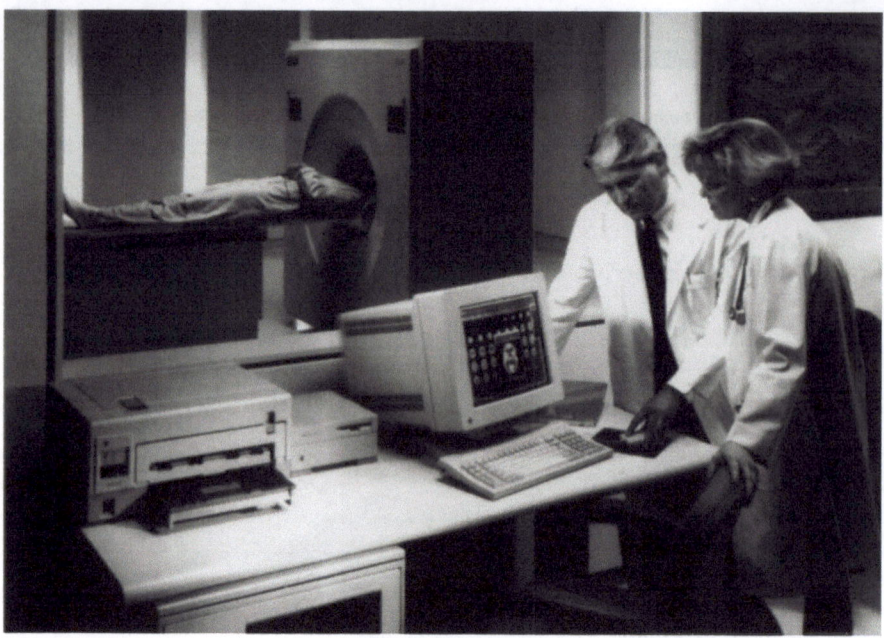

Figure 6

Siemens ECAT EXACT PET scanner

2.2.4 Advantages of PET Compared to SPECT

PET offers several advantages compared to single photon emission tomography (SPECT). These are the physical and biochemical properties of the positron emitter as well as the method of detection itself.

A SPECT system needs a collimator to detect the direction of the incoming gamma rays. The design of this collimator defines the sensitivity and the resolution of this system. Both parameters are related to each other and have to be optimized. In addition, the collimator forces a movement of the detector or the collimator itself to acquire all the projections needed for a complete data set. The volume has to be scanned sequentially.

In PET the coincidence defines the line of response (LOR). No additional collimator is needed. The resolution is only determined by the size of the detector and/or the size of its detecting element. The sensitivity of the device can be optimized independently. In modern PET scanners the detectors are placed in a circular fashion around the patient, covering the whole field of view simultaneously, or banks of detectors rotate with high speed around the patient, simulating a ring detector.

High resolution (e.g., a factor of 2–4 better than SPECT) and sensitivity (e.g., a factor of 10–100 better than SPECT) is possible with PET. In addition, the resolution and sensitivity are nearly constant within the entire field of view (FOV).

A certain portion of the gamma quanta being emitted are absorbed in the patient. An attenuation correction is therefore needed for quantitative imaging. In contrast to SPECT imaging a correct mathematical solution is possible. Transmission images with an external source allow the determination of the local distribution of the attenuation coefficient. This knowledge can be used to correct the emission data. As a result the image matrix can be displayed in absolute units (e.g., specific activity). Normalizing these units to the injected dose and to the weight of the patient allows the calculation of standard uptake values (SUV). The SUV can be used to compare the uptake of the tracer in different areas of the patient or between different patients.

The tracers used in PET are all very "biological". The labeling with ^{15}O, ^{11}C, ^{13}N, or ^{18}F does not change the structure of the biomolecules used. Taking into account the biochemical model of the metabolism of these tracers, even the metabolic rate of the tracer can be calculated. For this procedure blood samples are needed to determine the input function.

2.2.5 Quantitative PET

The above mentioned evaluation of quantitative PET requires a careful correction of all measured parameters, as there are:

2.2.5.1 Random Coincidences

Two events detected by two opposing detectors during the coincidence window may not originate from the same annihilation. Such a random coincidence will degrade the image quality and therefore has to be corrected. Random coincidences are proportional to the single rate of each detector and the length of the coincidence window. Knowing the exact rate of each detector and the length of each coincidence window allows the determination of the random coincidences. But, due to the total number of factors and the accuracy needed, this method is no longer used. A more effective way of correcting the prompt coincidences (e.g., the coincidences measured in the coincidence window) is by measuring the random coincidences directly within a delayed coincidence window of equal length. In this way random coincidences can be corrected in real time individually for every LOR.

2.2.5.2 Attenuation

A portion of the emitted 511-keV gamma rays are absorbed in the patient. This portion has to be corrected to obtain the correct distribution of the positron emitters. Attenuation can be corrected in PET by means of an external source. Most often ^{68}Ge/^{68}Ga-rod sources are used. For a transmission measurement these sources are extended from their lead shield into the FOV. Rotating around the patient, transmission data are acquired. These can be used to correct the emission data from this patient.

Recently ^{137}Cs-point sources have been used for the transmission measurement. In spite of being a single photon emitter with higher photon energy, these sources produce very acceptable transmission scans.

For both methods a segmentation of the transmission data sets improves the statistical accuracy of the correction significantly.

For brain imaging often a measured attenuation correction is not needed. By defining the contours of the brain a calculated attenuation map will provide correction factors with sufficient accuracy.

2.2.5.3 Scatter

A certain fraction of the events detected will be scattered within the patient. Although the design of the PET scanner reduces the effect of scatter by means of shields, septa, and energy discrimination, the remaining scatter has to be corrected. Whereas in standard 2D imaging easy mathematical models may be adequate, in the more sophisticated imaging situation with large angles of acceptance more complex models have to be used. These corrections reduce the effect of scattering significantly.

2.2.5.4 Dead Time

As every detector experiences dead time effects, these have to be evaluated carefully and, if possible, corrected. Standard correction schemes measure the rate of singles, true coincidences, random coincidences, and the detector lifetime in real time. Correction factors based on these measurements are applied to the data measured and the dead time effects can be neglected up to high count rates.

2.2.6 New Imaging Techniques

Recent developments in PET include 3D acquisition, iterative reconstruction, and new detector materials.

2.2.6.1 3D Acquisition

Standard PET scanners acquire data for each image slice individually (2D). The reconstruction is therefore easy, fast, and straightforward. Most often, filtered back projection is used. In addition, interslice septa can be added to reduce scatter effects significantly.

In 3D acquisition all possible coincidences are used to create the image. No septa are used. Therefore the sensitivity of 3D is a factor of 3–5 higher than for 2D (see Fig. 7). As data are no longer acquired individually for each slice, more sophisticated reconstruction algorithms have to be employed, such as PROMIS or FaVor. Rebinning the data into 2D data sets will increase the speed of reconstruction. Whereas methods like single or multislice rebinning (SSRB or MSRB, respectively) introduce significant non-isotropic resolution, Fourier rebinning (FORE) allows the conservation of the excellent intrinsic imaging characteristics of PET.

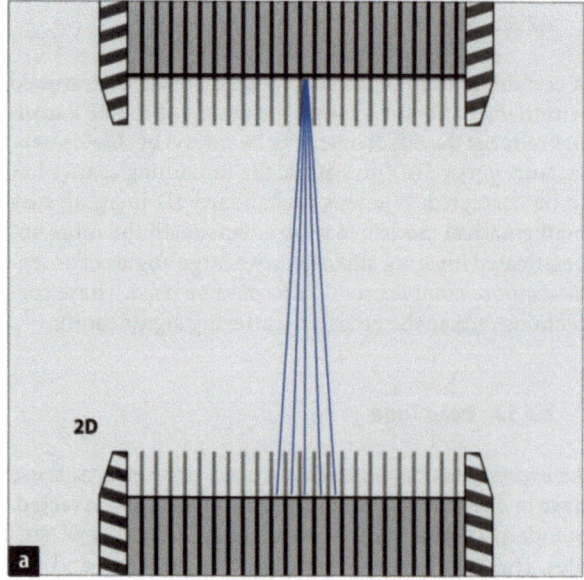

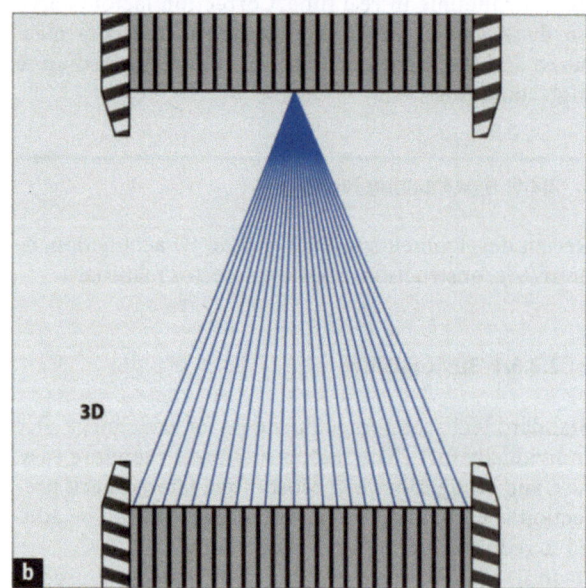

Figure 7 a, b

Comparison of 2D and 3D acquisition

2.2.6.2 Iterative Reconstruction

Filtered back projection is a fast and easy way to reconstruct PET data. Unfortunately high contrast and low image statistics may create significant striping artifacts in the reconstructed image. Iterative reconstruction is able to reconstruct images with fewer artifacts and higher contrasts. Improvements in computer power and new

Table 2. Characteristics of PET detectors

Parameter	NaI (Tl)	BGO	LSO
Density (g/cm3)	3.67	7.13	7.4
Mean free path (cm)	2.88	1.05	1.16
Index of refraction	1.85	2.15	1.82
Hygroscopic?	Yes	No	No
Rugged?	No	Yes	Yes
Decay time (ns)	230	300	40
Light output (relative)	100	15	75
Energy resolution (%)	7.8	10.1	<10

mathematical models allow today the use of iterative reconstruction in clinical routine. Most often OS/EM is used as a fast and effective method for the reconstruction of PET data.

2.2.6.3 New Detectors

NaI(Tl) is an ideal scintillator for low energy imaging but has a low stopping power for the 511-keV quanta. In addition it is hygroscopic and its count rate performance is limited. The use of PET with NaI(Tl) is therefore restricted to certain applications.

BGO's stopping power is adequate and BGO is not hygroscopic. But the decay constant for the scintillation light is similar to NaI(Tl). And its light output is relatively low.

The newly discovered scintillator lutetium-oxy-ortosilicate (LSO) combines all the characteristics needed for PET. It is fast, has a high light output, and the stopping power is comparable to that of BGO (see Table 2).

The first tests with this new scintillator justify the expectations for this material. PET scanners with this new detector will improve the imaging performance.

References

Derenzo SE (1979) Proceedings of the 5th Annual Conference on Positron Annihilation, Sendai, Japan

Hamacher K, Coenen HH, Stöcklin G (1986) Efficient stereospecific synthesis of non-carrier-added 2-[18F]- fluoro-2-deoxy-D-glucose using aminopolyether supported nucleophilic substitution. J Nucl Med 27:235–238

Warburg O (1931) The metabolism of tumors. Richard R. Smith, New York, pp 129–169

Normal Findings

H. Bender and H. Palmedo

3.1 Technique

- Overnight fasted patients
- Blood sugar <120 mg%
- Transmission scan: 7–10 min/bed position
- F-18-DG 370 MBq as intravenous bolus followed by a 10-ml saline flush
- Diuretic (Lasix 10 mg i. v. together with FDG)
- Oral hydration (0.7–1 l water)
- Resting period 60–90 min (separate, darkened room, lying)
- Emission scan: 10 min/bed position
- Image reconstruction: filtered backprojection, Hann filter, xyz-smoothing, decay and attentuation correction

3.2 Qualitative Image Assessment

- Intense physiological uptake is regularly observed in:
  - Brain (cortex, basal ganglia, cerebellum)
  - Kidney (pelvic area)
  - Urine bladder
- Intense physiological uptake is variably observed in:
  - Myocardium (non-fasted status, postchemotherapy)
  - Muscle (movement, tense patients)
  - Small muscles of the tongue
  - Distal ureters
  - Rectum
- Moderate physiological uptake is regularly observed in:
  - Mucosa of the head and neck area
  - Liver (mostly homogeneous, rarely spotty)
  - Spleen
  - Kidney (parenchyma)
- Moderate physiological uptake is variably observed in:
  - Larynx
  - Hilum of the lung
  - Ascending and thoracic aorta
  - Stomach wall
  - Gut (ascending and descending colon, rectum)
  - Bone marrow (unspecific BM activation due to infections or postchemotherapy: ribs, sternum, spine, pelvis)
- No uptake is regularly observed in:
  - Maxilla and mandible in the area of the roots of the teeth (gum)
  - Stomach content

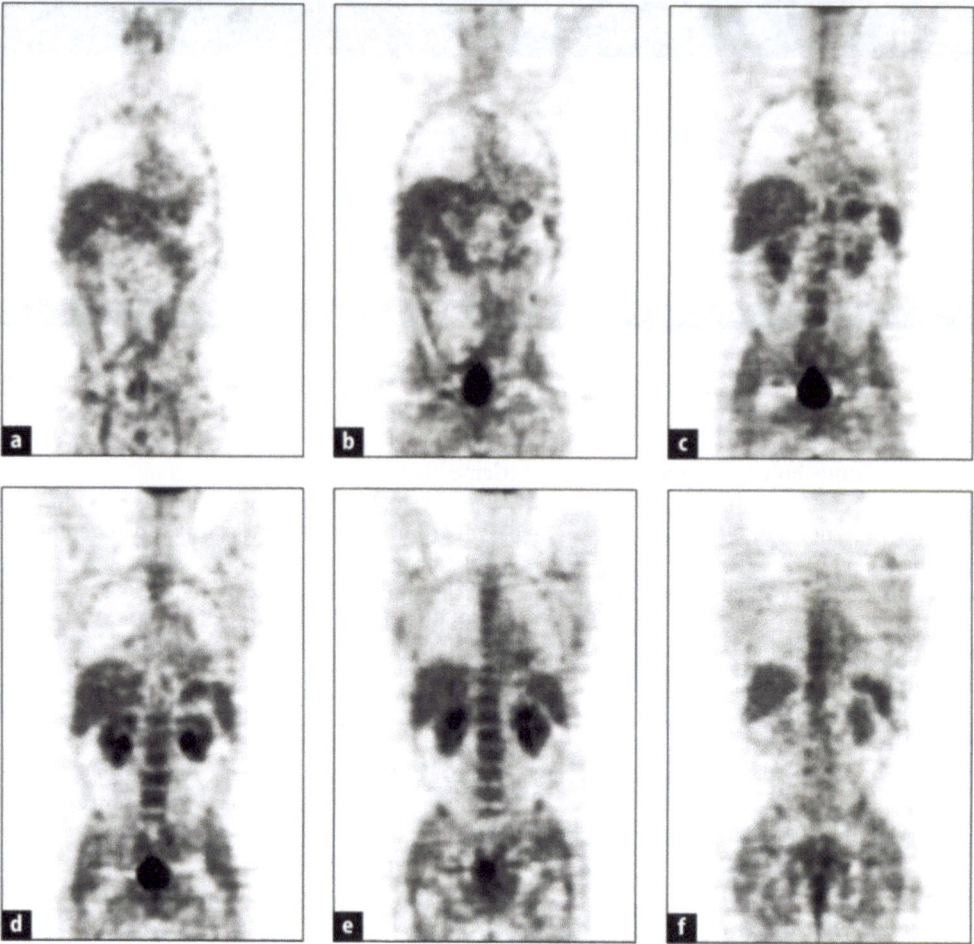

Figure 1 a–f

Series of coronal views of a normal patient (no evidence of disease). Physiological uptake can be seen with

- high intensity:
    - brain (cerebellum, **d**)
    - pelvis of both kidneys (**d–e**)
    - bladder (**b–e**)
- moderate intensity:
    - nasal/oval cavity (**a**)
    - liver (**a–f**)
    - spleen (**c–f**)
    - stomach (**b–c**)
    - gut (**a, b**)
    - bone marrow containing bones (spine, pelvis, stenum)
- minimal intensity:
    - mediastine including myocardium
- no uptake (background activity)
    - lung

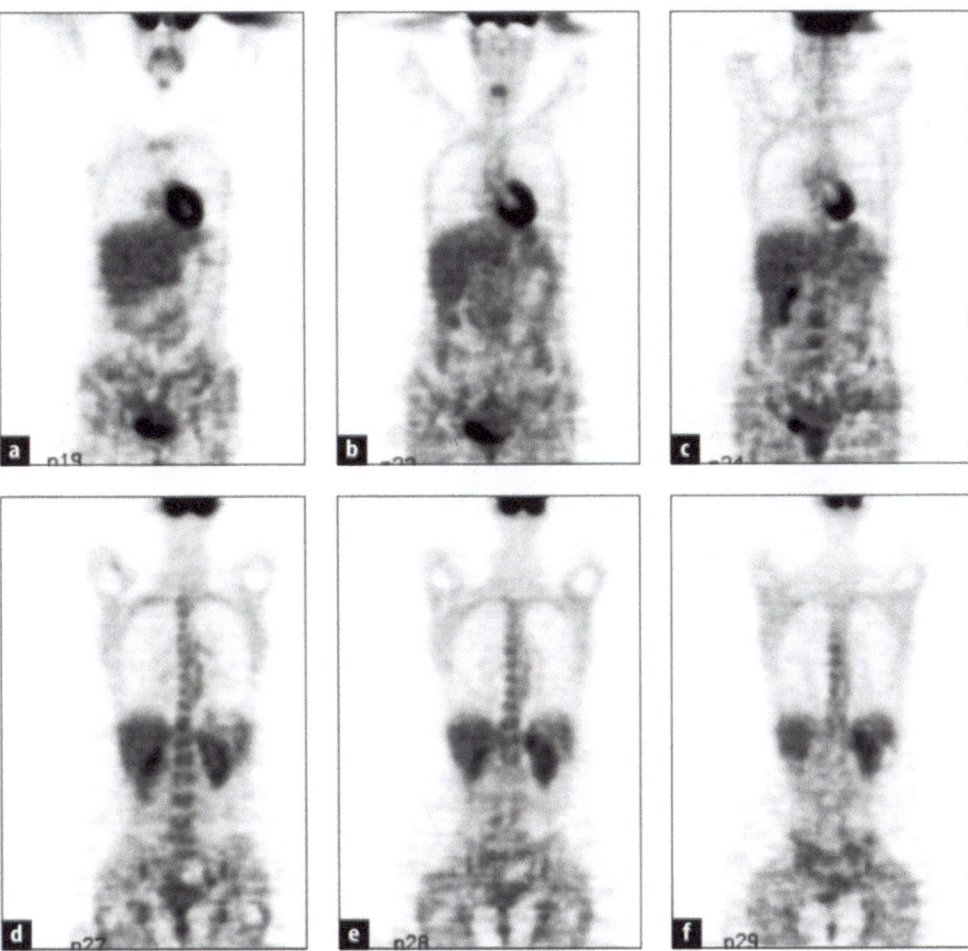

Figure 2 a–f

Normal variants as compared to Fig. 1 a–f.
- Intense uptake can be observed in myocardium (**a–c**).
- Moderate uptake in larynx (**b**).

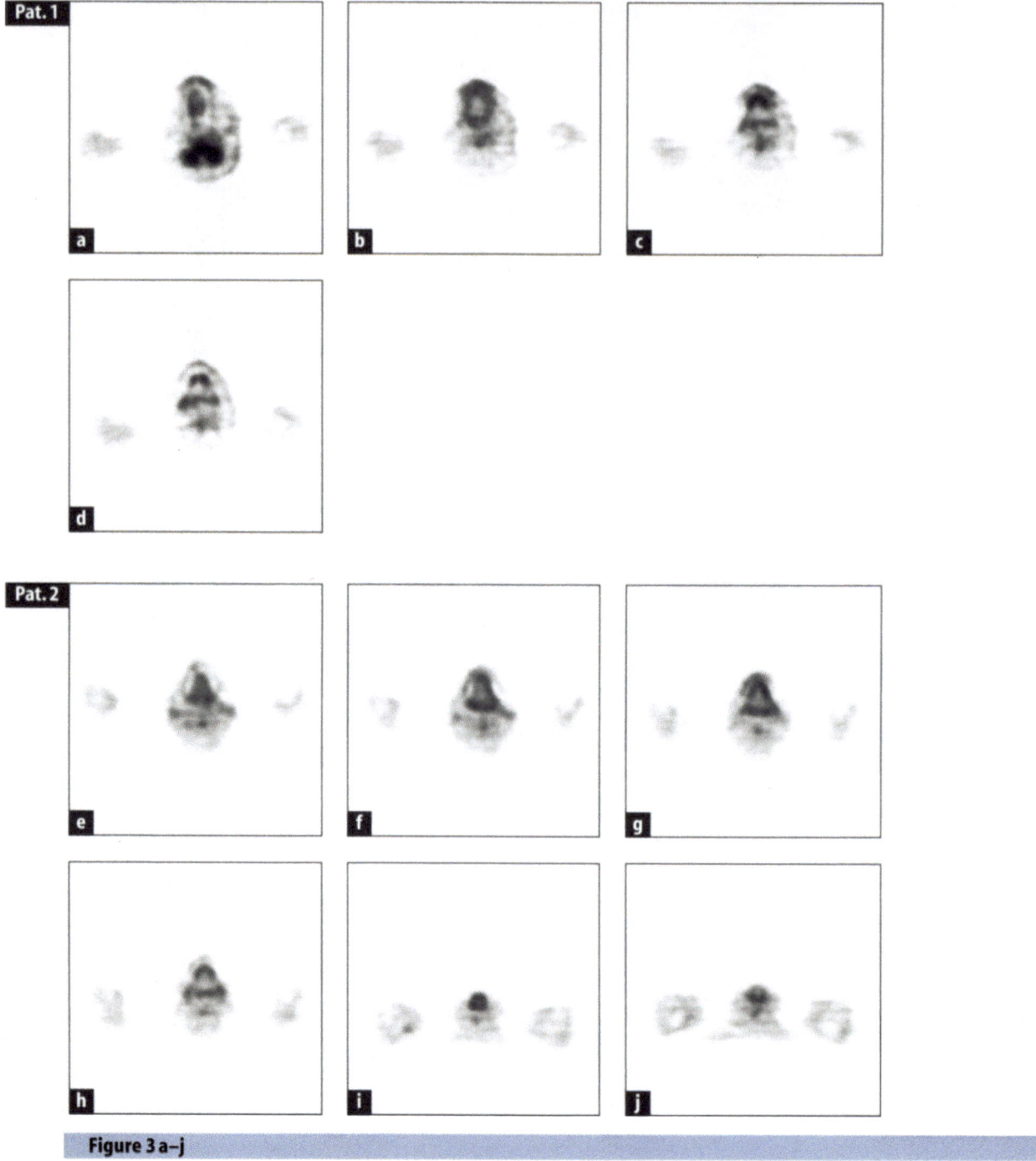

Figure 3 a–j

Series of transverse views of the head and neck region without the brain (disease-free patients).

Note: Intense uptake in the cerebellum (**a**), moderate uptake in the mucosa of the nasal/oral cavity (**a, b**), small muscles of the base of the tongue (**c–h**), Waldeyer's lymph nodes (**d**), parotis (**e**), and larynx (**i, j**).

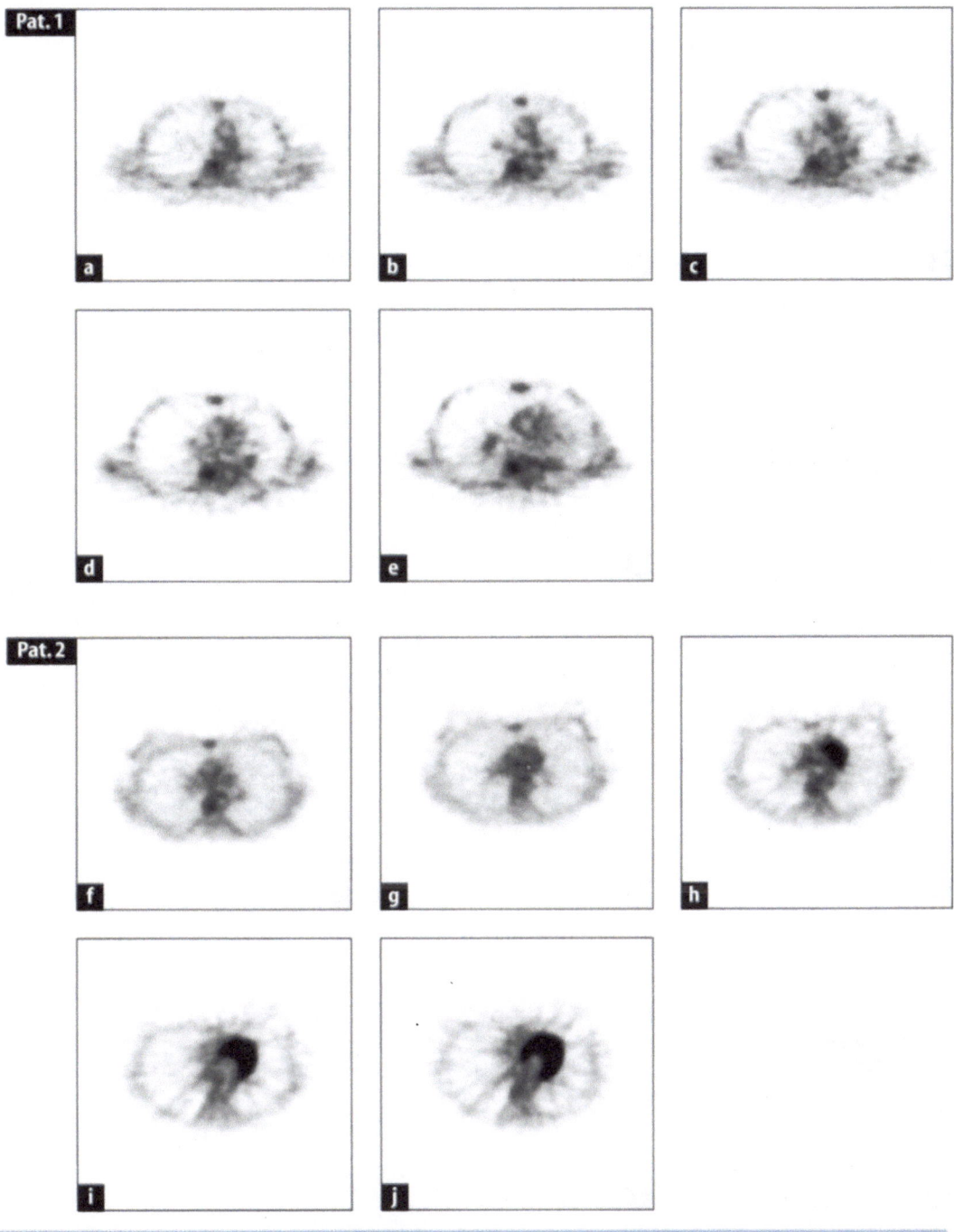

Figure 4 a–j

Series of transverse views of the thorax (no evidence of disease in this region).

Note: Intense uptake in the myocardium (**h–j**), moderate uptake in the mediastine (**a–j**), hilum of the lung (**b, d, e**) and sternum (**b–g**).

Figure 5 a–j

Series of transverse views of the upper abdomen (no evidence of disease).

Note: Intense uptake in the kidneys (**d, e, g–j**), moderate uptake (homogenous) in liver (**a–d, f–j**), spleen (**b–e**) and stomach (**b, c**), activity defect in the stomach content (**g–i**).

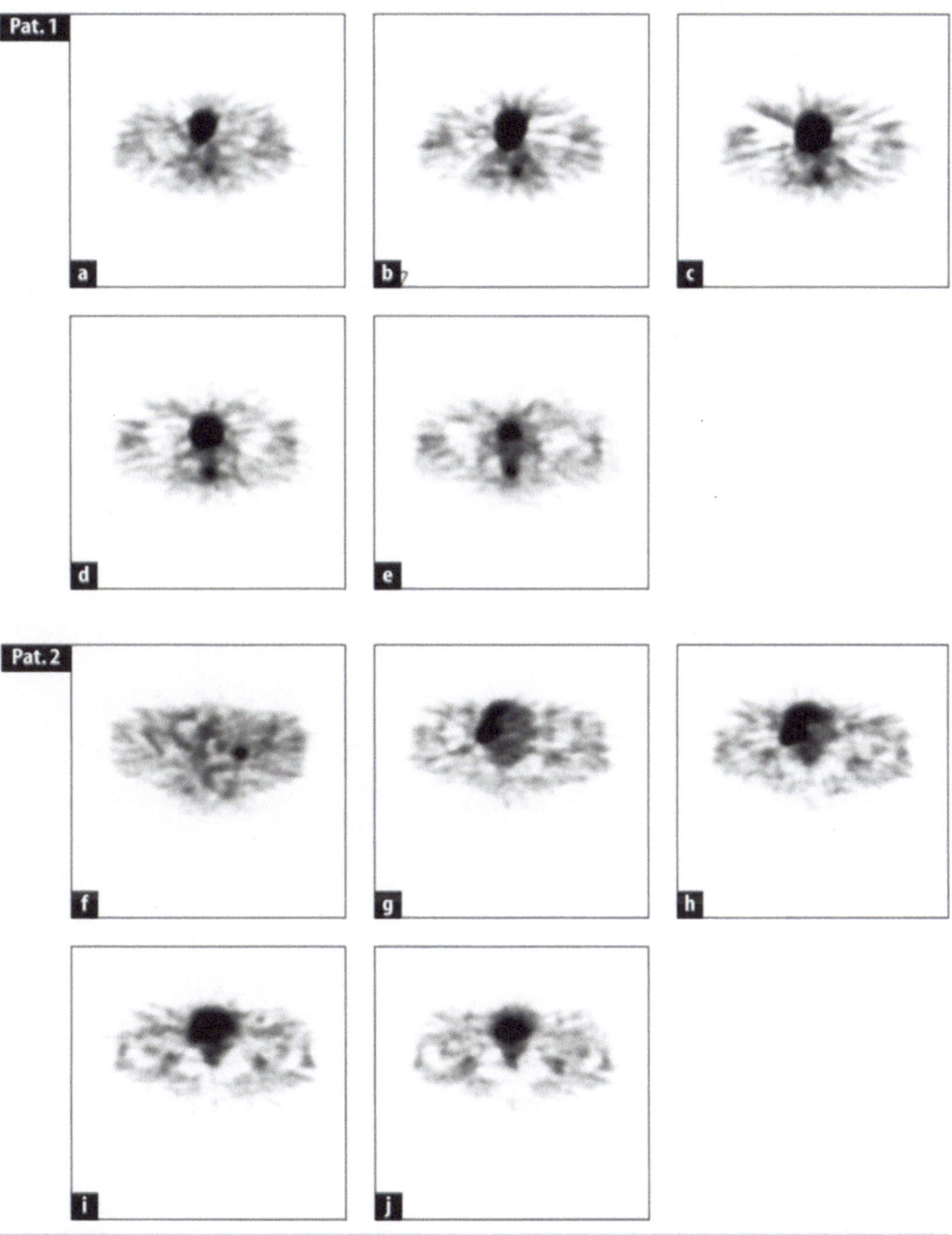

Figure 6 a–j

Series of transverse views of the pelvis.
Note: Intense uptake in rectum (**a–e**), irregular shaped urine bladder (**g–i**) due to displacement by the uterus (small urine depot in the left ureter (**f**).

Cancer of the Head and Neck

H.-J. Straehler-Pohl and H. Bender

Head and neck cancers represent roughly 3–5% of the total new cancer cases. In the United States 40,000 new cases are observed each year. The male-to-female ratio is 3:1. While head-and-neck tumors were primarily tumors of older males, a significant increase of the incidence has been observed in female and younger patients. Significant risk factors are nicotine and alcohol abuse. Characteristically, head and neck tumors often become occult for a long time either due to their primary localization of the tumor and/or due to a rather late consultation of a physician.

More than 90% of the tumors are histologically squamous cell carcinomas, which show avid glucose utilization.

4.1 Primary Tumor

Figure 1 a–c

Diagnosis: Cancer of the nasal cavity.

Patient and History: 72-year-old patient with a mass in the upper nasal cavity.

Technique: Transmission-corrected scans with a slice thickness of 4 mm, image reconstruction by filtered backprojection.

PET Results: Coronal (**a**), transverse (**b**) and sagittal (**c**) PET views show a large focus with an intense FDG accumulation in the nasal cavity.

Histology: Adenocarcinoma; pT3 N3 M0; G3.

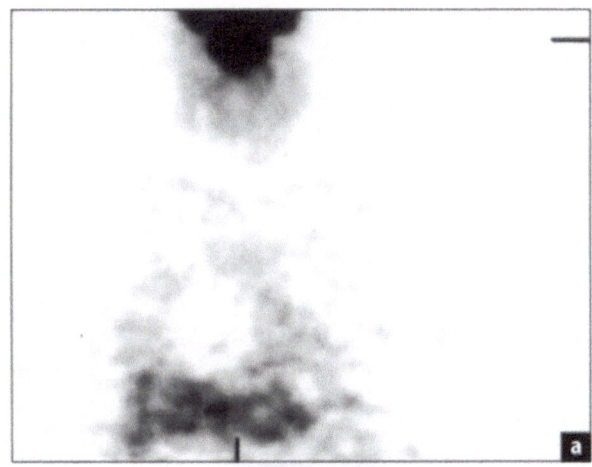

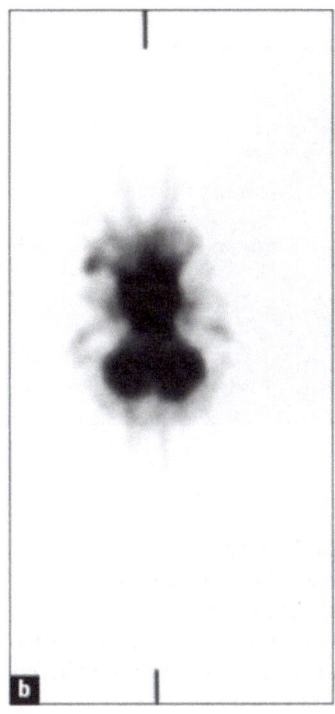

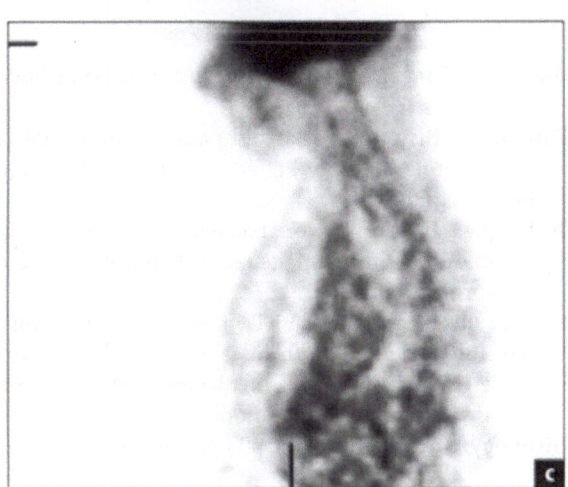

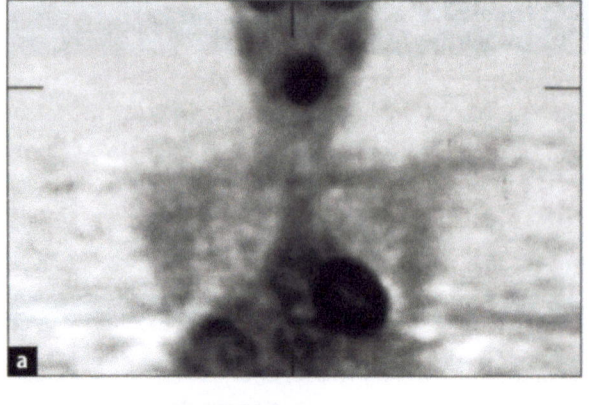
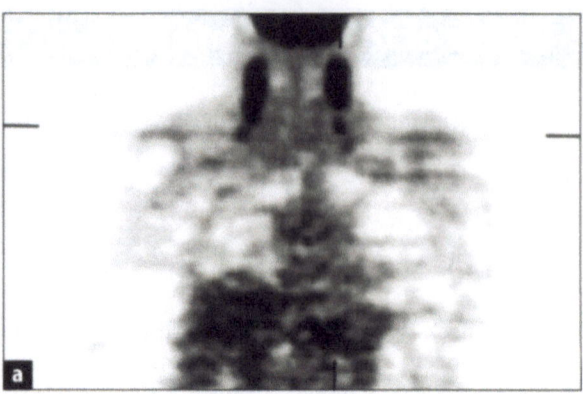
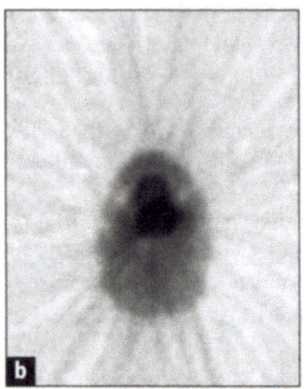
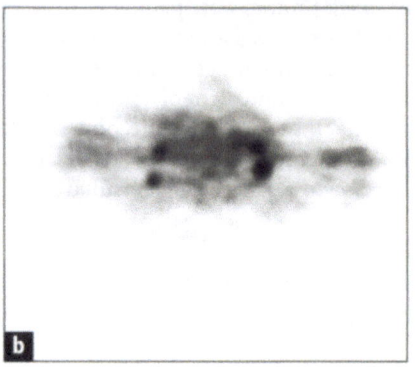
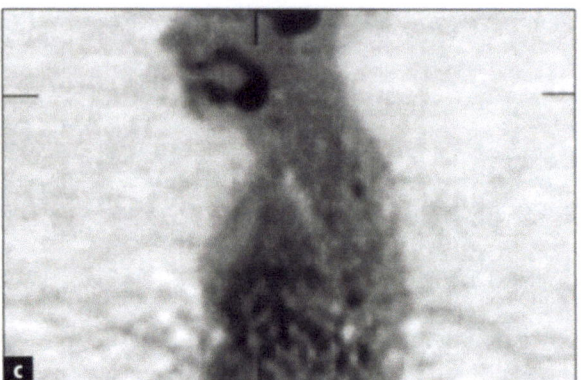

Figure 2 a–c

Diagnosis: Cancer of the oral cavity.
Patient and History: 56-year-old patient with a tumor suspicious mass in the oral cavity.
Technique: Transmission-corrected scans with a slice thickness of 4 mm, image reconstruction by filtered backprojection.
PET Results: Coronal (**a**), transverse (**b**) and sagittal (**c**) PET views show a large focus with an intense FDG accumulation in the oral cavity.
Histology: Squamous cell carcinoma; pT3 N0 M0; G3.

Figure 3 a, b

Diagnosis: Cancer of the nasal cavity with lymph node metastases.
Patient and History: 72-year-old patient with a mass in the upper nasal cavity. Patient was referred for lymph node staging.
Technique: Transmission-corrected scans with a slice thickness of 4 mm, image reconstruction by filtered backprojection.
PET Results: Coronal (**a**) PET images show a string of multiple foci along both sides of the neck; the transverse (**b**) images reveal involvement of the ventral and dorsal jugular lymph node groups.
Histology: Adenocarcinoma; pT3 N3 M0; G3.

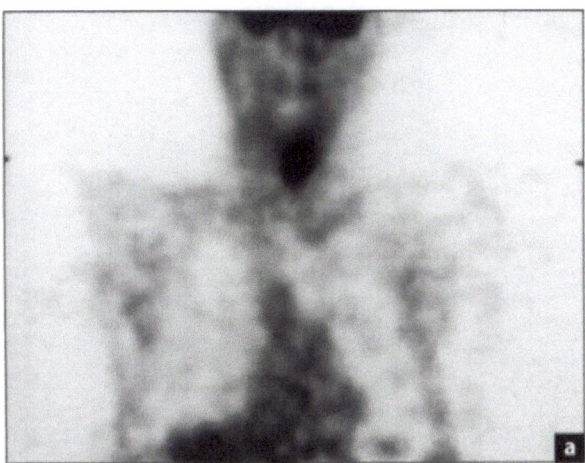

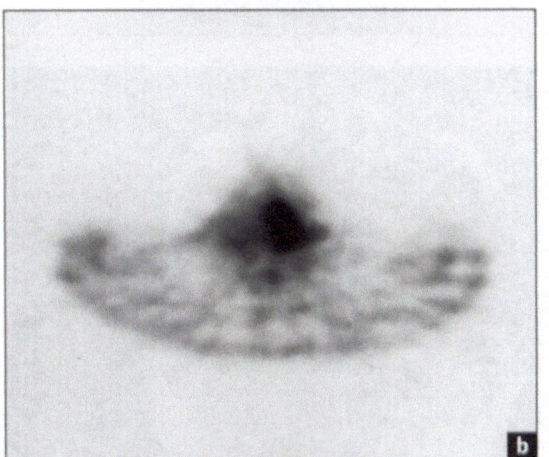

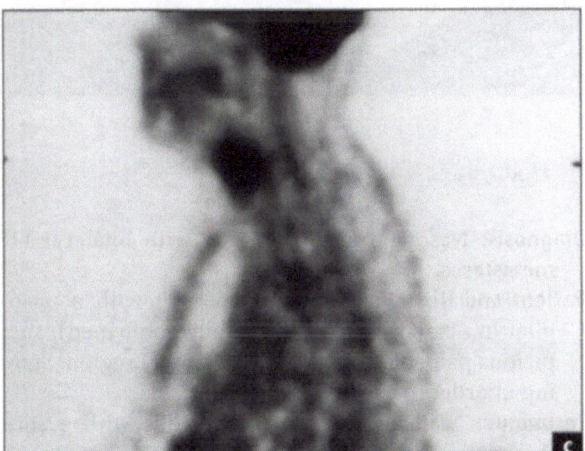

Figure 4 a–c

Diagnosis: Larynx cancer.

Patient and History: 71-year-old patient with suspected larynx carcinoma.

Technique: Transmission-corrected scans with a slice thickness of 4 mm, image reconstruction by filtered backprojection.

PET Results: Coronal (**a**), transverse (**b**) and sagittal (**c**) PET views show a large focus with an intense FDG accumulation in projection on the left part of the larynx.

Histology: Squamous cell carcinoma; pT4 N1 Mx; G3.

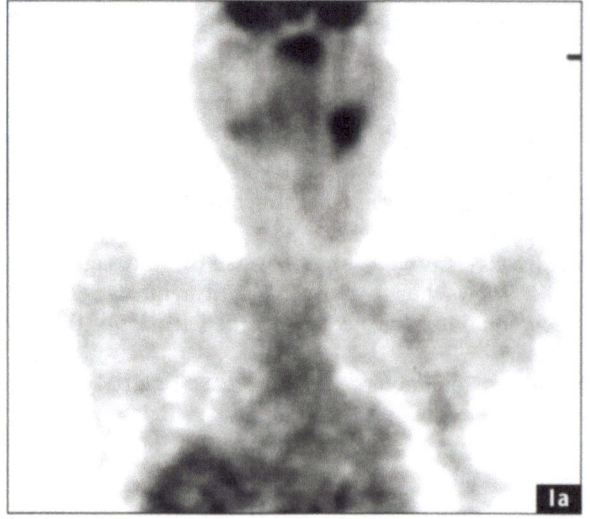
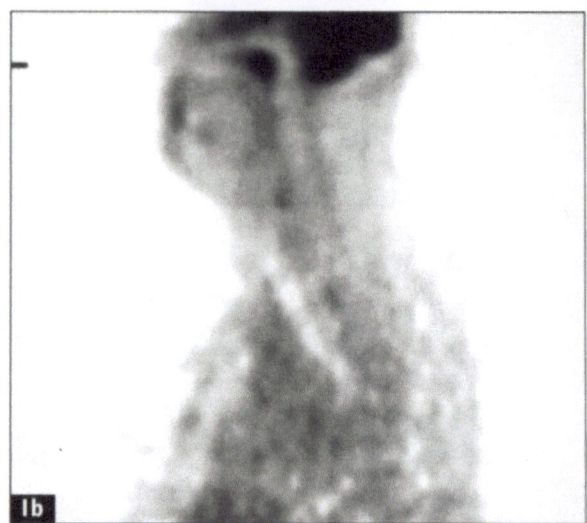
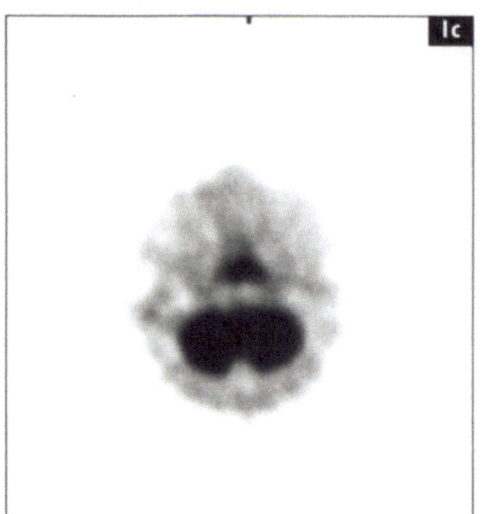
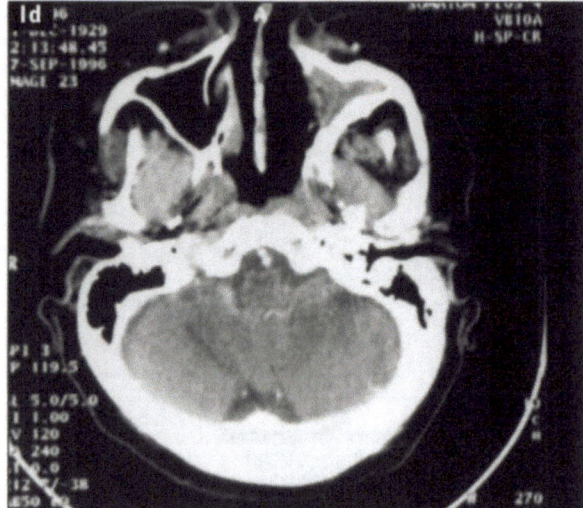

4.2 Lymph Node Metastases

Figure 5 a–d (I and II)

Diagnosis: Nasopharynx carcinoma with bilateral LN metastases.

Patient and History: 69-year-old patient with a nasopharynx carcinoma (histologically confirmed); suspicious palpable LN on the left cervical region. Staging in order to exclude distant metastases.

Technique: Transmission-corrected scans with a slice thickness of 4 mm, image reconstruction by filtered backprojection.

PET Results: Series I: The coronal (**a**), sagittal (**b**), and transaxial (**c**) views show one focus in projection on the upper nasopharynx. The CT scan (**d**) shows a tissue formation, which corresponds to the PET finding.

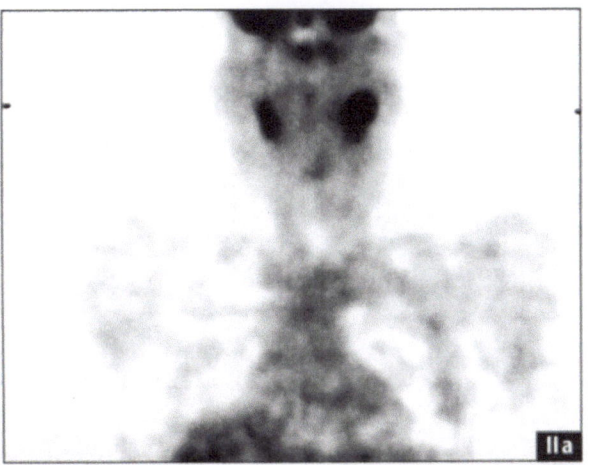
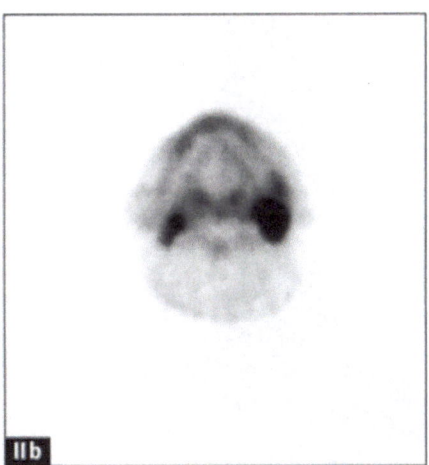
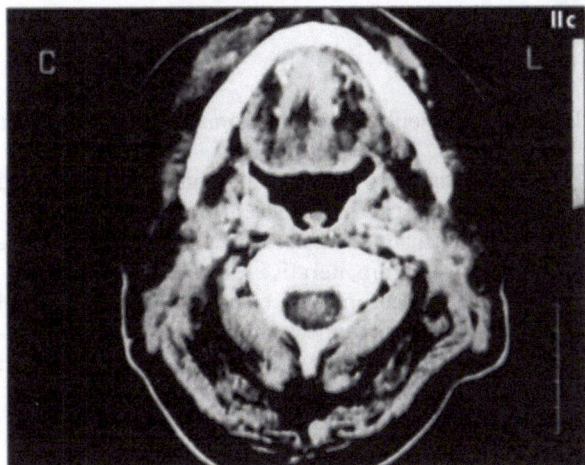

Series II: The coronal (**a**) and transaxial (**c**) views show bilateral cervical foci (left>>right). The CT scan (**c**) with contrast enhancing agent shows a tissue formation on the left side, which corresponds to the PET finding, but which was considered normal on the right side.

Cave! Due to differences in image angle PET and CT slices do not completely correspond.

Histology: Squamous cell carcinoma.

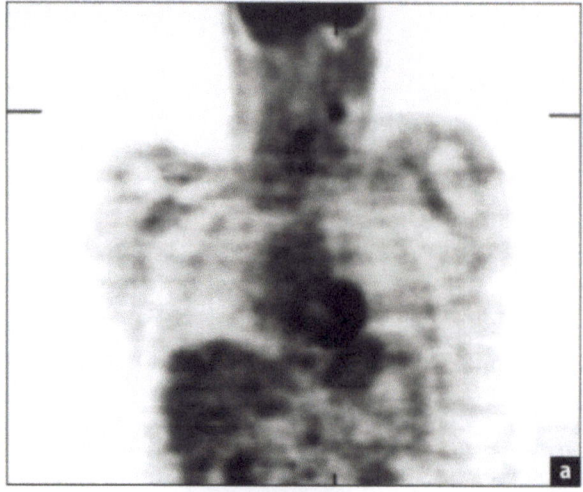

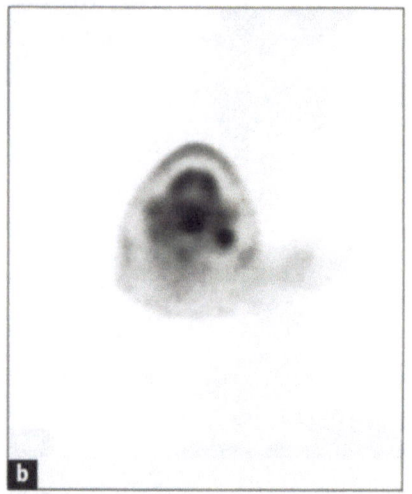

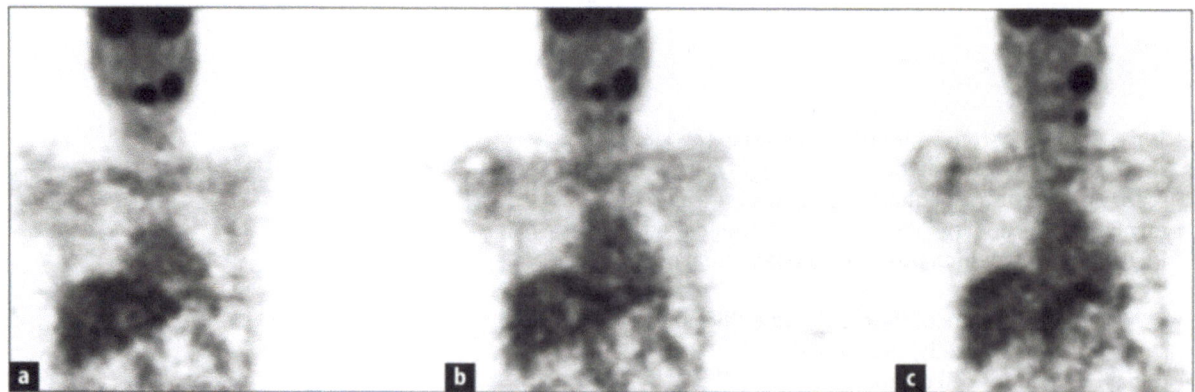

Figure 6 a–c

Diagnosis: Hypopharynx carcinoma with lymph node metastases.

Patient and History: 55-year-old patient with a confirmed hypopharynx carcinoma. Preoperative staging.

Technique: Transmission-corrected scans with a slice thickness of 4 mm, iterative image reconstruction.

PET Results: The coronal (**a**), transaxial (**b**) and sagittal (**c**) views show one of two small foci in the left, middle cervical region. No other lymph node or distant metastases were detected.

Histology: Squamous cell carcinoma; pT3 N2 M0.

Figure 7 a–c

Diagnosis: Oropharynx cancer with lymph node metastases.

Patient and History: 65-year-old patient with a tumor suspected mass in the left neck.

Technique: Transmission-corrected scans with a slice thickness of 4 mm, image reconstruction by filtered backprojection.

PET Results: The series of coronal (**a–c**) views shows (*I*) a large focus on the upper left neck, corresponding to the palpable mass, (*II*) a small focus in the lower left neck, corresponding to a prior unknown lymph node metastasis, and (*III*) a small focus in the oral cavity, suspected to be the primary tumor. No lymph node metastases were detected in the right neck.

Histology: Squamous cell carcinoma; pT2 N1 M0.

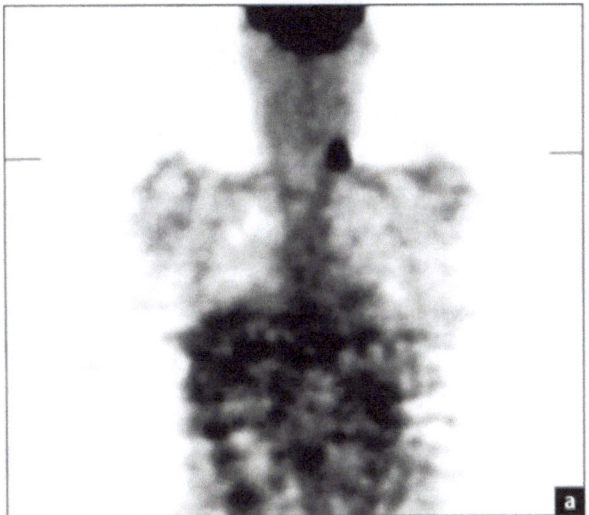

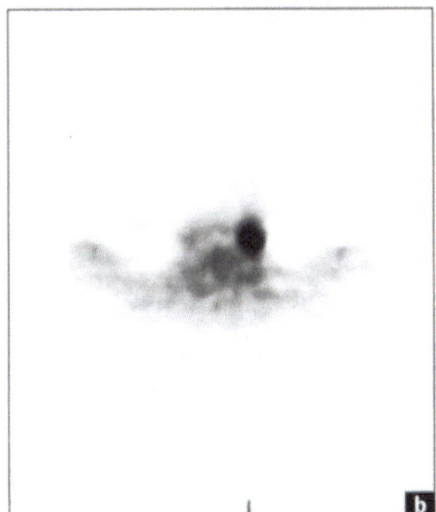

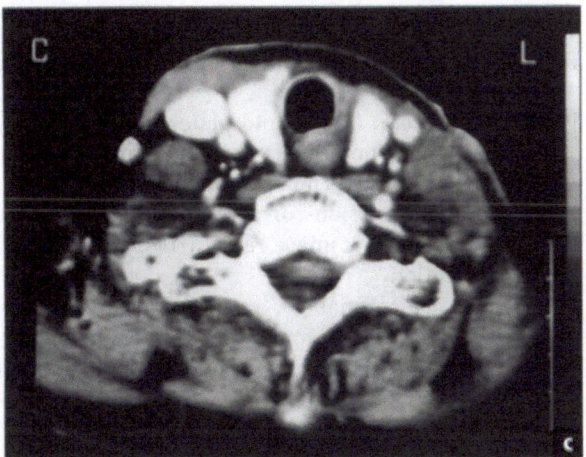

Figure 8 a–c

Diagnosis: Oropharynx carcinoma with a solitary lymph node metastasis.

Patient and History: 56-year-old patient with a hypopharynx carcinoma (8/97). About 3 months after surgery the patient developed a palpable mass in the left supraclavicular region. Restaging to exclude distant metastases.

Technique: Transmission-corrected scans with a slice thickness of 4 mm, image reconstruction by filtered backprojection.

PET Results: The coronal (**a**) and transaxial (**b**) PET views show a large focus in the left supraclavicular region, corresponding to the palpable mass. The CT study (**c**) with contrast enhancing agent confirms a tumor in the same region. No other tumor sites (distant metastases) could be identified.

Histology: Squamous cell carcinoma; pT4 N2 M0.

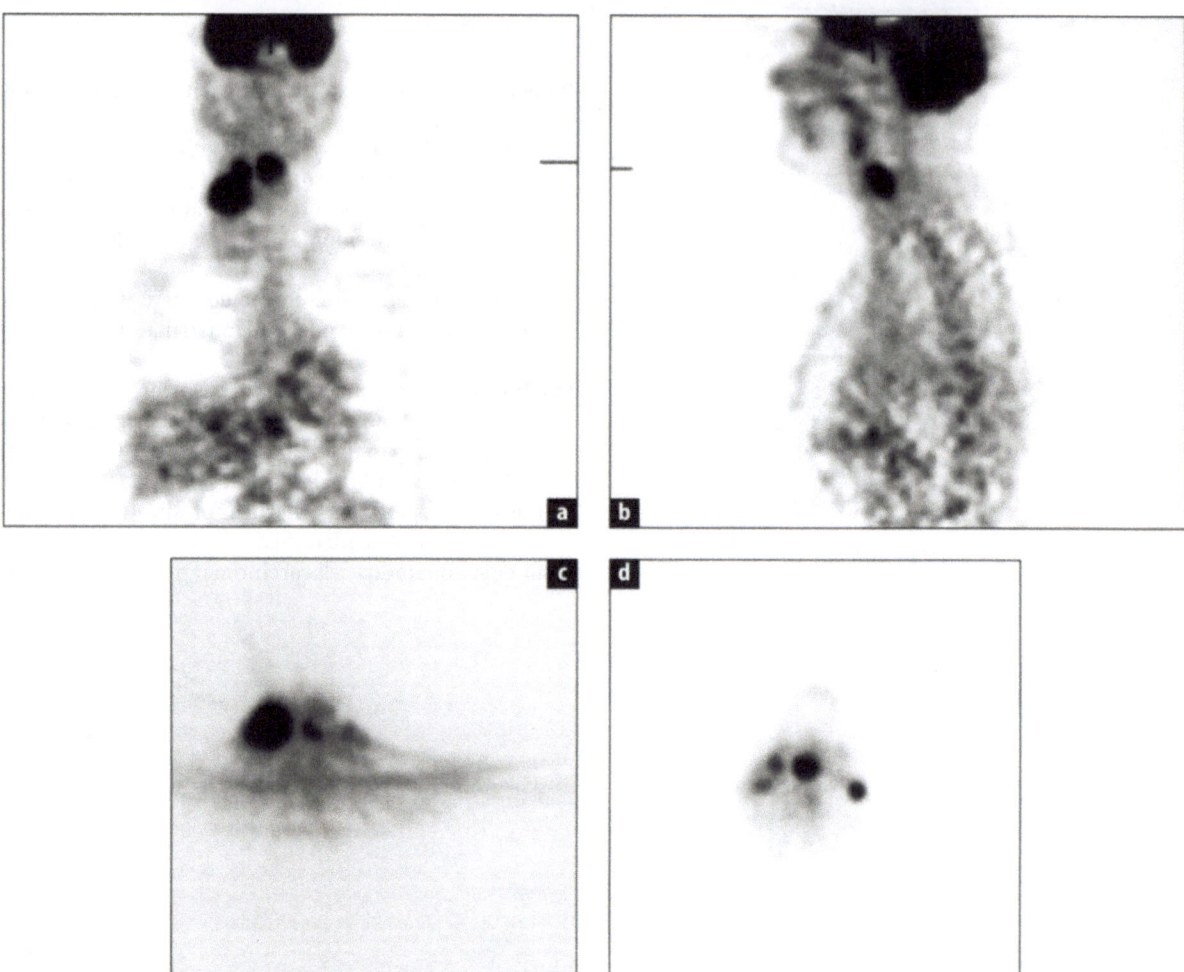

Figure 9 a–d

Diagnosis: Hypopharynx carcinoma with bilateral lymph node metastases.

Patient and History: 65-year-old patient with a hypopharynx carcinoma and a large cervical lymph node metastasis on the right side. Staging to exclude distant metastases.

Technique: Transmission-corrected scans with a slice thickness of 4 mm, image reconstruction by filtered backprojection.

PET Results: The coronal (**a**) view shows two larger foci. The central one corresponds to the known primary tumor and the right cervical focus to the palpable mass (LN metastases). The transaxial views reveal lymph node involvement of the right (**c**) and the left (**d**) cervical LN groups.

Histology: Squamous cell carcinoma.

Figure 10 a–c ▶

Diagnosis: Cancer of unknown primary (CUP syndrome).

Patient and History: 68-year-old patient with a solitary cervical lymph node metastasis (adenocarcinoma). No evidence of the primary tumor site.

Technique: Transmission-corrected scans with a slice thickness of 4 mm, image reconstruction by filtered backprojection.

PET Results: The coronal (**a**), transaxial (**b**) and sagittal (**c**) views show a small focus in projection on the dorsal, middle mediastine. The finding could be confirmed by CT and proved to be a central bronchial carcinoma. No lymph node metastases were detected in the right cervical region. Note the diffuse uptake of FDG in the bone marrow (spine) as a result of the prior chemotherapy (bone marrow activation).

Histology: Non-small cell lung carcinoma (adenocarcinoma).

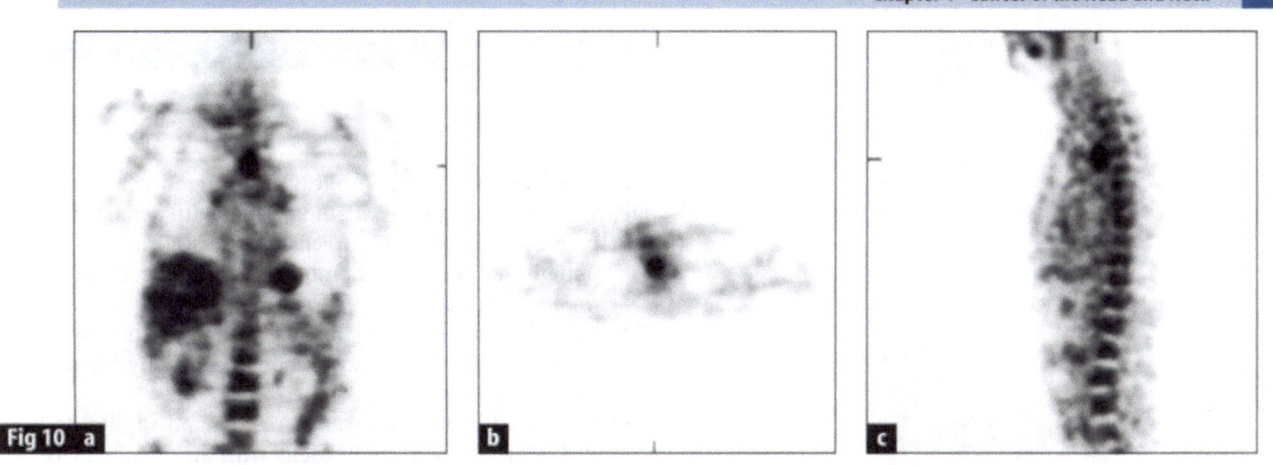

Fig 10 a b c

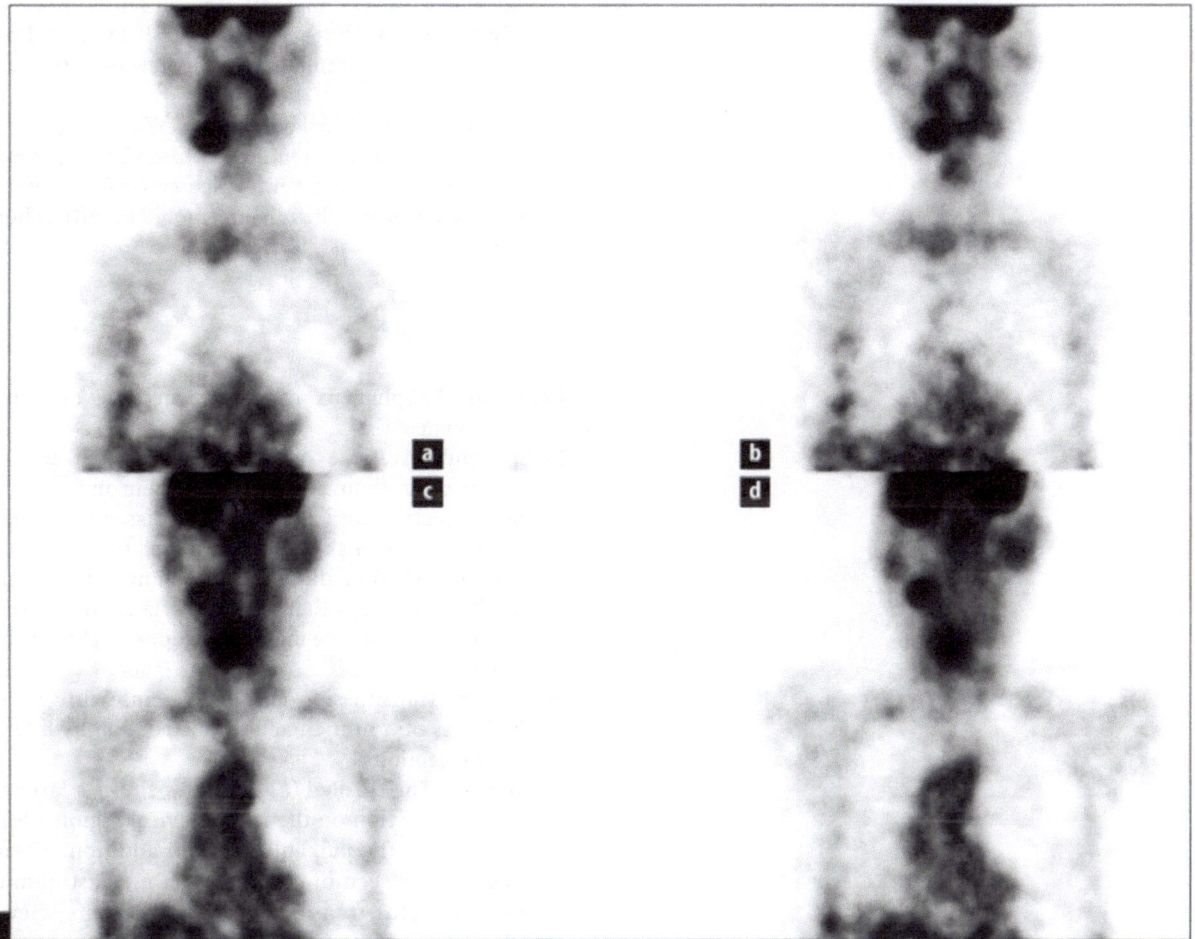

Fig 11

Figure 11 a–d

Diagnosis: Cancer-of-unknown primary (CUP syndrome).

Patient and History: 58-year-old patient with recurrent cervical lymph node metastases; cancer of unknown primary (CUP syndrome).

Technique: Transmission-corrected scans with a slice thickness of 4 mm, image reconstruction by filtered backprojection.

PET Results: The series of coronal (**a–d**) views shows (*I*) a small focus on the upper right neck, corresponding to the palpable lymph node, and (*II*) a larger focus in projection on the right part of the larynx, suspected to be the primary tumor. No lymph node metastases were detected in the left cervical region.

Histology: Squamous cell carcinoma; pTx N2a Mx.

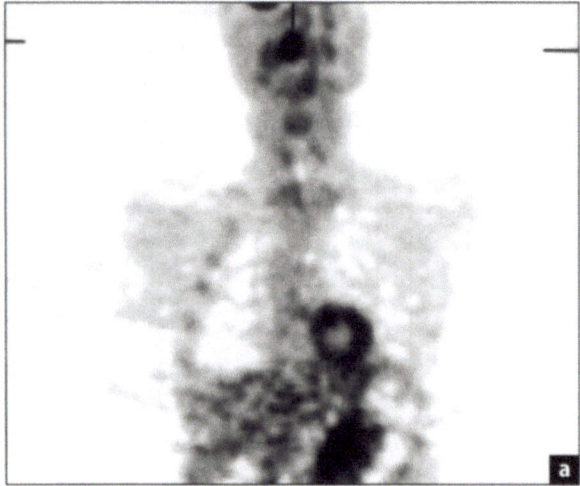

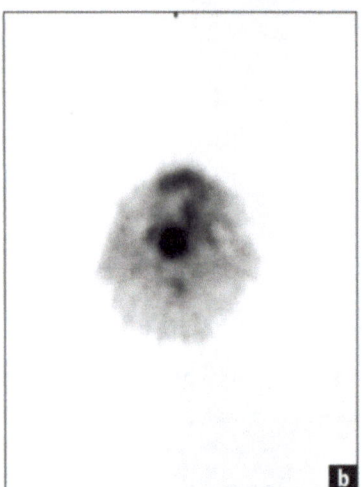

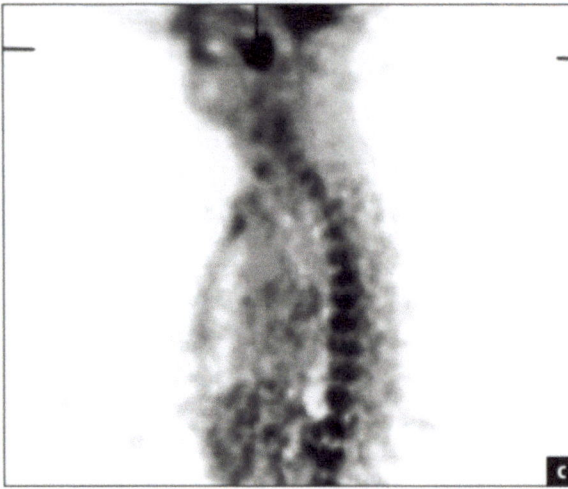

4.3 Recurrence

Figure 12 a–c

Diagnosis: Cancer of the oral cavity/recurrence.

Patient and History: 72-year-old patient with a mass suspicious for a tumor recurrence in the oral cavity. The patient had received chemotherapy 6 weeks prior to the PET study.

Technique: Transmission-corrected scans with a slice thickness of 4 mm, image reconstruction by filtered backprojection.

PET Results: Coronal (**a**), transverse (**b**) and sagittal (**c**) PET views show a small focus with an intense FDG accumulation in the upper oral cavity. The FDG PET was able to reveal bilateral cervical lymph node involvement (not shown). The sagittal (**c**) view shows diffuse tracer accumulation in the sternum, spine and the stomach.

Histology: Squamous cell carcinoma; pT4 N3 M0; G3.

Cave! Chemotherapy can induce diffuse FDG accumulation in the bone marrow, which can either obscure bone metastases or be misinterpreted as diffuse bone metastases.

Figure 13 a–c ▶

Diagnosis: Oropharynx cancer (recurrence of lymph node metastases).

Patient and History: 65-year-old patient with an oropharynx carcinoma (12/97); treatment included tumor resection and lymph node dissection. About 6 months later, a skin metastasis was removed; conventional staging did not detect any other tumor manifestation; another 3 months later, the patient developed a palpable mass in the upper right cervical region.

Technique: Transmission-corrected scans with a slice thickness of 4 mm, image reconstruction by filtered backprojection.

PET Results: The coronal (**a**) PET view shows a large focus in projection on the right cervical region, corresponding to the palpable mass. In addition, a small focus can be seen in the upper left mediastinum on the coronal (**a**), transaxial (**b**), and sagittal (**c**) views.

Histology: Squamous cell carcinoma; pT4 N2.

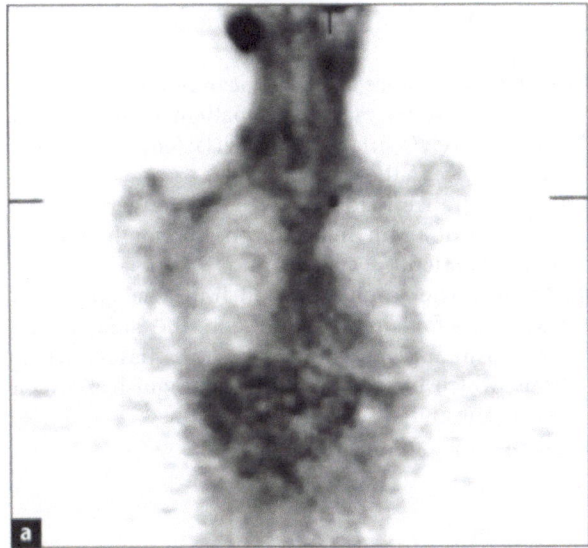

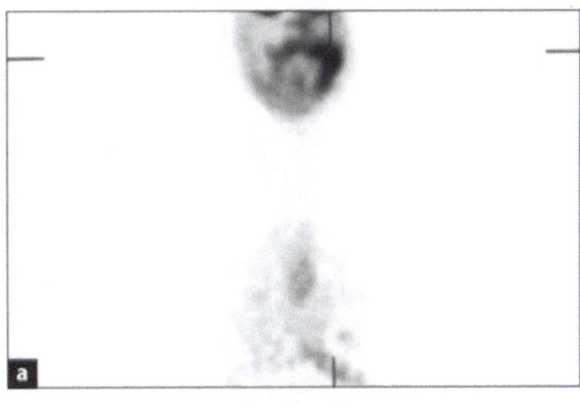

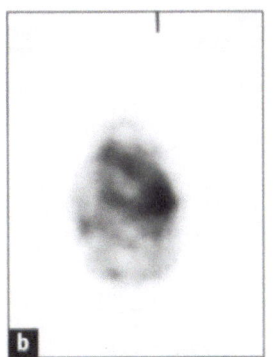

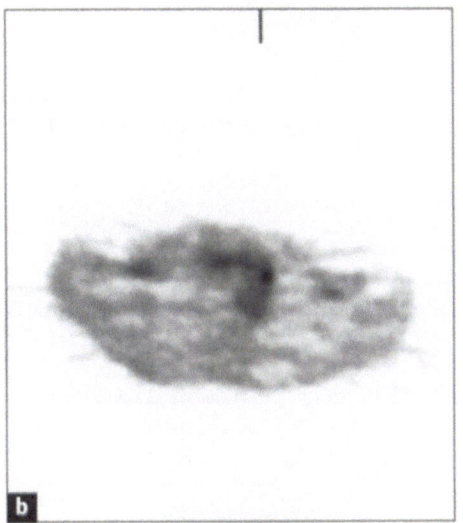

Figure 14 a, b

Diagnosis: Local recurrence of an oropharynx carcinoma.

Patient and History: 64-year-old patient with an oropharynx carcinoma (8/96); tumor resection and lymph node dissection; radiation therapy; local tumor recurrence (1/97) with extensive surgical revision; (3/97) suspicion of local tumor recurrence.

Technique: Transmission-corrected scans with a slice thickness of 4 mm, image reconstruction by filtered backprojection.

PET Results: The coronal (**a**) and transaxial (**b**) views show a larger focus in projection on the left oral cavity, corresponding to the former resection site.

Histology: Squamous cell carcinoma.

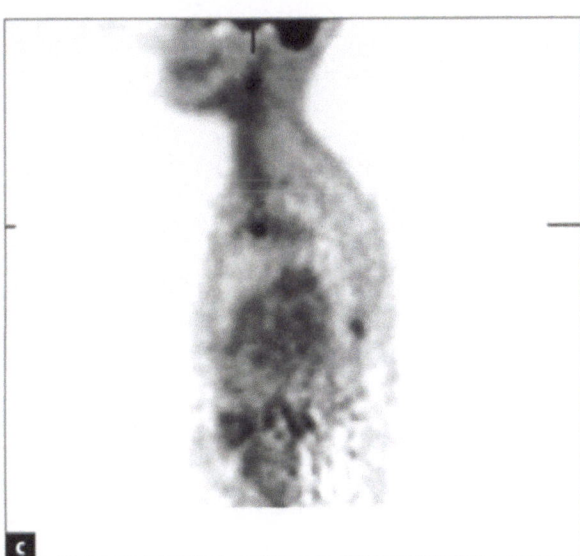

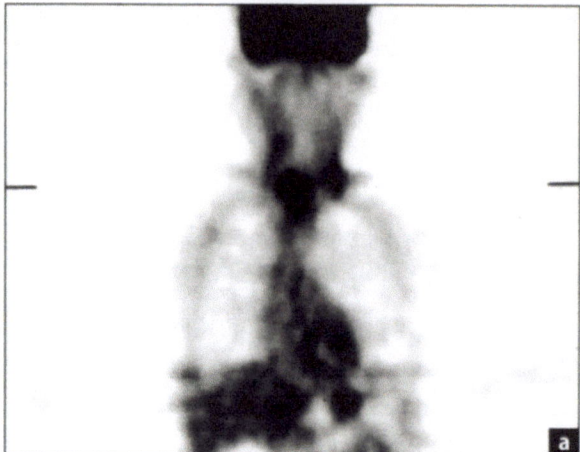

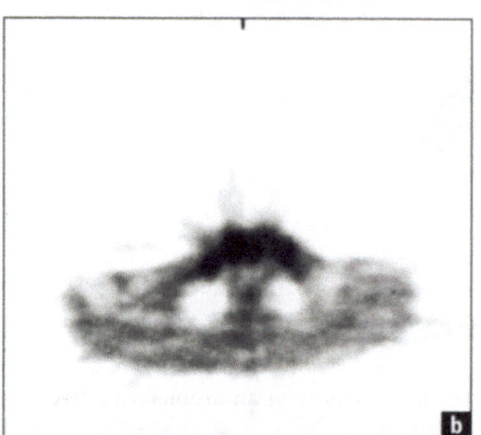

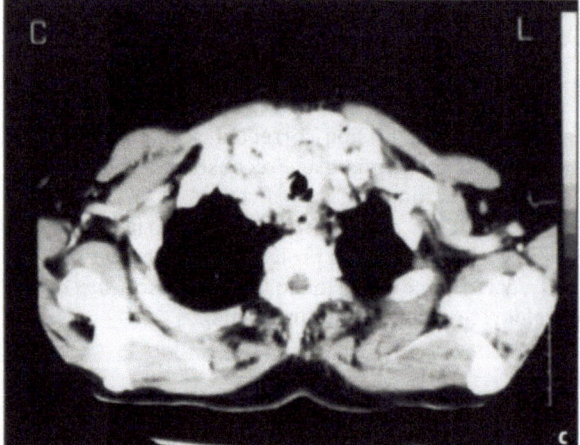

Figure 15 a–c

Diagnosis: Recurrence of a larynx carcinoma.

Patient and History: 73-year-old patient with a larynx carcinoma (12/95); laryngectomy; (11/96) suspicion of a recurrence in the stoma.

Technique: Transmission-corrected scans with a slice thickness of 4 mm, image reconstruction by filtered backprojection.

PET Results: The coronal (**a**) and transaxial (**b**) views show two foci in projection on the area of the tracheostoma. The CT scan (**c**) shows tissue formations, which cannot definitely distinguish between scar tissue and local recurrence.

Histology: Squamous cell carcinoma.

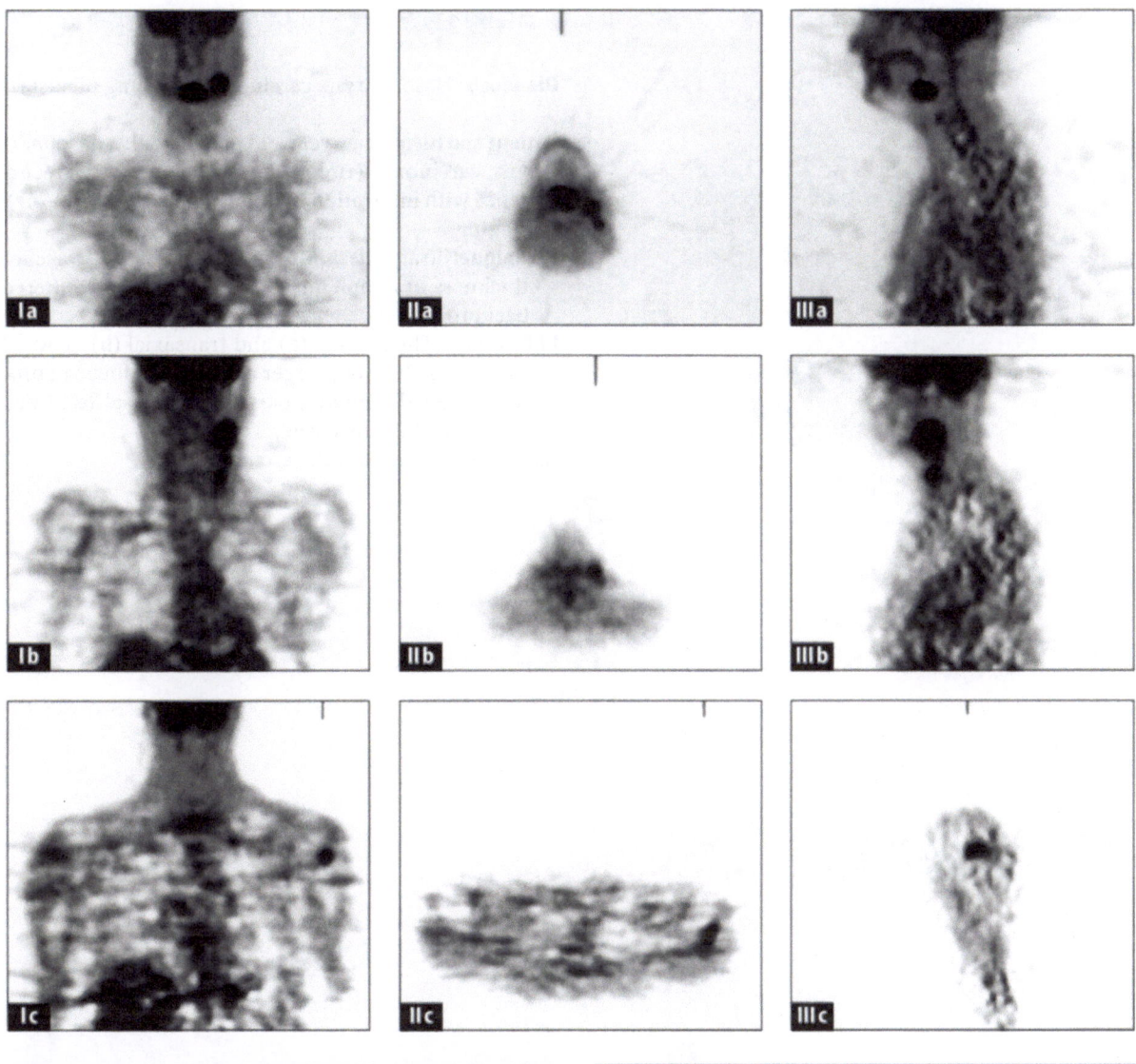

4.4 Distant Metastases

Figure 16 a–c

Diagnosis: Oropharynx carcinoma with lymph node and bone metastases.

Patient and History: 51-year-old patient with palpable cervical lymph nodes due to a confirmed oropharynx carcinoma.

Technique: Transmission-corrected scans with a slice thickness of 4 mm, image reconstruction by filtered backprojection.

PET Results: Series (**a–c**) of coronal (**I**), transaxial (**II**) and sagittal (**III**) PET views show a focus in projection on the primary (oropharynx) (**I–IIIa**), multiple left cervical foci (*LN*) (**I–IIIb**) and a solitary focus in the left humerus (**I–IIIc**).

Histology: Squamous cell carcinoma.

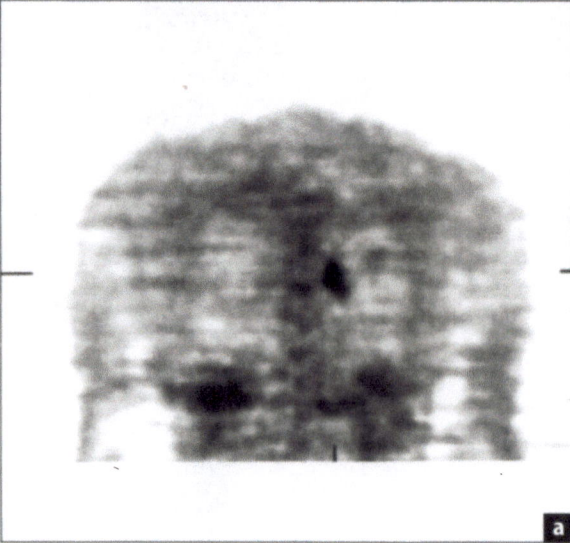

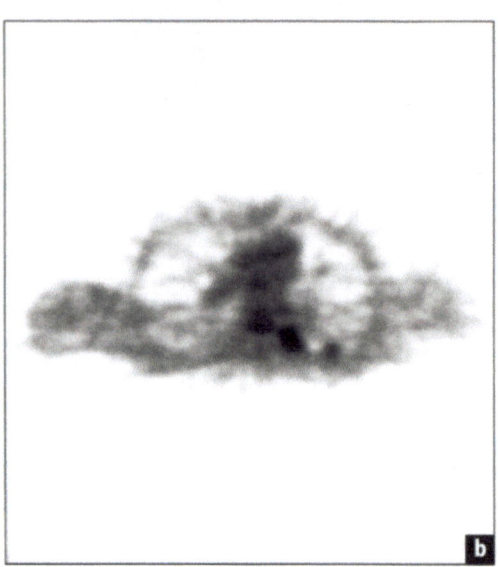

Figure 17 a, b

Diagnosis: Nasopharynx carcinoma with lung metastases.

Patient and History: 44-year-old patient with a nasopharynx carcinoma (11/96); suspicion of a local recurrence with infiltration into the maxillary sinus (4/97); staging.

Technique: Transmission-corrected scans with a slice thickness of 4 mm, image reconstruction by filtered backprojection.

PET Results: The coronal (**a**) and transaxial (**b**) views of the thorax show one larger and a minor focus in projection on the middle part of the dorsal left lung, paravertebrally localized.

Histology: Squamous cell carcinoma.

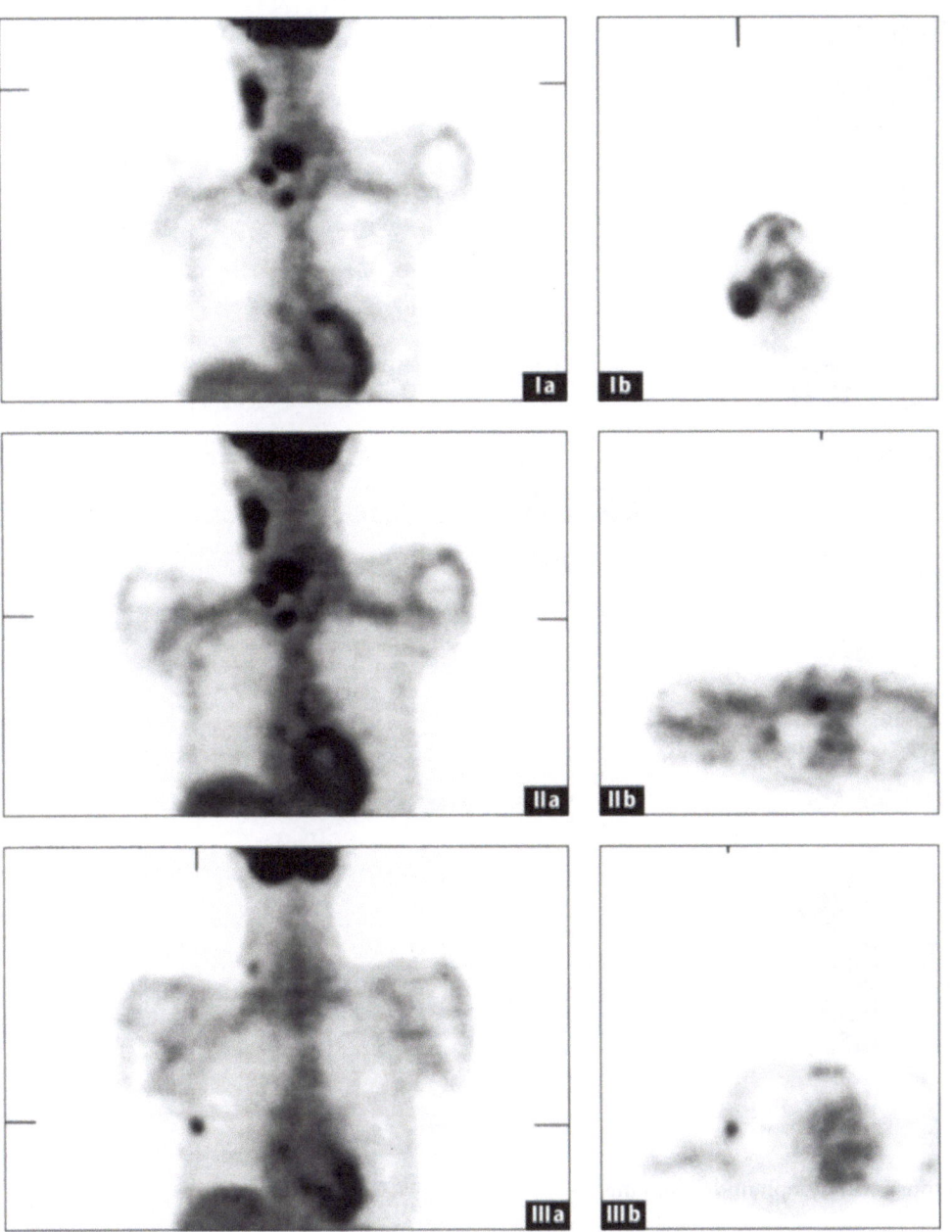

Figure 18 a, b

Diagnosis: Supraglottic larynx carcinoma with lymph node and lung metastases.

Patient and History: 56-year-old patient with a suspected supraglottic larynx carcinoma. Preoperative staging.

Technique: Transmission-corrected scans with a slice thickness of 6 mm, iterative image reconstruction.

PET Results: Series (I–III). The coronal (**a**) and transaxial (**b**) views show multiple foci along the right neck (**I–IIa**), including the suggested primary tumor (**I–IIa**), retroclavicular lymph nodes (**IIa, b**) and a small thoracic lesion, at the middle, right thorax wall (**IIIa, b**). The latter lesion cannot be differentiated as lung or bone metastasis.

Histology: Squamous cell carcinoma, cT2 N2 M1.

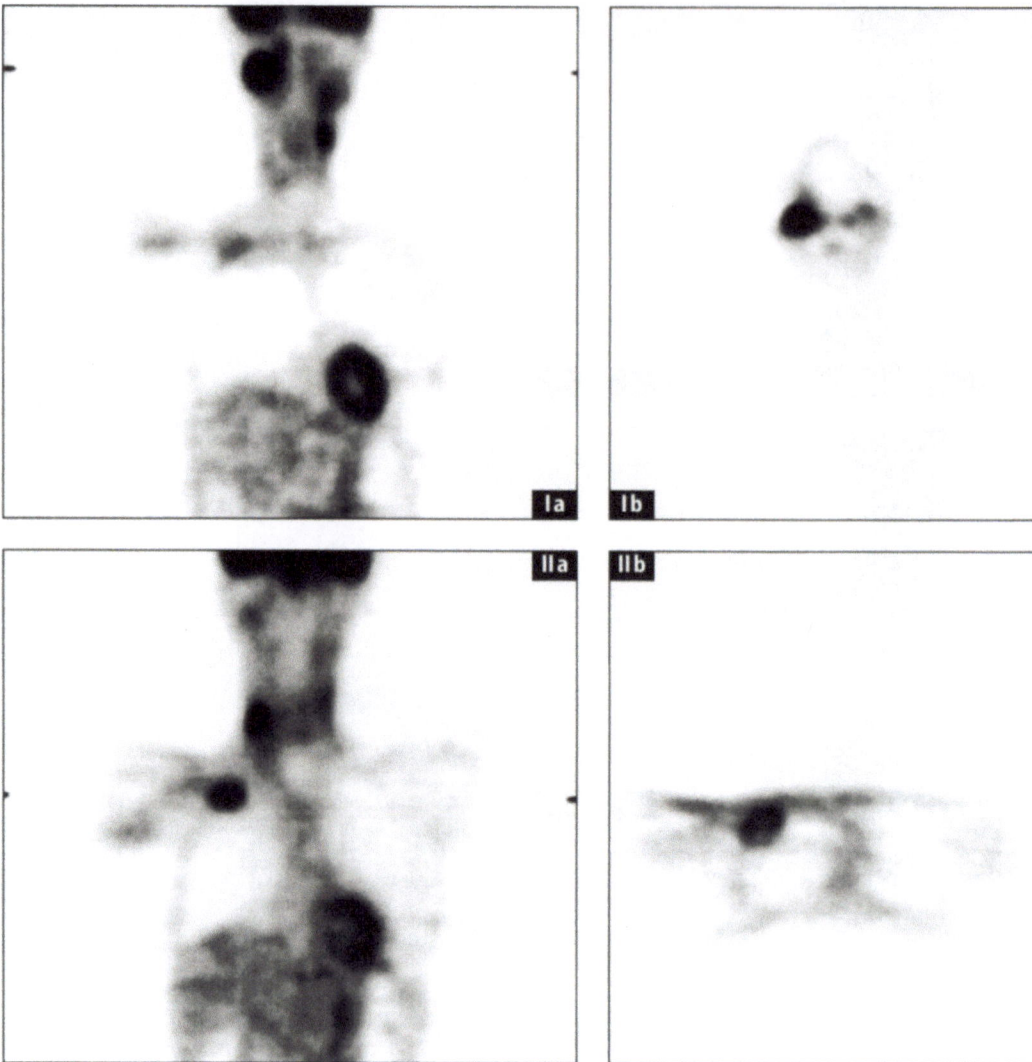

Figure 19 a, b

Diagnosis: Cancer of a tonsil with lymph node and lung metastases.

Patient and History: 76-year-old patient with a large palpable mass on the right upper neck and a suspicious lymph node in the supraclavicular region. Preoperative staging.

Technique: Transmission-corrected scans with a slice thickness of 4 mm, image reconstruction by filtered back projection.

PET Results: Series (I, II). The coronal (**a**) and transaxial (**b**) views show a focus in projection on the palpable mass and lymph node on the right neck (**I, II a**). In addition, PET revealed an unknown focus in the middle of the left neck and a focus in the apex of the right lung.

Histology: Adenocarcinoma, cT4 N2 M1.

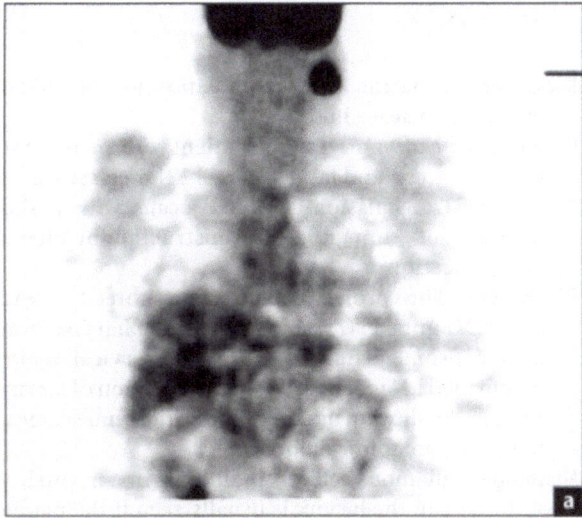

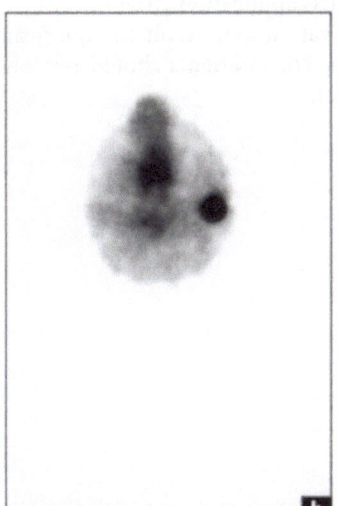

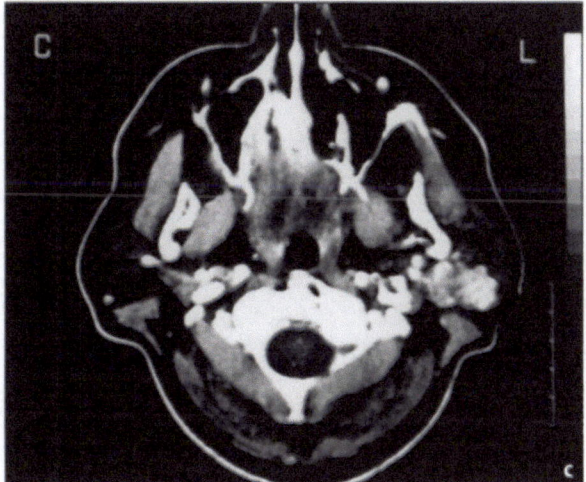

4.5 Pitfalls

Figure 20 a–c

Diagnosis: Palpable tumor-suspicious mass; grading?

Patient and History: 59-year-old patient with a palpable mass on the left mandibular region (parotis). Grading?

Technique: Transmission-corrected scans with a slice thickness of 4 mm, image reconstruction by filtered backprojection.

PET Results: The coronal (**a**) and transaxial (**b**) views show one area with an avid FDG accumulation in projection on the left parotic gland, corresponding to the palpable mass. The CT scan (**c**) with contrast enhancing agent shows a tissue formation, corresponding to the PET finding, and classified as a tumor. CT and PET proved to be false-positive.

Histology: Pleomorphic adenoma (benign).

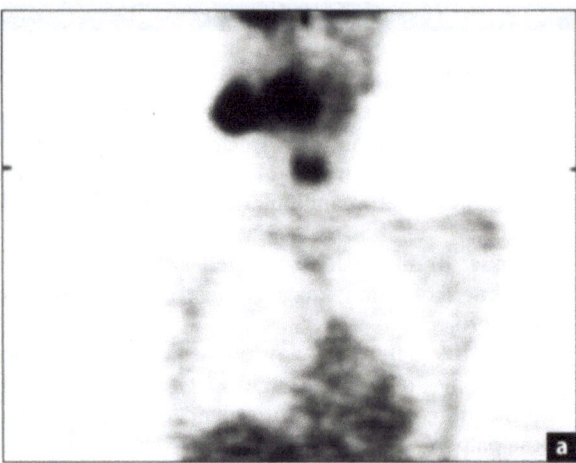

Figure 21 a, b

Diagnosis: Unspecific FDG accumulation, no evidence of malignant disease in the larynx.

Patient and History: 56-year-old patient with an oropharynx carcinoma and large cervical LN metastases.

Technique: Transmission-corrected scans with a slice thickness of 4 mm, image reconstruction by filtered backprojection.

PET Results: The coronal (**a**) view shows three foci with avid FDG uptake: (*I*) region of the oropharynx (confirmed primary tumor), (*II*) right cervical region (confirmed LN metastasis), and (*III*) region of larynx. The larynx shows a bilobular formation and seems to follow the anatomical borders.

Histology: Squamous cell carcinoma; larynx: normal.

Cave! Uptake in the larynx is usually seen if the patient talks or sings after FDG application. After injection of FDG, muscular activation can result in significant tracer accumulation. Thus patients should rest and asked to be kept quiet.

Malignant Melanoma

J. H. Risse, H. Palmedo and H. Bender

Malignant melanoma is becoming an increasingly common disease, and this tumor is showing the most rapid increase in number of new cases diagnosed. The incidence is doubling every 6–10 years. For example, in 1980, 1 in 250 individuals developed melanoma in the USA, projected to increase to 1 in 75 by the year 2000. Melanomas most commonly occur on the back, between the scapulae in men, and the lower extremities in women, but can be located anywhere on the body including eyes and ears.

In our experience, patients with malignant melanoma (MM) usually are referred to PET shortly after a suspicious skin lesion has been removed and histologically diagnosed as MM. Consequently, no primary MM is included in our series.

5.1 In Transit and Limited Nodal Metastases (AJCC Stage III)

Two microstaging methods have been used for localized melanoma, i. e., the total vertical height (Breslow) and the dermal layer invasion level (Clark). It has been clearly demonstrated that tumor thickness is a more accurate prognostic factor than level of invasion. According to the current American Joint Committee on Cancer (AJCC) staging system, stages I and II refer to localized melanoma. Stage III is defined as limited nodal metastases involving only one regional lymph node basin, or fewer than five in transit metastases without nodal metastases. In transit metastases are located between the primary melanoma and the first station regional nodal basin. Increasing stage numbers correlate inversely with survival.

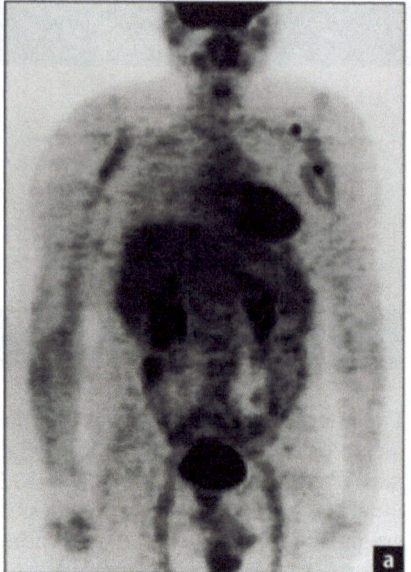
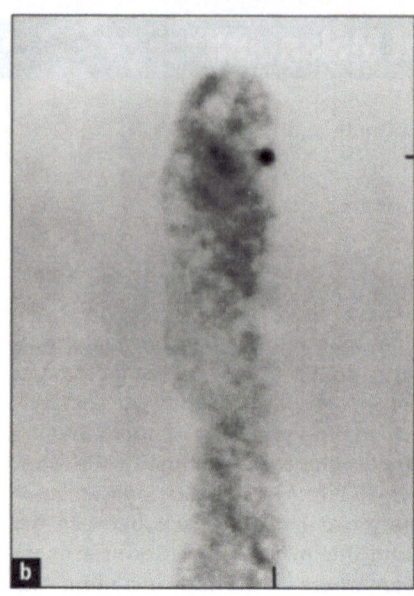
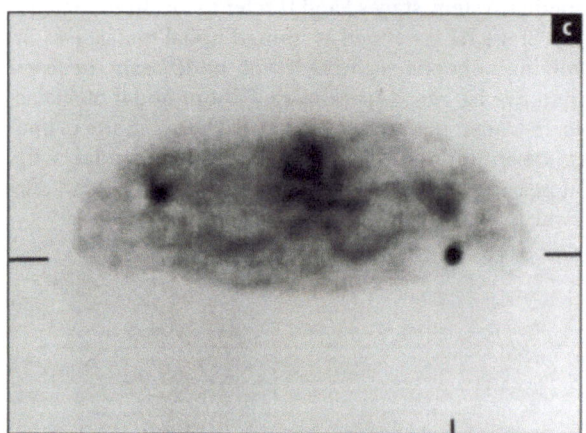
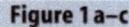

Figure 1 a–c

Patient and History: 52-year-old male with a history of MM in the left shoulder region 1 year ago. A first postoperative PET was unsuspicious. Four months ago, another PET proved left axillary lymph nodes which were removed immediately. After conventional chemotherapy PET restaging was performed.

Technique: 3D volume projection and transmission corrected emission scans with a slice thickness of 6 mm. Iterative reconstruction.

PET Results: In the projection view (**a**), two focal FDG accumulations are obvious in projection to the left shoulder and axilla region. On the transversal (**c**) and sagittal slice (**b**) the localization of the caudal lesion to the skin level is shown. Cranial lesion similar. Both lesions were categorized as in transit metastases. Note the good visualization of the greater vessels (see also Fig. 11).

◀ Figure 2

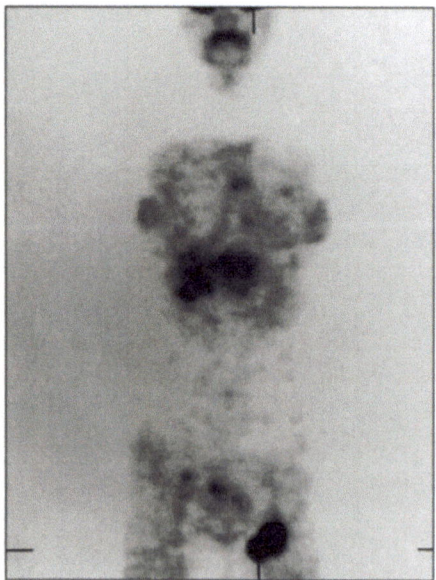

Patient and History: 50-year-old female with a MM at the left calf removed 1 day ago.

Technique: Transmission corrected emission scans with a slice thickness of 6 mm. Iterative reconstruction.

PET Results: There is an obvious FDG accumulation in the left inguinal region in this coronal slice. Detailed analysis demonstrated the binodal character of the lesion with a bigger lateral node. Quantitation yielded a standard uptake value (SUV) of 16.5 in that node, compared to a SUV of 6.6 in the cerebellum.

Figure 3 a–g

Patient and History: 78-year-old female without a cancer history but with a palpable mass in the left inguinal region. The first (preoperative) PET and two follow-ups are presented.

Technique: First PET: non-corrected emission scan, follow-up PETs: transmission corrected emission scans, all with a slice thickness of 6 mm. Reconstruction: Filtered back projection.

PET Results: In the preoperative PET, a solitary FDG accumulation is demonstrated in the left inguinal region (**a** coronal; **b** transversal slice). The mass was shown to be an inguinal lymph node by CT (**c** arrowhead), was removed, and proved to be a metastasis of a MM with unknown primary tumor localization. Five months later, the follow-up PET (**d** coronal; **e** sagittal) revealed a massive local progress without evidence of distant metastases. Another 2 months later, multiple hepatic (one example in the transversal plane; **f** left liver lobe) and pulmonary (**g**) lesions became evident. The primary tumor localization remained unknown.

Cave! There are massive artifacts in (**d**) and (**e**) due to paravasation in the right cubital vein such that no diagnosis could be made in this transversal body slice. The acquisition in this bed position was repeated with the right arm out of the field of view. In (**f**), the FDG accumulation in the right renal pelvis might be mistaken for another liver metastasis.

Fig. 3 d–g see page 40

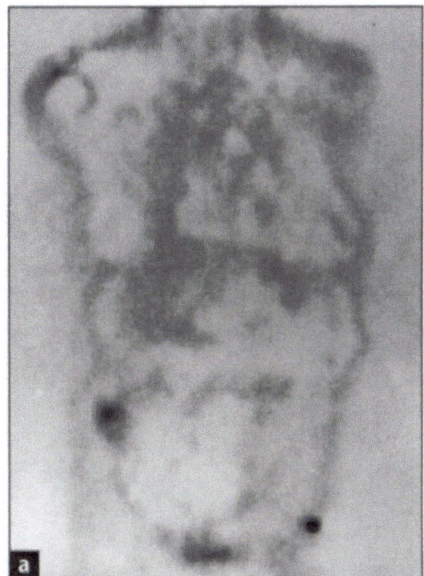

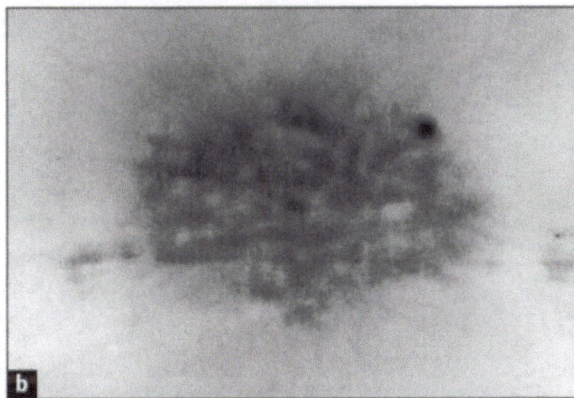

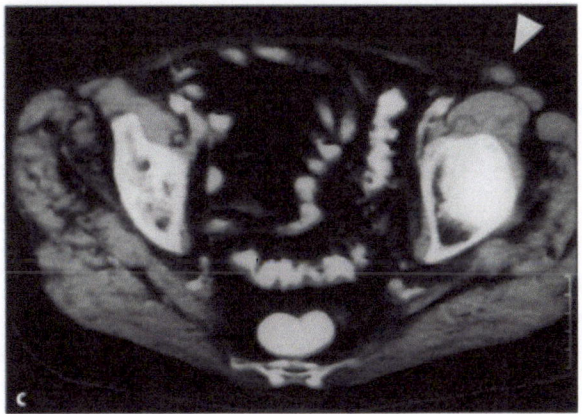

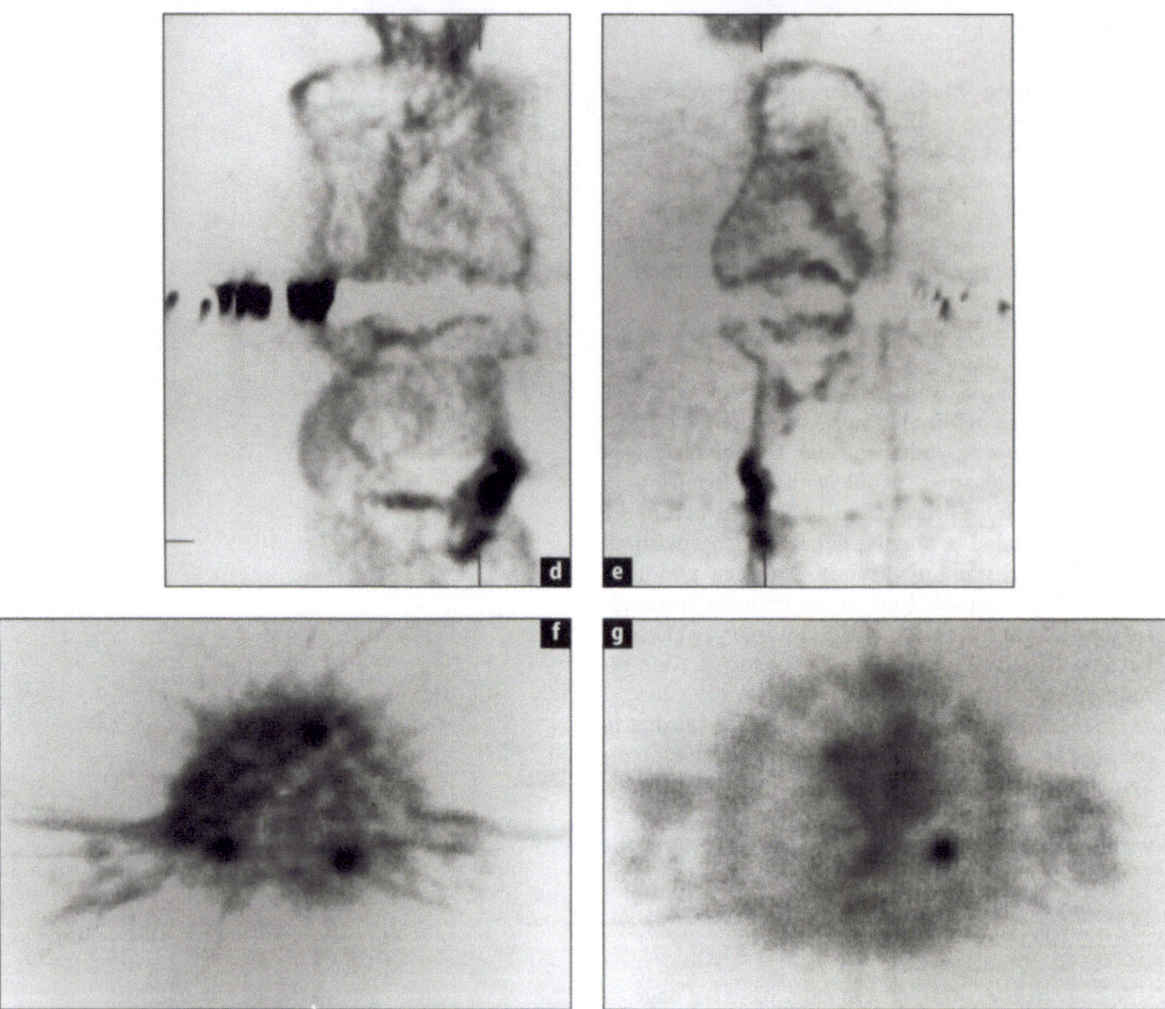

Figure 3 d–g

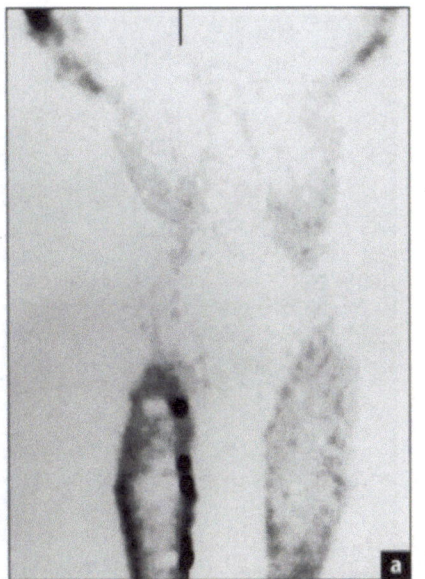
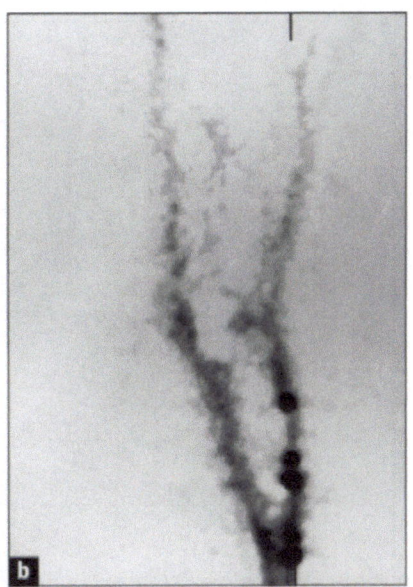
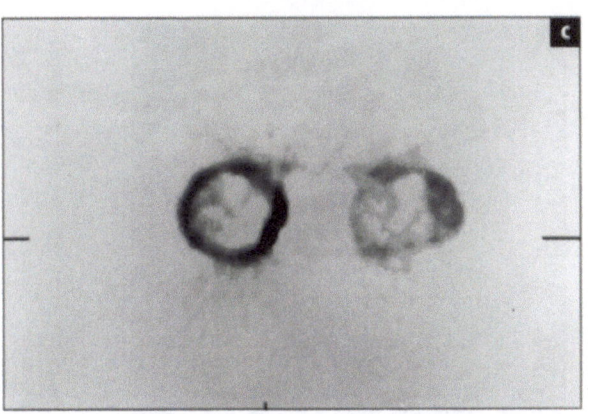
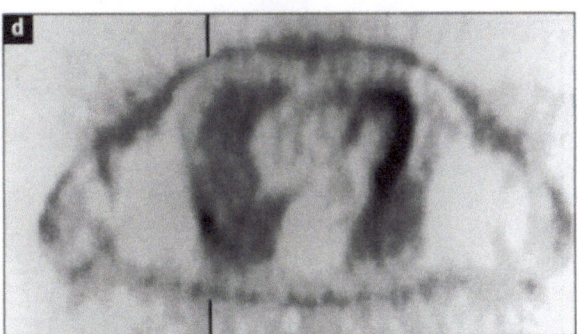

5.2 Distant metastases (AJCC Stage IV)

AJCC stage IV includes advanced regional or distant metastases. Melanoma can metastasize to almost every organ and tissue. In clinical series, the most frequent metastatic sites are (in decreasing order) the skin and lymph nodes, lungs, liver, brain, and bone. In contrast, the frequencies detected in autopsy series are much higher, culminating in the lungs, followed by the liver, skin, brain, gastrointestinal tract and other visceral sites. Generally, patients with systemic metastases have very poor prognoses with a mean survival of about 6 months. Nevertheless, patients with tumors in favorable sites, such as the lung or bone, do somewhat better.

Figure 4 a–d

Patient and History: 68-year-old male with a history of MM at the right calf 4 years ago. After 3 years, in transit and inguinal lymph node metastases were removed and followed by an unsuspicious PET 4 months later.

Technique: Non-corrected emission scans with a slice thickness of 6 mm. Iterative reconstruction.

PET Results: On the coronal (**a**) and sagittal (**b**) slice of the right leg, multiple focal FDG accumulations can be noted which imitate a string of pearls in a mediodorsal meridian of the calf. However, the transversal slice (**c**) shows that there are more lesions in all planes. Furthermore, PET revealed new pulmonary lesions (**d** transversal).

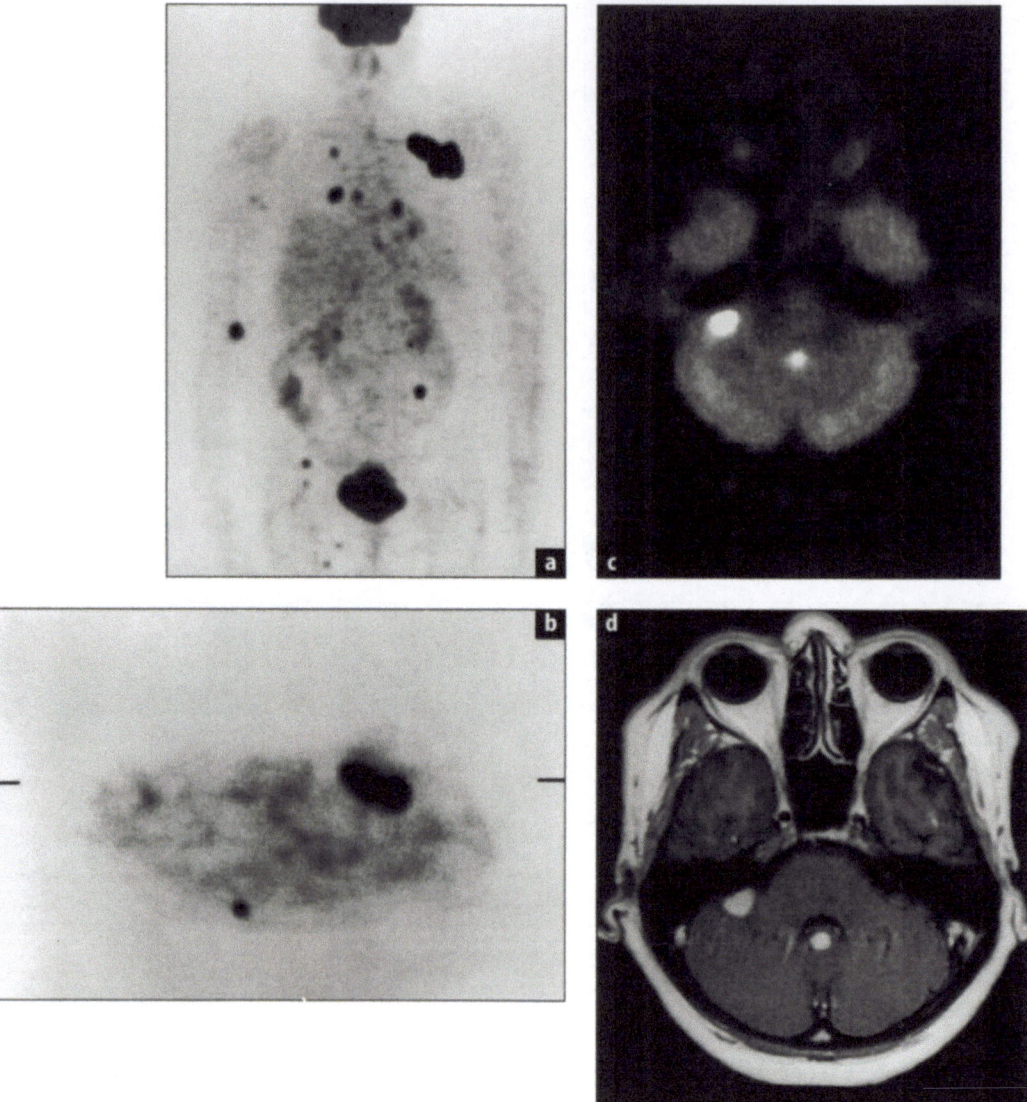

Figure 5 a–d

Patient and History: 55-year-old female with a history of MM in the left cubital region which was removed 4 years ago. A PET 3 months ago revealed multiple metastases throughout the body. After a conventional chemotherapy PET restaging was performed.

Technique: Whole body: 3D volume projection and transmission corrected emission scans with a slice thickness of 6 mm. Brain: transmission corrected emission scans with a slice thickness of 3 mm. Iterative reconstruction.

PET Results: In the projection view (**a**), multiple focal FDG accumulations are demonstrated in projection to the left axilla, thorax, abdomen, right cubital vein, right iliac region and thigh, and brain. The left axil-lary metastases shown on the transversal slice in (**b**) represent the sentinel lymph nodes as well as continuing lymph node groups. Additionally, a skin metastasis in the right scapular region can be identified. On the transversal slice in (**c**), two cerebellar metastases were detected which were proven by magnetic resonance imaging [MRI, in (**d**), here: gadolinium-enhanced transversal T1-weighted spin echo sequence].

Cave! There is no pathologic activity in the former primary tumor site at the left upper limb. The focal FDG accumulation in the right cubital vein region is due to local inflammation belonging to an i.v. line.

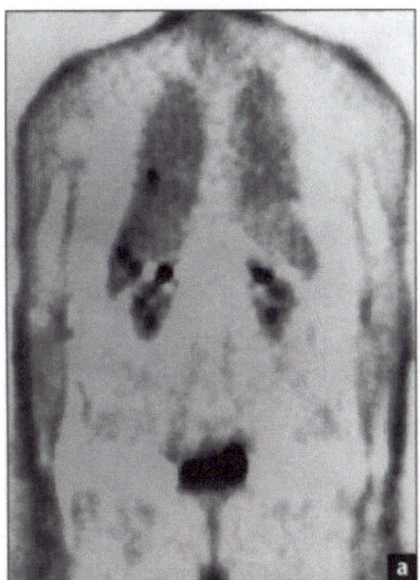

Figure 6 a–c

Patient and History: 68-year-old male with a history of MM in the right inferior scapula region 4 years ago.

Technique: Non-corrected emission scan with a slice thickness of 6 mm. Reconstruction: Filtered back projection.

PET Results: On the coronal slice (**a**), two focal FDG accumulations in the right liver lobe and a third lesion in the right lung can be identified. The CT of the thorax (**b**) showed the pulmonary lesion with a diameter of approximately 0.7 cm; in (**c**), one of the corresponding liver nodules to the PET findings can be seen (*arrow*). However, multiple further pulmonary and hepatic nodules ranging from 0.3 to 1.0 cm were detected by CT but not by PET.

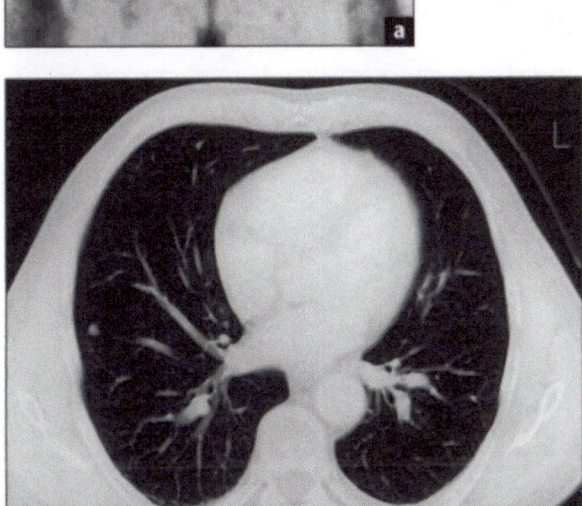

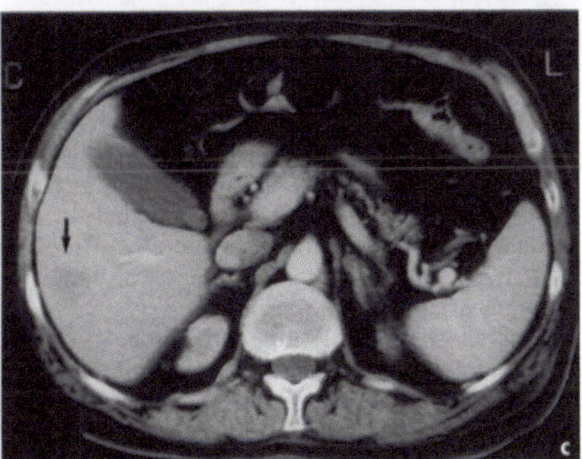

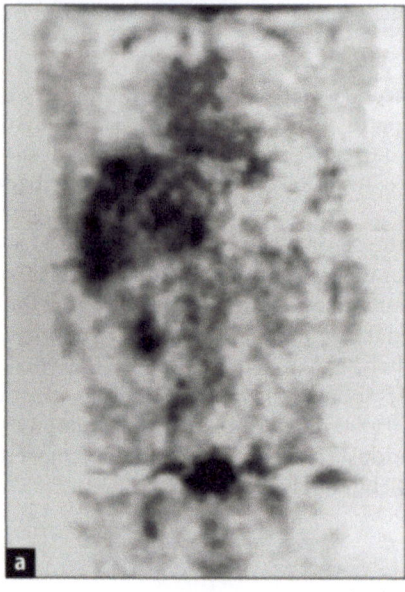

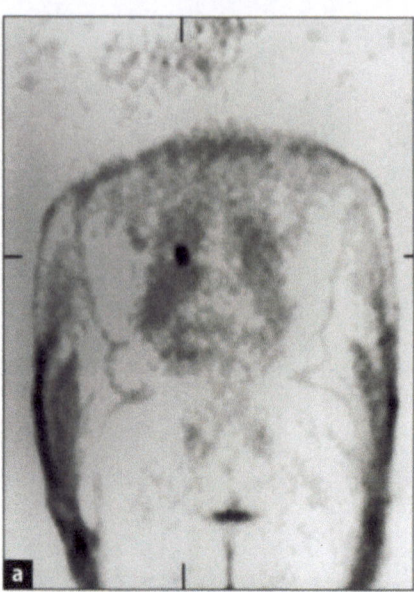

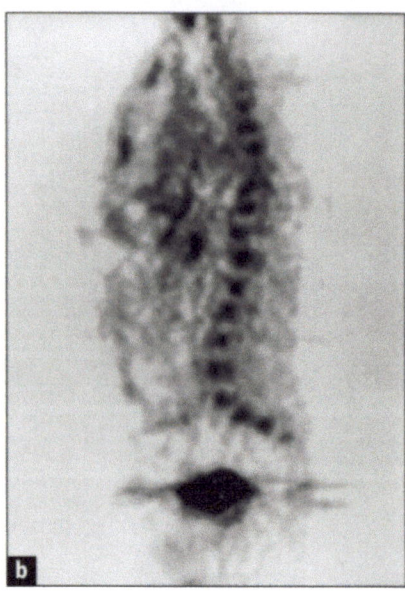

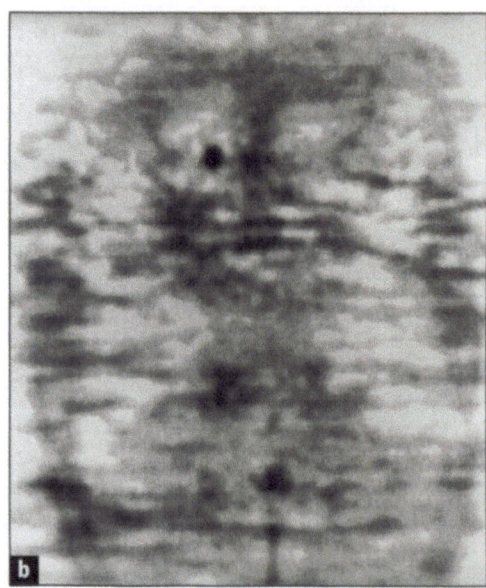

Figure 7 a, b

Figure 8 a, b

Patient and History: 82-year-old male with a history of MM at the right knee, excised 3 years ago.

Technique: Transmission corrected emission scans with a slice thickness of 6 mm. Filtered back projection.

PET Results: On the coronal slice (**a**), multiple focal FDG accumulations can be noted in the liver, right inguinal region, and paraaortic lymph nodes. On the sagittal slice (**b**), additional focal FDG accumulations are shown in the spine and sternum.

Cave! After chemotherapy, a bone marrow activation may mask or sometimes mimic skeletal metastases in PET. In this case, a bone marrow activation could be ruled out by bone marrow scintigraphy; all PET findings corresponded to bone metastases.

Patient and History: 65-year-old female with a history of a large MM at the right neck 1 year ago. A recent CT scan revealed suspicious pulmonary nodules.

Technique: Transmission corrected and non-corrected emission scans with a slice thickness of 6 mm. Filtered back projection.

PET Results: The coronal slices (**a, b**) show one focal FDG accumulation in the right lung. Note the different presentation in the non-corrected emission scan (**a**) and the transmission corrected emission scan (**b**).

Cave! Note the typical linear enhancement of the lateral forearms in the non-corrected emission scan which disappears after transmission correction. The focal FDG accumulation at the right wrist represents a little paravasation.

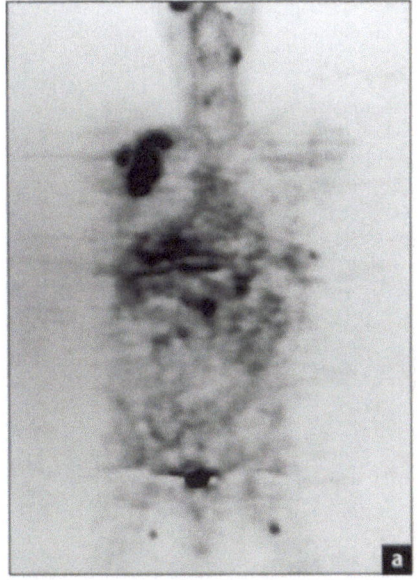
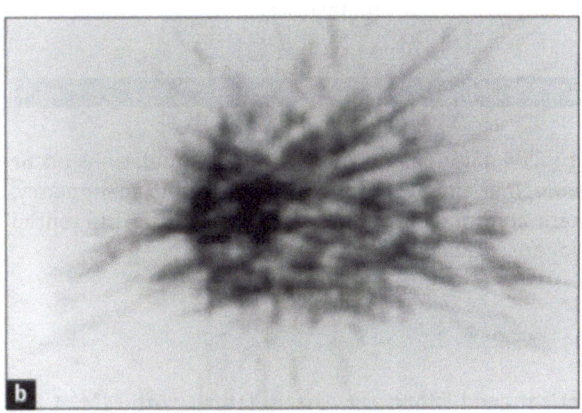
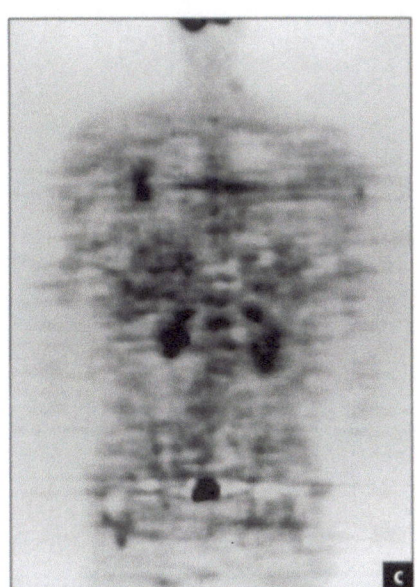
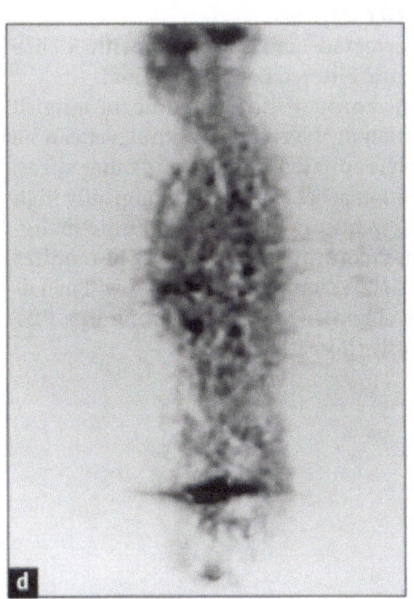
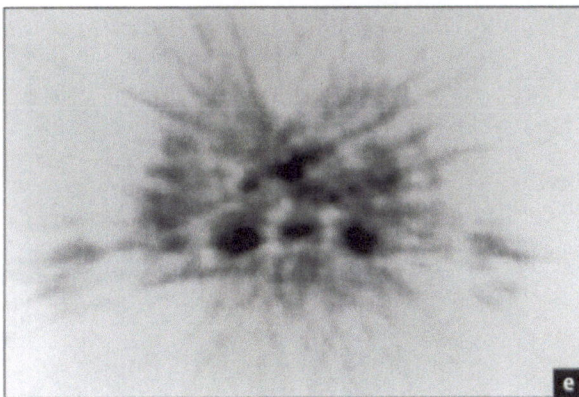

Figure 9 a–e

Patient and History: 67-year-old male with a palpable mass in the right axilla and a history of MM between the scapulae which was removed 24 years ago, followed by radiation.

Technique: Transmission corrected emission scans with a slice thickness of 6 mm. Filtered back projection.

PET Results: On the coronal slice (**a**), massive FDG accumulations in the right axilla are obvious which involve the thoracic wall and right lung as well. Additionally, multiple focal FDG accumulations are demonstrated in the liver, paraaortic region, left neck, and both inguinal sides. The liver lesions are better delineated in the transversal plane (**b**).

Additionally, multiple inhomogeneous lesions in the spine can be identified (**c** coronal, **d** sagittal, **e** transversal plane). In (**e**), a focal FDG accumulation between the renal pelvis on both sides is shown which belongs to the spine. Paraaortic accumulations represent lymph node metastases.

5.3 Pitfalls

In PET imaging in oncology, FDG accumulations occur in normal situations which might mimic malignancy. Some common pitfalls are presented and the differential diagnoses discussed.

Figure 10 ▶

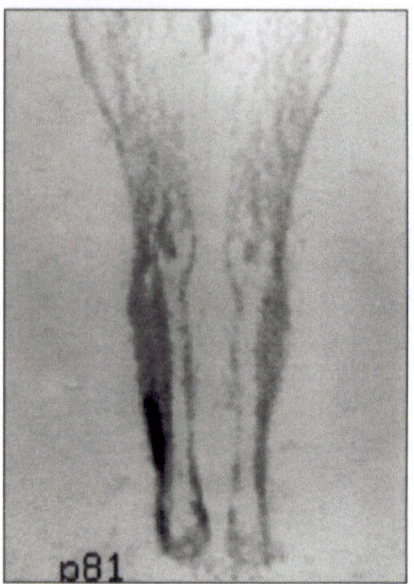

Patient and History: 72-year-old female with MM at the right calf, excised 6 days ago.

Technique: Non-corrected emission scans with a slice thickness of 6 mm. Filtered back projection.

PET Results: On the coronal slice a significant longish FDG accumulation at the right calf skin level can be identified which is apparent for about 15 other slices.

Cave! Recent operation areas show a pathologically high glucose utilization and may therefore mimic malignancy. Since local control of a primary MM requires wide local excision, a significant skin area will usually demonstrate obvious FDG accumulation in a PET performed shortly thereafter.

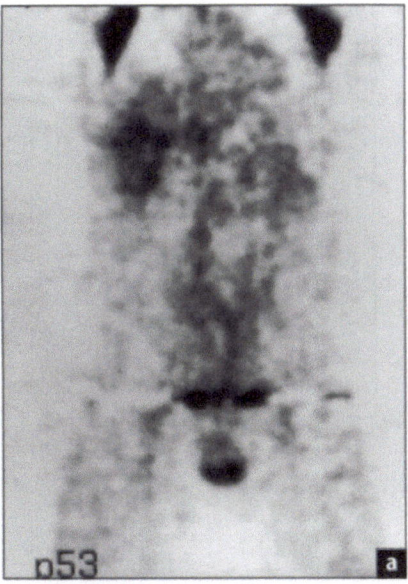

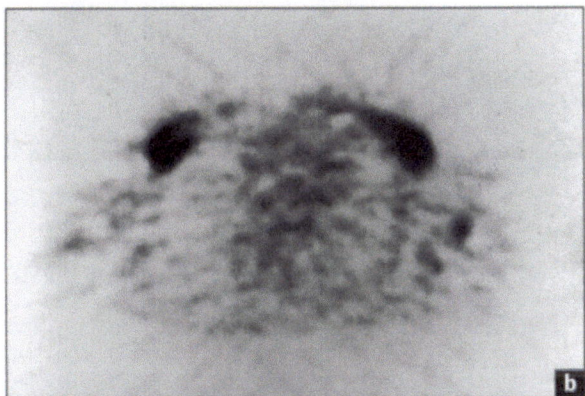

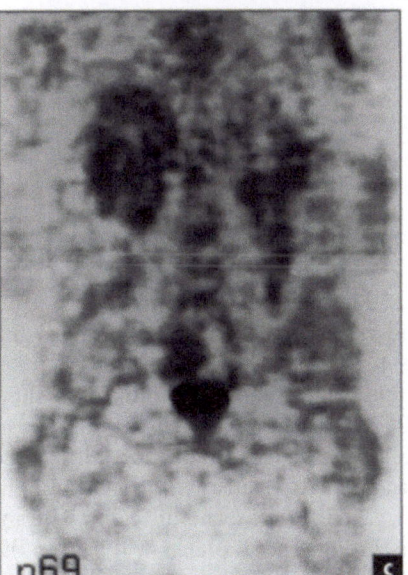

Figure 11 a–c

Patient and History: 40-year-old male with a history of MM at the right thigh, excised 3 days ago.

Technique: Transmission corrected emission scans with a slice thickness of 6 mm. Filtered back projection.

PET Results: On the coronal slice (**a**), a symmetrical triangular FDG accumulation in the lateral thoracic walls can be identified. On the transversal slice (**b**), the localization in the ventral thoracic wall is demonstrated. The configuration is typical for the pectoralis muscles. The patient used crutches because of his recent thigh operation. In the left axilla, another focal FDG accumulation can be noted; the coronal slice (**c**) shows that this is a tubular structure thought to be a vessel. There was no evidence of malignancy in this PET.

Cave! Patients after recent operation of the lower limbs may need crutches; when not used to this walking aid, some muscle groups such as the pectoralis muscles will be highly activated and therefore show a significant FDG accumulation, mimicking malignancy. Of course, the symmetric appearance in typical muscle compartments, together with the pertinent history, will lead to the correct diagnosis. Vessels are not unlikely to be visualized in a PET scan; if detected in a perpendicular plane, a vessel may appear as a "hot spot" and mimic malignancy. A plane showing the long axis will reveal the tubular character and lead to the correct diagnosis (see also Fig. 1).

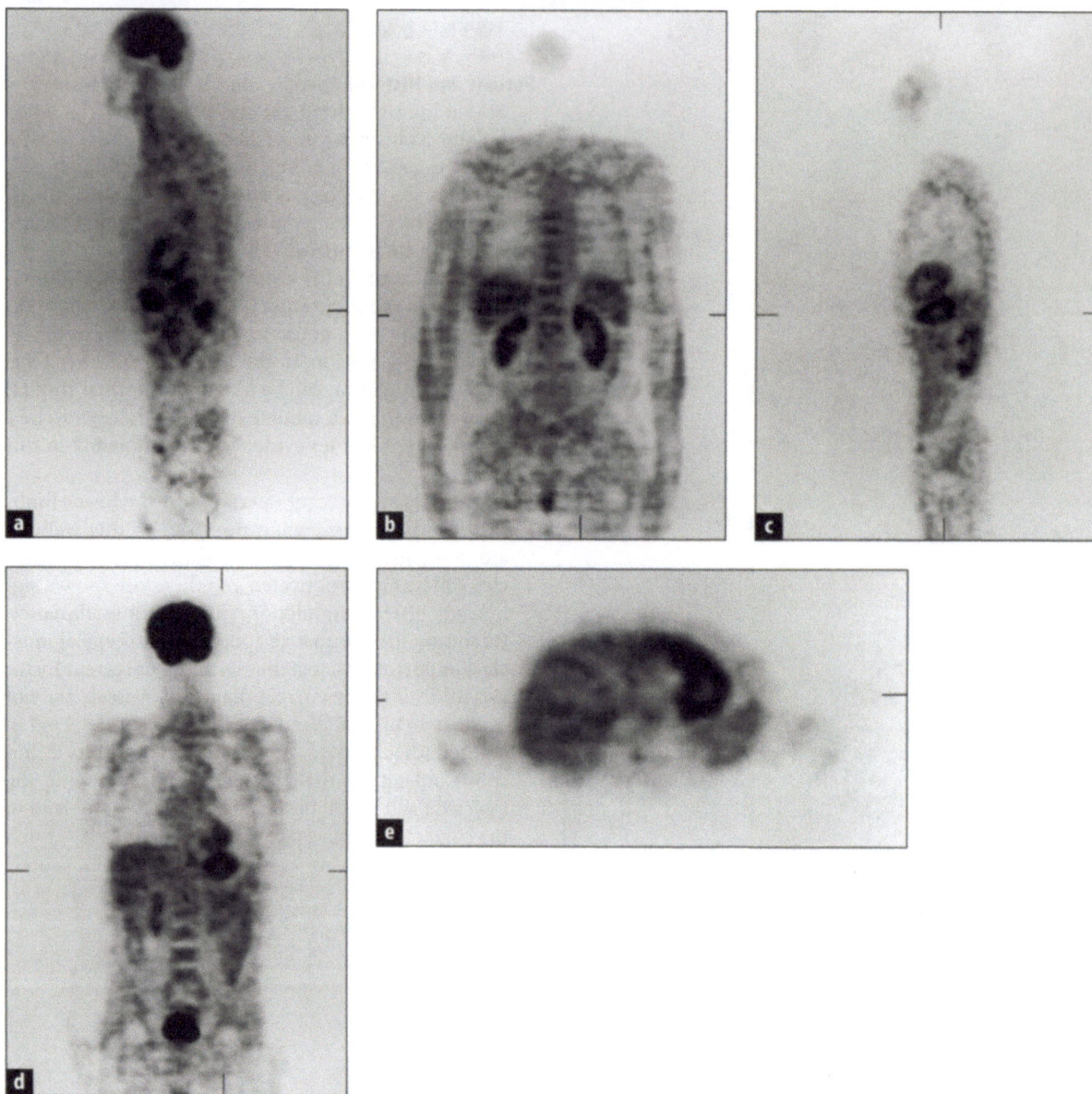

Figure 12 a–e

Patient and History: 67-year-old male with a history of MM at the right forehead, removed 3 days ago.

Technique: Transmission corrected emission scans with a slice thickness of 6 mm. Iterative reconstruction.

PET Results: On the sagittal slice (**a**), three FDG accumulations in the upper abdomen below the heart apex can be noted. The most posterior lesion turned out to be the medial part of the upper pole of the left kidney in the coronal slice (**b**). The two remaining lesions were shown to represent parts of the digestive tract, i.e., stomach and duodenum, in a more lateral sagittal slice (**c**) and in the corresponding coronal (**d**) and transversal (**e**) planes.

Cave! The gastrointestinal tract is not unlikely to show significant FDG accumulations which may appear as one or many focal lesions as well as a more diffuse uptake. Typical accumulation sites are the gastroesophageal junction, gastric fundus, and the colon. The anatomic course throughout all planes will lead to the correct diagnosis.

References

1. Balch CM, Reintgen DS, Kirkwood JM, Houghton A, Peters L, Ang KK (1997) Cutaneous melanoma. In: DeVita VT Jr, Hellman S, Rosemberg SA (eds) Cancer. Principles and practice of oncology, 5th edn. Lippincott-Raven, Philadelphia, pp 1947–1995

2. Balch CM, Milton GW (eds) (1985) Cutaneous melanoma: clinical management and treatment results worldwide. Lippincott, Philadelphia

3. Wagner JD, Schauwecker D, Davidson D, Coleman JJ 3rd, Saxman S, Hutchins G, Love C, Hayes JT (1999) Prospective study of fluorodeoxyglucose-positron emission tomography imaging of lymph node basins in melanoma patients undergoing sentinel node biopsy. J Clin Oncol 17:1508–1515

4. Kamel IR, Kruskal JB, Gramm HF (1998) Imaging of abdominal manifestations of melanoma. Crit Rev Diagn Imaging 39:447–486

5. Kim DG, Kim CY, Paek SH, Lee DS, Chung JK, Jung HW, Cho BK (1998) Whole-body [18F]FDG PET in the management of metastatic brain tumours. Acta Neurochir Wien 140:665–673

6. Holder WD Jr, White RL Jr, Zuger JH, Easton EJ Jr, Greene FL (1998) Effectiveness of positron emission tomography for the detection of melanoma metastases. Ann Surg 227:764–769

7. Macfarlane DJ, Sondak V, Johnson T, Wahl RL (1998) Prospective evaluation of 2-[18F]-2-deoxy-D-glucose positron emission tomography in staging of regional lymph nodes in patients with cutaneous malignant melanoma. J Clin Oncol 16:1770–1776

8. Rinne D, Baum RP, Hor G, Kaufmann R (1998) Primary staging and follow-up of high risk melanoma patients with whole-body 18F-fluorodeoxyglucose positron emission tomography: results of a prospective study of 100 patients. Cancer 82:1664–1671

9. Wagner JD, Schauwecker D, Hutchins G, Coleman JJ 3rd (1997) Initial assessment of positron emission tomography for detection of nonpalpable regional lymphatic metastases in melanoma. J Surg Oncol 64:181–189

10. Damian DL, Fulham MJ, Thompson E, Thompson JF (1996) Positron emission tomography in the detection and management of metastatic melanoma. Melanoma Res 6:325–329

11. Larcos G, Maisey MN (1996) FDG-PET screening for cerebral metastases in patients with suspected malignancy. Nucl Med Commun 17:197–198

12. Reske SN, Bares R, Büll U, Guhlmann A, Moser E, Wannenmacher MF (1996) Clinical value of positron emission tomography (PET) in oncologic questions: results of an interdisciplinary consensus conference. Nuklearmedizin 35:42–52

13. Blessing C, Feine U, Geiger L, Carl M, Rassner G, Fierlbeck G (1995) Positron emission tomography and ultrasonography. A comparative retrospective study assessing the diagnostic validity in lymph node metastases of malignant melanoma. Arch Dermatol 131:1394–1398

14. Steinert HC, Huch Boni RA, Buck A, Boni R, Berthold T, Marincek B, Burg G, von Schulthess GK (1995) Malignant melanoma: staging with whole-body positron emission tomography and 2-[F-18]-fluoro-2-deoxy-D-glucose. Radiology 195:705–709

15. Boni R, Boni RA, Steinert H, Burg G, Buck A, Marincek B, Berthold T, Dummer R, Voellmy D, Ballmer B, et al. (1995) Staging of metastatic melanoma by whole-body positron emission tomography using 2-fluorine-18-fluoro-2-deoxy-D-glucose. Br J Dermatol 132:556–562

16. Gritters LS, Francis IR, Zasadny KR, Wahl RL (1993) Initial assessment of positron emission tomography using 2-fluorine-18-fluoro-2-deoxy-D-glucose in the imaging of malignant melanoma. J Nucl Med 34:1420–1427

Colorectal Cancer

E. Abella-Columna and P. E. Valk

In 1996, 134,000 new cases of colorectal carcinoma were diagnosed in the United States. About 70 % of these patients underwent resection with curative intent, but only two-thirds of them will be cured of their disease. About one-third of colorectal cancers recur after curative surgery [1], and most patients with recurrent tumor die of the disease. In a small fraction of patients, recurrence is limited to a single accessible site, and is amenable to surgical cure. Potentially resectable tumor that is localized to the liver is found in approximately 5 % [2] and resectable pulmonary metastases are found in 1–2 % of all patients who are diagnosed with colorectal cancer. In cancer of the rectum and sigmoid colon, a further 5 % of all patients develop pelvic recurrence that is amenable to resection with curative intent [3].

Diagnosis of recurrence and appropriate selection of patients for surgery is hindered by the low sensitivity of computerized tomography (CT) for early metastasis [4] and by the non-specificity of pelvic abnormalities that are detected by CT after resection of rectal tumors [5]. CT commonly fails to diagnose metastasis to the peritoneum, mesentry and lymph nodes, and underestimates extent of hepatic involvement. Also, differentiation of postsurgical changes from tumor recurrence is often equivocal. For detection of hepatic metastasis, CT superior mesenteric artery portography is more sensitive than conventional CT, but has a high false-positive rate, thereby lowering the positive predictive value [6].

Despite careful preoperative staging by CT, approximately 50 % of patients who are thought to have resectable hepatic metastasis are found to have non-resectable disease at surgery [7, 8]. Furthermore, the 5-year disease-free survival after attempted curative resection is only 20–40 % [7, 9], indicating that most patients have residual tumor that remains undetected, even after operative evaluation. More accurate preoperative staging would reduce the frequency of surgery for non-resectable recurrence, and more sensitive initial detection of recurrence might increase the rate of resectability at diagnosis.

6.1 Sensitivity and Specificity of PET vs. CT

Evaluations of FDG PET for initial diagnosis of recurrent colorectal cancer and for preoperative assessment of recurrence have demonstrated higher sensitivity and specificity than CT. Four direct comparisons of the two modalities in a total of 306 patients [10–13] showed overall sensitivity for all sites of recurrence of 95 % for PET and 66 % for CT. Sensitivity for detection of hepatic recurrence was 95 % and 83 % for PET and CT respectively, and for pelvic recurrence, 97 % and 63 % respectively.

Valk et al. also compared sensitivity and specificity of PET and CT by site of recurrence, and determined the 95 % confidence interval for the difference between the two modalities for each site (Table 1) [13]. PET was significantly more sensitive than CT overall. The largest difference between the two modalities was found in the abdomen and pelvis, where over one-third of sites that

Table 1. Sensitivity of PET and CT by sites of tumor recurrence

Site	PET		CT		Difference (95 % CI)
Liver	54/57	(95%)	48/57	(84%)	11% (−1%–22%)
Pelvis	30/31	(97%)	21/31	(68%)	29% (9%–49%)
Abdomen	22/28	(79%)	13/28	(46%)	33% (11%–54%)
Retroperitoneum	12/12	(100%)	7/12	(58%)	42% (10%–74%)
Lungs	16/17	(94%)	16/17	(94%)	0% (−19%–19%)
Other	12/12	(100%)	4/12	(33%)	67% (36%–98%)
Total	146/157	(93%)	109/157	(69%)	24% (16%–32%)

were true positive by PET were false negative by CT. CT also had ten false positive findings in the abdomen and pelvis, compared to three by PET. In the liver, the difference between the modalities was less at 11%, and resulted mainly from difficulty in differentiating benign from malignant abnormalities by CT. PET was also more specific than CT, but the difference between the two modalities was smaller.

Delbeke et al. [12] compared PET and CT to CT portography, which is more invasive and more expensive than PET or CT alone. For detection of hepatic metastasis, PET was more accurate than CT or CT portography (92%, 78% and 80% accuracy respectively). CT portography had a higher sensitivity than PET (97% vs. 91%), but PET had much higher specificity. More importantly, PET diagnosed unsuspected extrahepatic recurrence in 28% of patients.

6.2 Preoperative Staging of Recurrent Tumor

The impact of PET findings on preoperative staging of patients with recurrent tumor has been evaluated in five studies [13–17]. In each study, whole-body FDG PET imaging was performed in patients who were thought to have resectable recurrence following demonstration of limited tumor at a single site by conventional imaging. PET demonstrated recurrence in at least one undetected site in 15–32% of studies. In all studies taken together, PET demonstrated unsuspected metastasis in 66/279 patients (24%). In a management algorithm where recurrence at more than one site is treated as non-resectable, this would translate into avoidance of non-indicated surgery by demonstration of non-resectable tumor in 24% of patients.

An assessment of the effect of preoperative PET imaging on cost of patient management was carried out by Valk et al. [13], who evaluated PET in a treatment algorithm where limited tumor at a single site was considered resectable, while tumor at more than one site was considered non-resectable. They determined the rate of detection of unsuspected tumor at other sites in a prospective clinical study, and modeled the effect on cost on the basis of Medicare reimbursement rates. A PET cost of $1800 was assumed. The cost of avoided surgery exceeded the cost of PET studies, resulting in a net saving of $3003 per patient. Gambhir et al. used decision analysis to evaluate the impact of PET on the cost of managing a larger group, consisting of all patients with colorectal cancer who were found to have serum CEA elevation at some point in their illness [18]. In this broader use of PET, they determined savings of $220 with no significant change in life expectancy.

6.3 Diagnosis of Recurrent Tumor

Whole-body FDG PET imaging is also valuable for evaluation of patients who are thought to have possible recurrence on the basis of clinical findings or elevated serum CEA level. No direct comparison of PET and CT has been done in such patients, but two groups have evaluated patients with elevated serum CEA level and negative CT findings, with similar results. Flanagan et al. demonstrated PET sensitivity of 100% and specificity of 71% [19], while Valk et al. found sensitivity of 93% and specificity of 92% in these patients [13]. Most importantly, both groups found PET-positive recurrence in two-thirds of CT-negative patients with serum CEA elevation. Bender et al. have also compared PET and CT for routine follow-up of colorectal cancer patients, and demonstrated the advantages of PET in that setting as well [20].

6.4 Preoperative Staging of Primary Tumor

There has been only one report of the use of FDG PET for preoperative staging of primary colorectal cancer. Abdel-Nabi et al. evaluated 48 patients with primary tumors, and identified the tumor itself in all cases [21]. PET and CT fared equally poorly for detection of local lymph node involvement, both with a sensitivity of 29%, but PET was more sensitive than CT for detection of hepatic metastasis. The use of imaging for preoperative staging of primary colorectal cancer remains controversial, but it is apparent from this study and from the assessments of PET in recurrent tumor that if such staging is to be undertaken, it should be performed with PET. Low sensitivity for detection of local lymph node metastasis is of limited clinical importance, since these nodes are evaluated as part of the surgical procedure, while more sensitive detection of hepatic metastasis allows resection of such lesions in a single surgical procedure, when appropriate.

6.5 Indications for PET Imaging

- Whole-body FDG PET should be used as the first diagnostic procedure when recurrence of colorectal cancer is suspected.
- If PET is to be used in a more limited fashion, the following represent minimum indications for its use:
  - Preoperative staging of recurrent tumor.
  - Rising serum CEA level or clinical suspicion of recurrence and negative CT findings.
  - Equivocal abnormality by CT imaging.

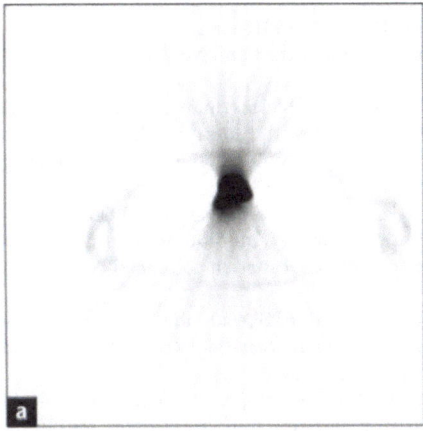

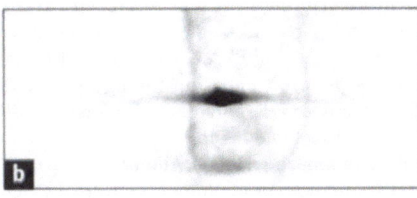

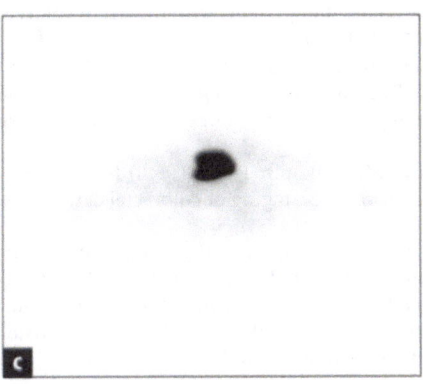

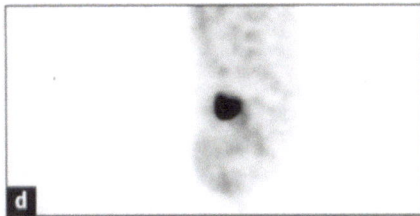

Figure 1a–d

Non-attenuation corrected transverse (**a**) and sagittal (**b**) images of the pelvis, demonstrating high bladder activity and associated positive (anteroposterior) and negative (lateral) reconstruction artifact. Images reconstructed with attenuation correction and iterative reconstruction (**c**) and (**d**) show elimination of bladder artifact

6.6 Technical Issues

1. Attenuation correction of images is important in colorectal cancer because of artifacts that are seen in non-corrected images of high-activity structures, including the renal collecting systems and the bladder. In non-corrected images, inequality of detected activity in low attenuation A-P projections and high attenuation lateral projections of the body produces positive and negative image artifacts (Fig. 1a,b), which may obscure lesion uptake. This problem can be avoided by attenuation correction of images (Fig. 1c,d). Attenuation correction is most effective in eliminating artifacts when used in combination with iterative image reconstruction methods, but is sufficiently effective for clinical purposes even when filtered backprojection is used. Bladder catheterization and irrigation represent efforts at dealing with the problem of image distortion resulting from high urinary activity, and such invasive procedures can be avoided by using attenuation correction of pelvic images.

2. Visual interpretation is the basis of reading PET images. The semiquantitative, standardized uptake value (SUV) (tissue uptake in μCi/ml, divided by injected dose in mCi/kg) is of little use in image interpretation, but may serve for more objective reporting of the activity in a lesion.

3. Physiologic uptake: In general, normal tissue uptake can be differentiated from abnormal uptake by the visible distribution of activity. Intestinal uptake is variable from patient to patient, and esophageal and gastric uptake are also commonly seen. The distribution of such uptake is generally linear and can be shown to follow the expected pattern, best seen in the coronal or sagittal planes. Uptake is also usually seen at colostomy sites. In 134 validated studies of colorectal cancer patients, there were only three instances of false-positive focal pelvic activity, which could have represented unrecognized focal intestinal uptake [13]. Urinary activity is also readily identifiable on the basis of distribution pattern.

References

1. August DA, Ottow RT, Sugarbaker PH (1984) Clinical perspectives on human colorectal cancer metastases. Cancer Metastasis Rev 3:303–324
2. Ballantyne GH, Quin J (1993) Surgical treatment of liver metastases in patients with colorectal cancer. Cancer 71 [Suppl]:4252–4266
3. Turk PS, Wanebo HJ (1993) Results of surgical treatment of nonhepatic recurrence of colorectal carcinoma. Cancer 71 [Suppl]:4267–4277
4. Steele GJ (1993) Standard postoperative monitoring of patients after primary resection of colon and rectum cancer. Cancer 71 [Suppl]:4225–4235
5. Kelvin FM, Maglinte DD (1987) Colorectal carcinoma: a radiologic and clinical review. Radiology 164:1–8
6. Peterson MS, Baron RL, Dodd GD III, et al. (1992) Hepatic parenchymal perfusion detected with CTPA: imaging-pathologic correlation. Radiology 183:149–155
7. Steele GJ, Bleday R, Mayer RJ, Lindblad A, Petrelli N, Weaver D (1991) A prospective evaluation of hepatic resection for colorectal carcinoma metastases to the liver: gastrointestinal tumor study group protocol 6584. J Clin Oncol 9:1105–1112
8. Saenz NC, Cady B, McDermott WVJ, et al. (1989) Experience with colorectal carcinoma metastatic to the liver. Surg Clin North Am 69:359–368
9. Hughes KS, Simon R, Songhorabodi S, et al. (1988) Resection of the liver for colorectal carcinoma metastases: a multi-institutional study of indications for resection. Surgery 103:278–288
10. Schiepers C, Penninckx F, De Vadder N et al. (1995) Contribution of PET in the diagnosis of recurrent colorectal cancer: comparison with conventional imaging. Eur J Surg Oncol 21:517–522
11. Ogunbiyi OA, Flanagan FL, Dehdashti F, et al. (1997) Detection of recurrent and metastatic colorectal cancer: comparison of positron emission tomography and computed tomography. Ann Surg Oncol 4:613–620
12. Delbeke D, Vitola JV, Sandler MP, et al. (1997) Staging recurrent metastatic colorectal carcinoma with PET. J Nucl Med 38:1196–1201
13. Valk PE, Abella-Columna E, Haseman MK, et al. (1999) Whole-body PET imaging with F-18-fluorodeoxyglucose in management of recurrent colorectal cancer. Arch Surg 134:503–511
14. Beets G, Penninckx F, Schiepers C, et al. (1994) Clinical value of whole-body positron emission tomography with [18F]fluorodeoxyglucose in recurrent colorectal cancer. Br J Surg 81
15. Vitola JV, Delbeke D, Sandler MP, et al. (1996) Positron emission tomography to stage metastatic colorectal carcinoma to the liver. Am J Surg 171:21–26
16. Lai DT, Fulham M, Stephen MS, et al. (1996) The role of whole-body positron emission tomography with [18F]fluorodeoxyglucose in identifying operable colorectal cancer. Arch Surg 131:703–707
17. Flamen P, Stroobants S, Cutsem EV, et al. (1999) Additional value of whole-body positron emission tomography with fluorine-18-2-fluoro-2-deoxy-D-glucose in recurrent colorectal cancer. J Clin Oncol 17:894–901
18. Gambhir SS, Valk P, Shepherd J, Hoh C, Allen M, Phelps ME (1997) Cost effective analysis modeling of the role of FDG-PET in the management of patients with recurrent colorectal cancer. J Nucl Med 38:9
19. Flanagan FL, Dehdashti F, Ogunbiyi OA, Siegel BA (1998) Utility of FDG PET for investigating unexplained plasma CEA elevation in patients with colorectal cancer. Ann Surg 227:319–323
20. Bender H, Metten M, Willkomm P, et al. (1998) Tumor markers and FDG-PET in the restaging of colorectal carcinoma. Eur J Nucl Med 25:942
21. Abdel-Nabi H, Doerr RJ, Lamonica DM, Cronin VR, Galantowicz PJ, Carbone GM, Spaulding MB (1998) Staging of primary colorectal carcinomas with fluorine-18 fluorodeoxyglucose whole-body PET: correlation with histopathologic and CT findings. Radiology 206:755–760

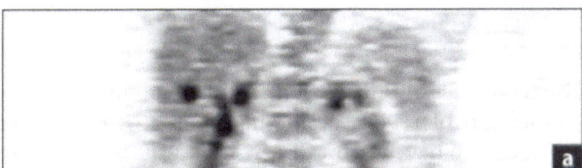

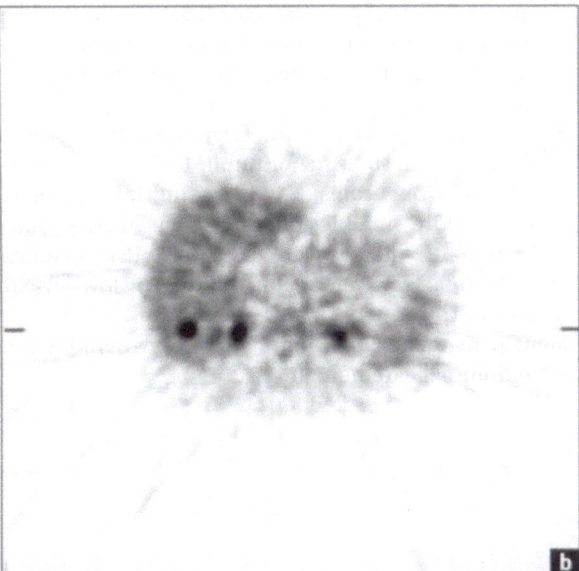

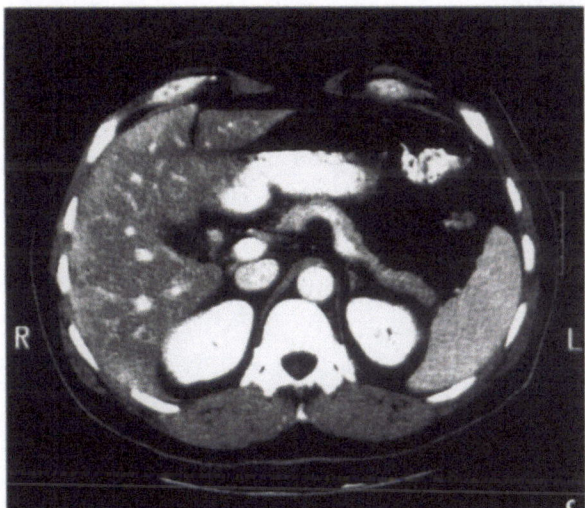

Figure 2 a–c

History: 52-year-old man, who had undergone right hemicolectomy for carcinoma of the ascending colon 1 year earlier, was found to have a rising serum CEA level [13]. CT scan of the abdomen showed mild fatty infiltration of the liver, with no change from a previous scan 4 months earlier. PET study to evaluate CEA elevation.

Technique: Non-corrected whole-body imaging, with attenuation-corrected imaging of the abdomen.

PET Findings: Coronal (**a**) and transverse (**b**) PET images of the liver show a hypermetabolic focus in the posterior right lobe of the liver, characteristic of hepatic metastasis. The corresponding arterial-phase CT image (**c**) shows no abnormality, and later-phase images were also normal. CT-negative metastatic foci were also seen in two other PET image sections.

Cave! Similarity of abnormal hepatic foci to foci of excreted activity in the adjacent renal calyces and pelvis.

Management and Follow-up: Repeat CT imaging 8 weeks later showed six hepatic lesions up to 1 cm in diameter, consistent with metastatic disease. Chemotherapy was commenced.

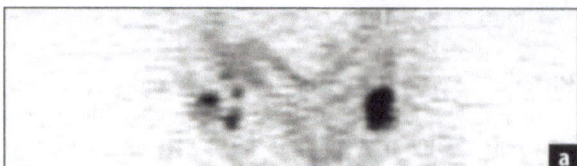

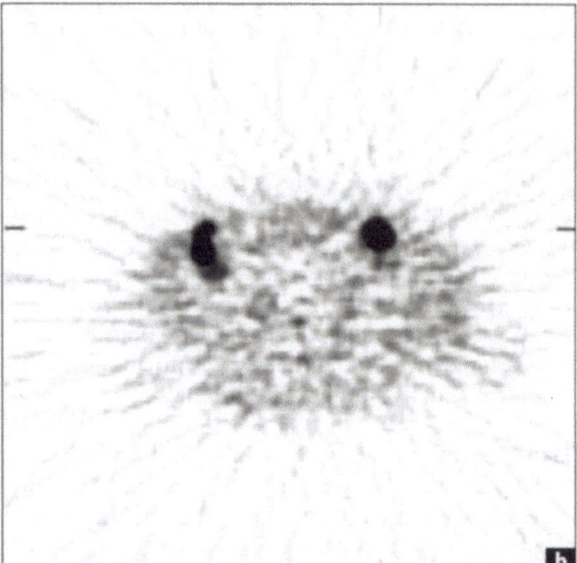

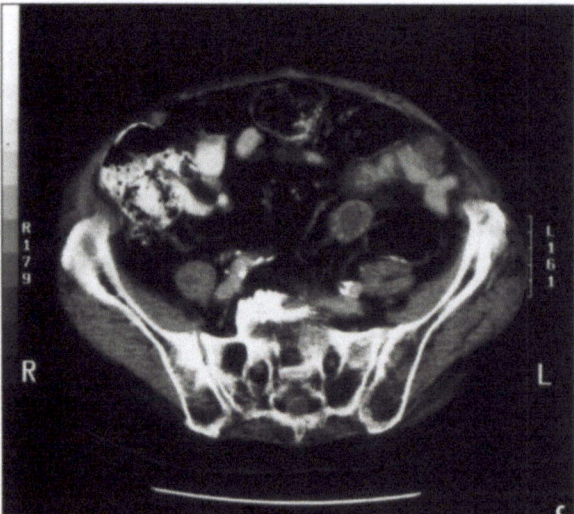

Figure 3 a–c

History: An 89-year-old woman, who had undergone resection of rectal carcinoma 14 months earlier, was found to have serum CEA rising to 27. CT scan of the abdomen and pelvis showed no evidence of recurrent tumor. PET study to evaluate serum CEA elevation.

Technique: Non-corrected whole-body imaging, with attenuation-corrected imaging of the abdomen and pelvis.

PET Findings: Coronal (**a**) and transverse (**b**) images of the abdomen show major tumor foci in the right and left lower quadrants, as well as multiple smaller lesions. More small lesions were seen in other image sections. CT image (**c**) at same level as (**b**) was normal

Cave! Normal transverse colon outlined by low-level uptake of tracer (**a**).

Management and Follow-up: Laparotomy demonstrated abdominal carcinomatosis.

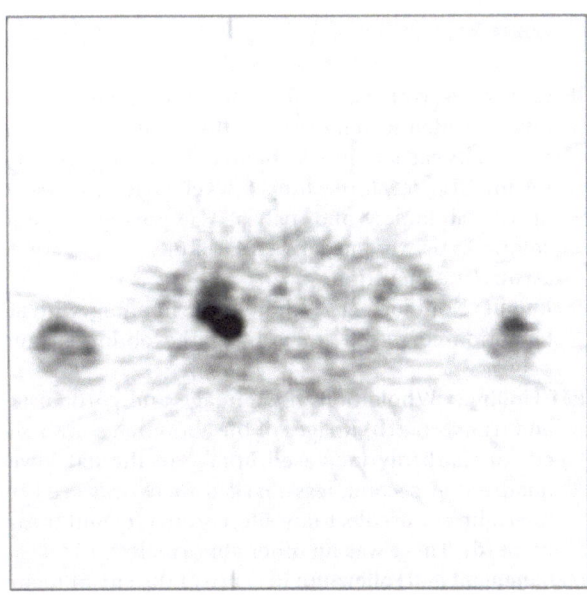

Figure 4

History: 74-year-old woman, who had undergone resection of carcinoma of rectosigmoid colon 3 years earlier, and a cecal carcinoma 1 year earlier. She was now found to have an increasing serum CEA level, which reached 22.7. CT scans of the abdomen and pelvis showed no evidence of recurrence. PET study to evaluate CEA elevation.

Technique: Non-corrected whole-body imaging, with attenuation-corrected imaging of the abdomen and pelvis.

PET Findings: Transverse PET image (shows a focus of markedly increased uptake in the right lower quadrant of the abdomen. Whole-body images showed no other abnormality.

Management and Follow-up: Laparotomy showed a locally recurrent tumor mass at the site of previous cecal resection. There was no other evidence of tumor, and the mass was resected. One month after surgery serum CEA level was normal at 1.8.

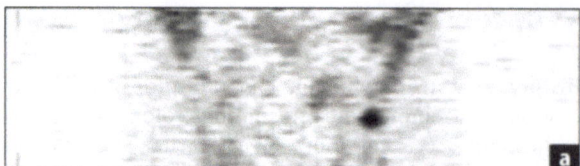

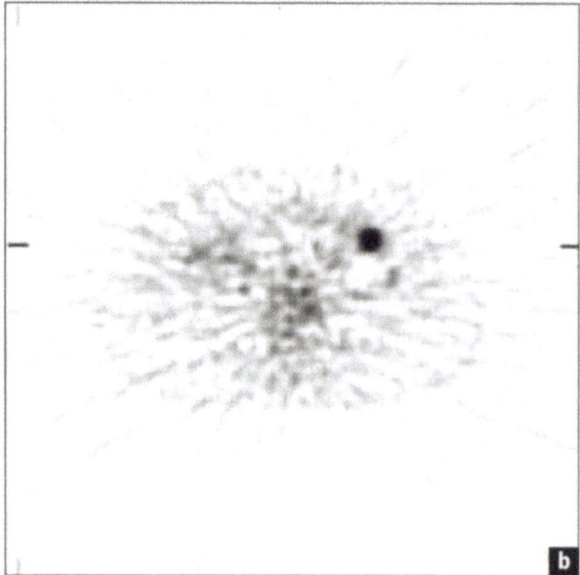

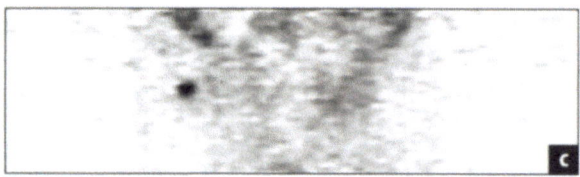

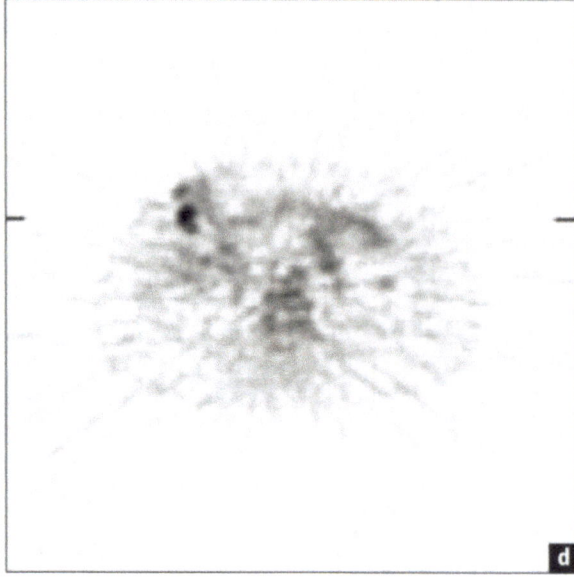

Figure 5 a–d

History: 53-year-old man who had undergone colectomy for adenocarcinoma of the transverse colon 18 months earlier. He was found to have an increasing serum CEA level, reaching a level of 10.9. CT scan of the abdomen and pelvis, CT portogram and colonoscopy were negative. PET study to investigate serum CEA elevation.

Technique: Non-corrected whole-body imaging, with attenuation-corrected imaging of the abdomen and pelvis.

PET Findings: Whole body PET image and coronal (**a**) and transverse (**b**) images of the abdomen show a focus of markedly increased uptake in the left lower quadrant. A second, less-marked focus was seen on the right, at the colostomy site, coronal (**c**) and transverse (**d**). There was no other abnormality.

Management and Follow-up: Because of the site of recurrence, curative resection was not considered appropriate. Laparotomy was performed 4 months later, when the patient developed intestinal obstruction, and abdominal carcinomatosis was found.

Cave! (i) Focal uptake is commonly seen at colostomy sites, probably as a result of inflammation, and need not represent tumor. (ii) The patient may already have had more extensive tumor at the time of the PET scan than the scan demonstrated. When a group of 40 patients underwent laparotomy after PET had demonstrated a single focal recurrence, 7 patients (17%) were found to have more extensive, non-resectable tumor. Most commonly, undiagnosed diffuse peritoneal or pelvic sidewall tumor spread was found, in addition to a PET-positive tumor mass. When tumor grows in thin layers, PET commonly fails to resolve the tumor in its smallest dimension.

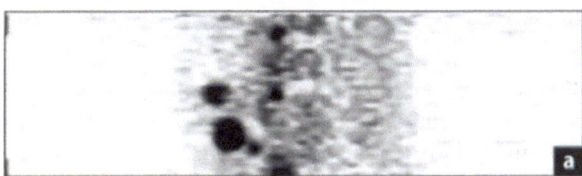

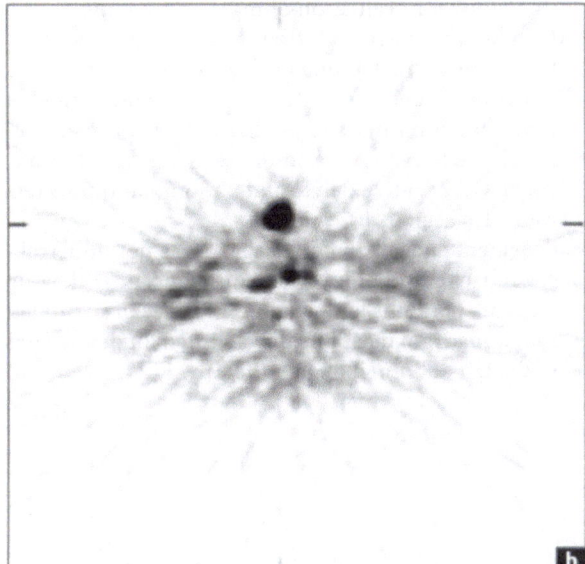

Figure 6 a, b

History: 59-year-old man who was found to have serum CEA elevation to 56.8 ng/ml, 1 year after resection of colon carcinoma, with subsequent demonstration of hepatic metastasis by CT. CT showed no evidence of recurrence elsewhere in the abdomen or pelvis. PET study for preoperative evaluation.

Technique: Non-corrected whole-body imaging, with attenuation-corrected imaging of the abdomen and pelvis.

PET Findings: Sagittal (**a**) and transverse (**b**) PET images of the abdomen show multiple abdominal and retroperitoneal tumor foci, in addition to the known hepatic tumor, which was also positive by PET.

Cave! Low-activity lumbar intervertebral disks aid in anatomic localization of lesions in sagittal image (**a**).

Management: Surgery was not performed.

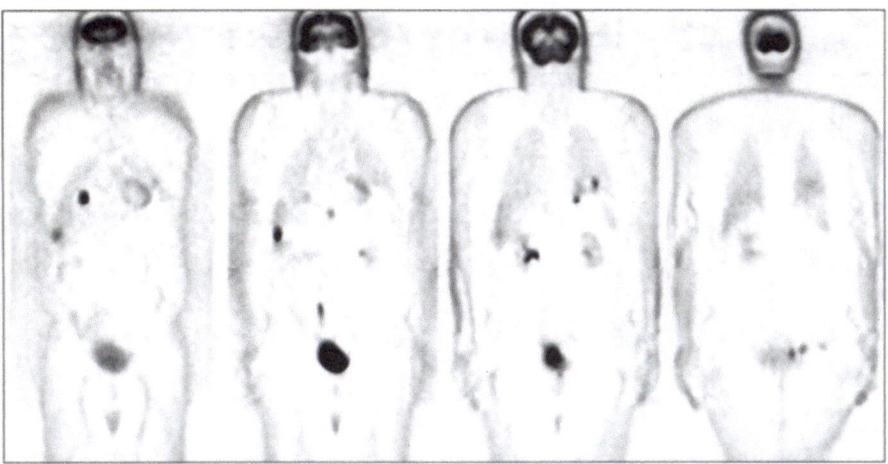

Figure 7/Case 6

History: 62-year-old man, who underwent resection of rectal carcinoma 5 years earlier, was found to have two abnormalities in the liver on CT, consistent with metastatic tumor. CT of the pelvis showed post-treatment changes, unchanged from a previous CT 9 months earlier. Chest CT examination was not performed. PET study for preoperative evaluation, prior to possible resection of hepatic metastases.

Technique: Non-corrected whole-body imaging and attenuation-corrected imaging of upper abdomen and pelvis.

PET Findings: Coronal whole-body PET images show foci of increased uptake in the liver, left lung and left pelvis, characteristic of metastasis.

Management: Surgery was not performed. The patient was treated by chemotherapy.

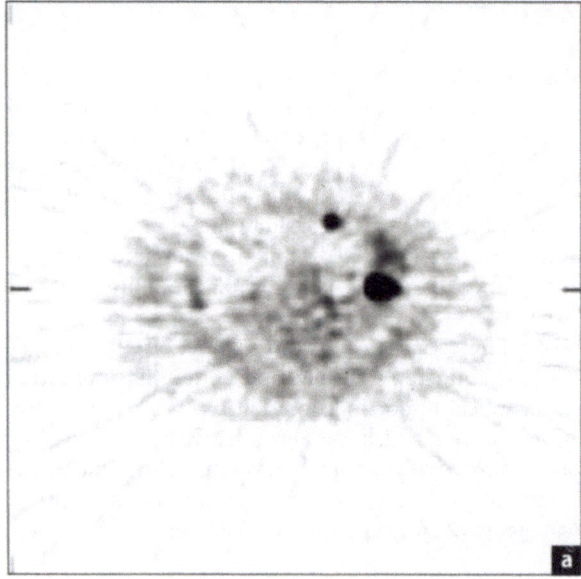

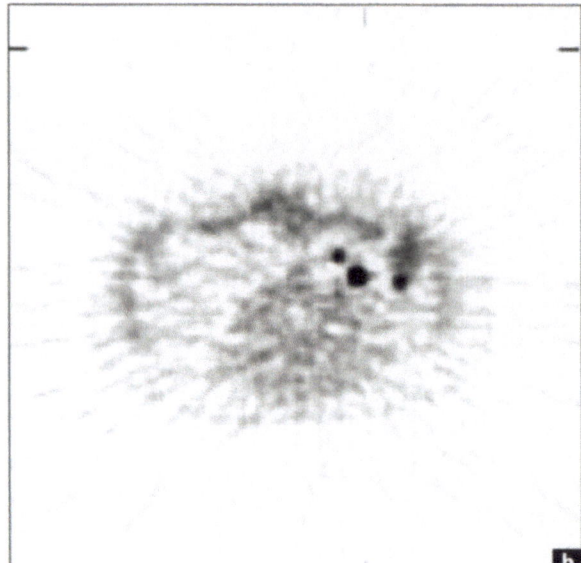

Figure 8 a, b

History: 70-year-old man, who had undergone resection of descending colon carcinoma 2 years earlier, was found to have a 3 × 1.5-cm mass on CT, close to the site of resection. No other lesions were seen. Preoperative PET study for evaluation of mass and staging.

Technique: Non-corrected whole-body imaging, with attenuation-corrected imaging of the abdomen.

PET Findings: Transverse PET image (**a**) showed the left lower quadrant mass to be markedly hypermetabolic, characteristic of tumor recurrence. Multiple, small, CT-negative pelvic and abdominal tumor foci were also seen (**a, b**).

Management and Follow-up: Surgery was not undertaken and chemotherapy was commenced. Follow-up CT scan 4 months later showed increase in size of left lower quadrant mass and development of new lesions in the left abdomen during therapy.

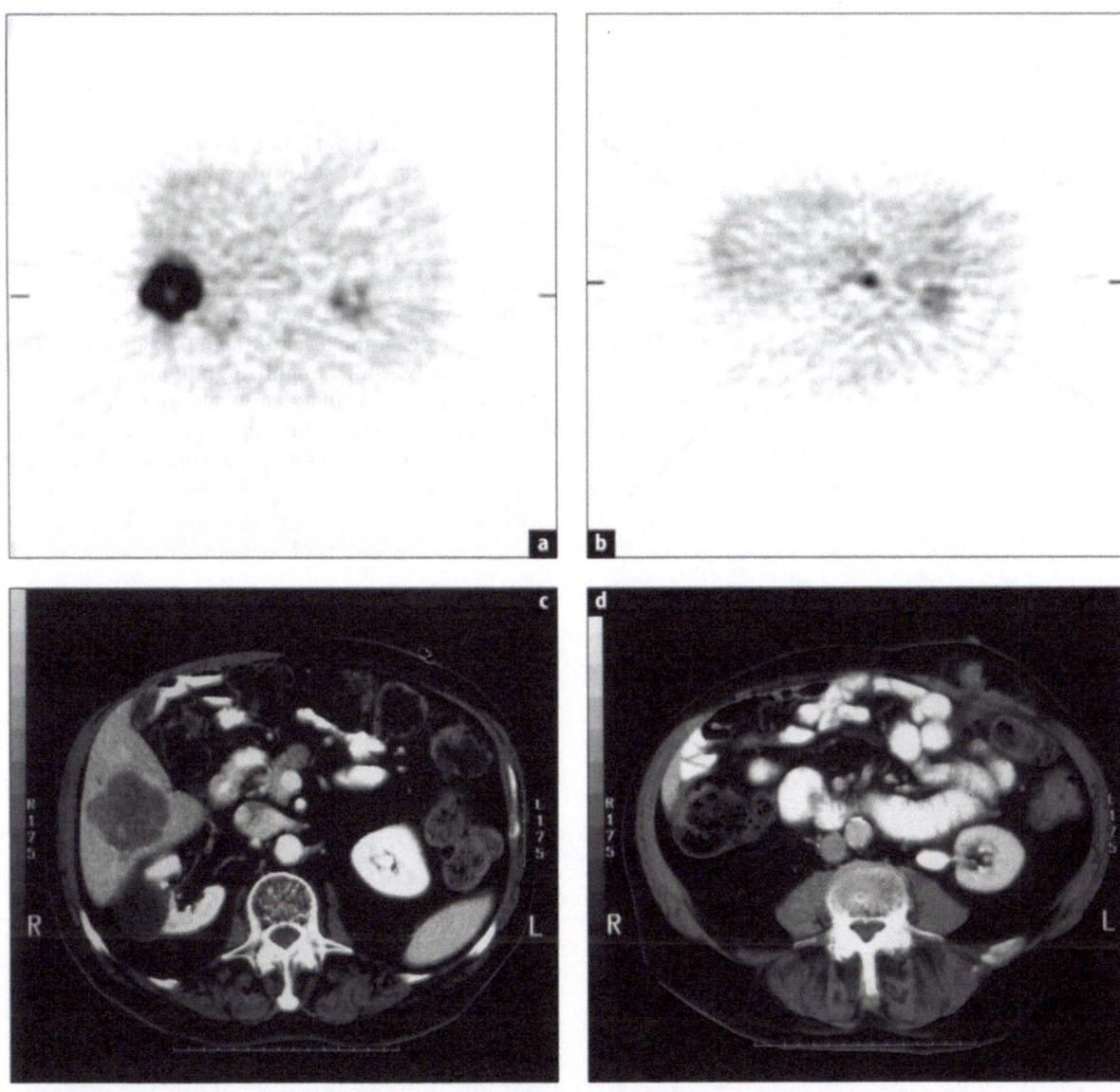

Figure 9 a–d

History: 72-year-old man, treated by irradiation and chemotherapy for locally recurrent rectal carcinoma. One year later, follow-up CT of the pelvis and abdomen showed solitary hepatic metastasis, with no evidence of residual pelvic tumor or tumor at other sites. Preoperative PET study to evaluate patient for possible hepatic resection.

Technique: Non-corrected whole-body imaging, with attenuation-corrected imaging of upper abdomen and pelvis.

PET Findings: Transverse PET images show a hypermetabolic mass in the posterior right lobe of the liver (**a**) and a small retroperitoneal focus of increased uptake, which is characteristic of retroperitoneal lymph node metastasis. Corresponding CT images show the hepatic lesion (**c**), but no retroperitoneal abnormality is apparent (**d**). Pelvic PET images were normal.

Management: Surgery was not performed, and the patient was treated by chemotherapy.

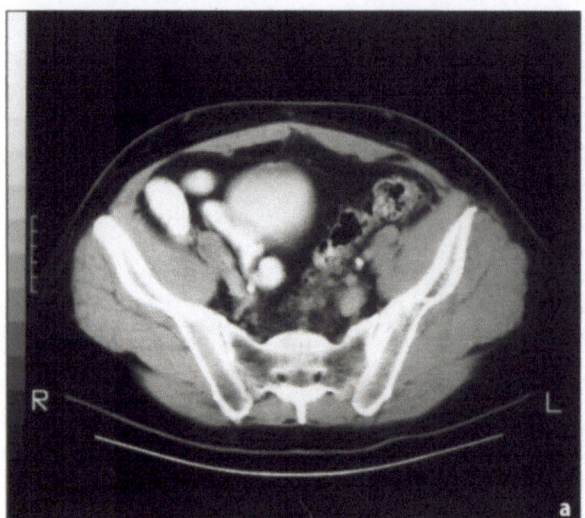

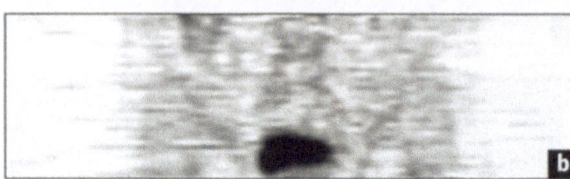

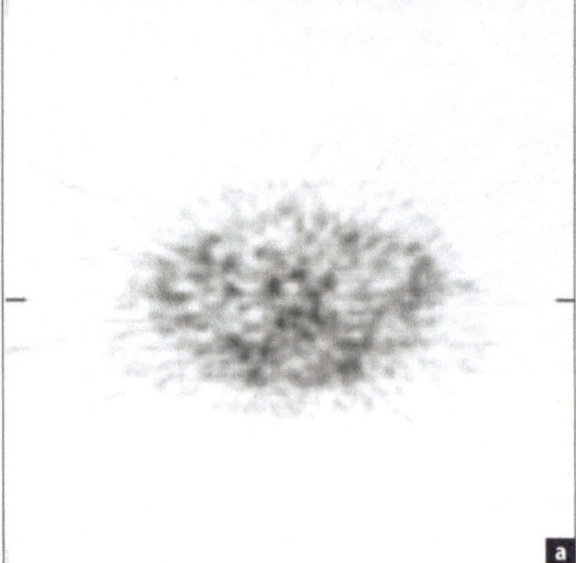

Figure 10 a–c

History: 59-year-old man, who had undergone resection of a sigmoid carcinoma 16 months earlier, was found to have left iliac lymph node enlargement on CT examination (**a**). PET study to evaluate lymphadenopathy.

Technique: Non-corrected whole-body imaging, with attenuation-corrected imaging of the abdomen and pelvis.

PET Findings: Coronal (**b**) and transverse (**c**) PET images of the pelvis at the level of the CT lesion showed no abnormality, indicating benign lymphadenopathy. Whole-body PET images were also normal.

Management and Follow-up: During 18 months of clinical follow-up, the patient remained well without treatment. Serum CEA level remained between 0.7 and 1.1.

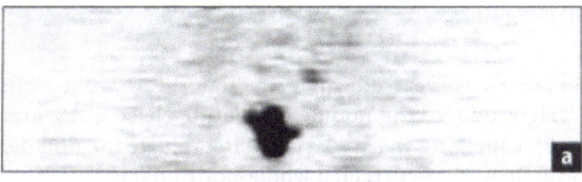

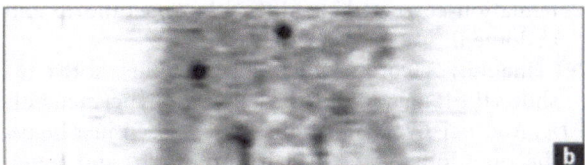

Figure 11 a, b

History: 70-year-old woman who was found to have rectal carcinoma by sigmoidoscopic biopsy. CT scan of the abdomen and pelvis showed lymph nodes measuring less than 1 cm in the presacral and left pararectal regions. There was no evidence of hepatic metastasis. The serum CEA level was 86 ng/ml. PET study for preoperative staging of primary tumor.

Technique: Non-corrected whole-body imaging, with attenuation-corrected imaging of the abdomen and pelvis.

PET Findings: Coronal image of the pelvis (**a**) shows markedly elevated uptake in the primary rectal tumor. Small tumor foci were seen in the presacral region and the left pelvic outlet, and one of these is also seen in (**a**). Coronal image of the liver (**b**) shows two metastatic foci, and multiple other foci were seen in other image sections.

Management and Follow-up: Patient underwent abdominoperineal resection. Histologic examination showed involvement of 5/6 proximal and 20/20 distal rectal lymph nodes. Liver biopsy was positive for metastasis.

Cave! Apparent low activity of lymph node metastasis in (**a**), compared to primary and hepatic lesions, resulting from small lesion size (under 1 cm in this case). A PET scanner with intrinsic resolution of 5 mm full-width half-maximum (FWHM) has a reconstructed image resolution of 8 mm FWHM or more, depending on reconstruction method. At this resolution, the actual activity of a lesion will be accurately depicted in the image only if the lesion measures at least 20 mm in all dimensions. A smaller lesion will be "blurred" and will appear larger than it actually is, so that its activity will appear diminished.

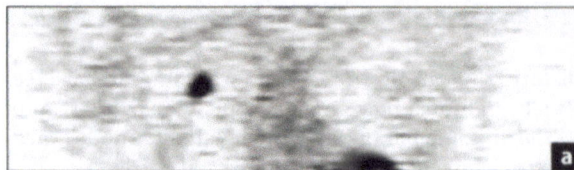

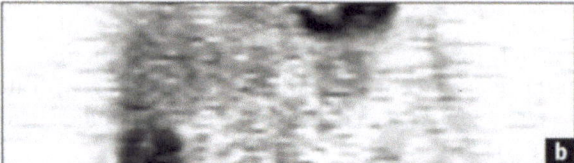

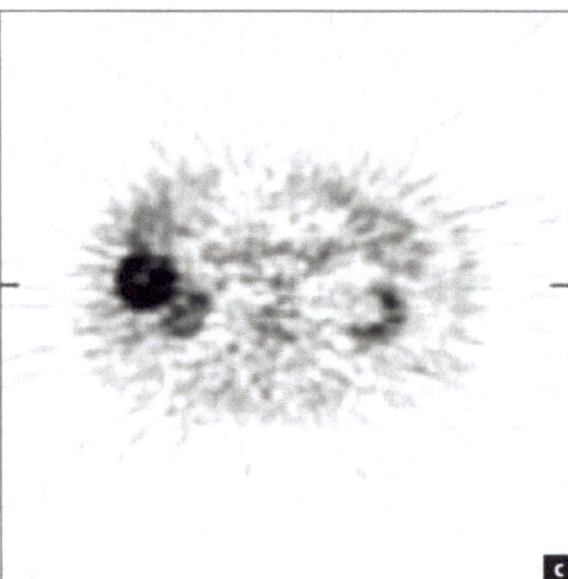

Figure 12 a–c

History: A 66-year-old man was found to have a 2-cm right upper lung nodule on routine chest X-ray, and PET imaging was undertaken to evaluate the nodule.

Technique: Non-corrected whole-body imaging, with attenuation-corrected imaging of the upper thorax and abdomen.

PET Findings: A coronal PET image of the thorax (**a**) shows the lung nodule to be markedly hypermetabolic. Another hypermetabolic mass is seen just below the right lobe of the liver in coronal (**b**) and transverse (**c**) PET images of the abdomen. Whole-body PET images showed no other abnormalities.

Histologic Diagnosis: Biopsy of the lung nodule demonstrated squamous cell carcinoma, and the patient underwent right upper lobectomy. At laparotomy, the abdominal mass was found to be a primary adenocarcinoma of the ascending colon, and this also was resected. No metastases from either tumor were found.

Cave! Primary colorectal cancer may be seen in previously treated patients who are undergoing evaluation for tumor recurrence, and are found to have a second primary lesion rather than recurrent tumor.

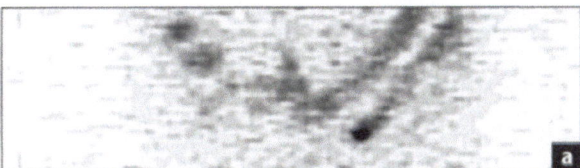

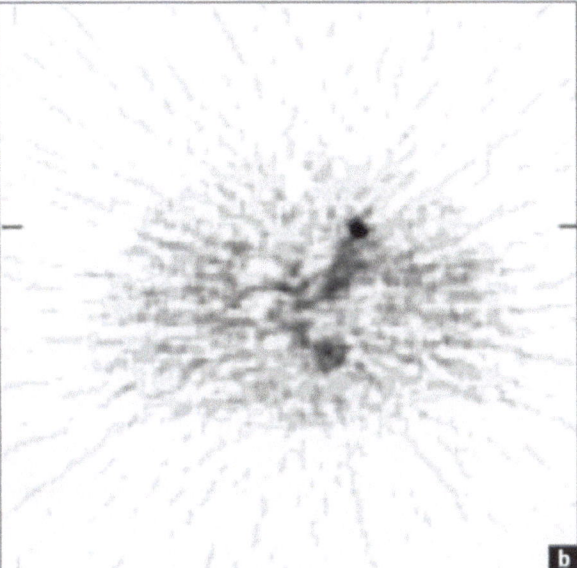

Figure 13 a, b

History: 82-year-old woman who had undergone right hemicolectomy for cecal carcinoma 2 years earlier. She was found to have an increasing serum CEA level, reaching a level of 15.3. CT scan of the abdomen and pelvis showed fatty change of the liver only. Colonoscopy with biopsy showed no evidence of tumor. PET study to investigate serum CEA elevation.

Technique: Non-corrected whole-body imaging, with attenuation-corrected imaging of the abdomen and pelvis.

PET Findings: Whole-body images and subsequent attenuation-corrected coronal (**a**) and transverse (**b**) images of the pelvis show a small hypermetabolic focus in the left hemipelvis, which appears to lie along the course of the descending/sigmoid colon. There was no other abnormality.

Follow-up: Exploratory laparotomy revealed no abnormality in the descending/sigmoid colon, or elsewhere in the pelvis. Seven months after the PET study the patient died of unrelated causes.

Cave! Further history that was obtained after the laparotomy revealed that a small polyp had been found colonoscopy at 40 cm, and that multiple biopsies had been obtained of this lesion, 4 days pre-PET. These showed no evidence of malignancy. Increased FDG uptake may occur with postoperative tissue healing, and it may be that postbiopsy healing of the polyp was responsible for the focal hypermetabolism in this case. This was the most marked false-positive focal abnormality that was seen in a series of 134 validated PET studies for recurrent colorectal cancer. Out of a total of five false-positive PET findings, three were in the pelvis.

Thyroid Cancer

F. Grünwald

The annual incidence of malignant thyroid tumors is about 4/100,000 in women and 1.5/100,000 in men. The most frequent forms are tumors with follicle cell differentiation (papillary and follicular carcinoma) and those with C-cell differentiation (medullary thyroid cancer, MTC). In most cases, thyroid carcinomas with follicle cell differentiation (differentiated carcinoma, DTC) have a good prognosis, even in the presence of lung metastases. Therefore, thyroid cancer is a rare cause of cancer-associated death. Nevertheless, an early detection of tumor recurrence is essential for therapy planning.

7.1 Primary Tumor/Preoperative Staging

In contrast to other organ systems, FDG-PET is not useful for thyroid cancer detection prior to surgery in most cases, especially in areas with a high incidence of thyroid nodules, since the specificity becomes too low. Nevertheless, if a "hot lesion" in the thyroid gland is seen in a PET study performed for other reasons, further examination is necessary to exclude malignancy (Fig. 1). In some cases with known carcinoma, particularly in MTC, a preoperative PET scan can be useful for lymph node staging.

7.2 Differentiated Thyroid Cancer

The blood level of thyroglobulin (Tg) is the most important parameter during treatment and follow-up of DTC. If recurrence is suspected, iodine-131 scintigraphy is the functional imaging technique of choice since this method allows the evaluation of therapy options. In patients with DTC who have had normal Tg values after thyroidectomy and ablative ^{131}I therapy, presenting with elevated Tg values during follow-up, suggesting recurrence, in whom iodine-131 scintigraphy WBS is negative (particularly Hürthle cell carcinomas and poorly differentiated cancers), functional imaging techniques are necessary to detect tumor sites to plan further therapeutic steps. In iodine-negative tumors, FDG-PET has a sensitivity of about 85%. In patients with known iodine-positive tumor sites, FDG-PET is useful to detect additional (iodine-negative) sites (Fig. 2).

Thyroid hormone treatment should not be withdrawn before FDG-PET imaging. It is recommended to perform FDG-PET when no major masses of benign remnant tissue are expected because it might be difficult to differentiate remnant tissue from local recurrence.

7.2.1 Local Recurrence/Lymph Node Metastases

Particularly papillary thyroid cancer is associated with lymph node metastases, which do not affect prognosis significantly. In many cases it is not possible to differentiate recurrence from local metastatic disease; therefore both entities are often summarized with respect to imaging techniques. Besides the cervical lymph nodes, the mediastinum is involved predominantly in lymph node metastases. The main pitfalls are unspecific FDG uptake in the larynx (Fig. 3) (especially if the patient talks after tracer injection), in the thymus (which must not be misinterpreted as mediastinal lymph node metastases) and in cervical muscles (Fig. 4) (particularly if the patient is not relaxed after tracer injection).

7.2.2 Distant Metastases (Figs. 5, 6)

The lung and bones are affected most frequently by distant metastases. In contrast to many other malignant diseases, patients suffering from distant metastases have a good chance of cure, particularly in diffuse lung metastases, if these are iodine-positive. With respect to subsequent therapy, FDG-PET can be used to localize single metastases prior to surgery or radiotherapy and multiple metastases before starting a redifferentiation therapy with retinoic acid.

7.3 Medullary Thyroid Cancer

MTC occurs either as sporadic (about 75 % of all patients) or as hereditary tumor disease (multiple endocrine neoplasia, MEN) type 2A and 2B as well as hereditary MTC).

7.3.1 Local Recurrence/Lymph Node Metastases

In contrast to differentiated thyroid cancer, lymph node staging has a major influence on the prognosis of MTC, lymph node dissection being essential during primary surgery. The rate of known malignancy prior to surgery is higher than in differentiated thyroid cancer; therefore the presurgical evaluation has more clinical relevance. In some cases, the origin of malignancy cannot be determined initially (differential diagnosis, e.g., lung cancer, lymphoma; Fig. 7); nevertheless it is very important to define tumor extent exactly before planning surgical procedures.

7.3.2 Distant Metastases

Calcitonin (sensitivity improved by pentagastrin test) and CEA are the most important tumor markers in the follow-up of medullary thyroid cancer. There are several tracers for functional imaging (mIBG, In-octreotide, DMSA, anti-CEA), but the detection of tumor tissue is difficult in many cases, especially if the metastatic sites are < 10 mm in diameter. If multiple distant metastases occur in MTC, the prognosis is poor, since chemotherapy and radiotherapy are rarely successful.

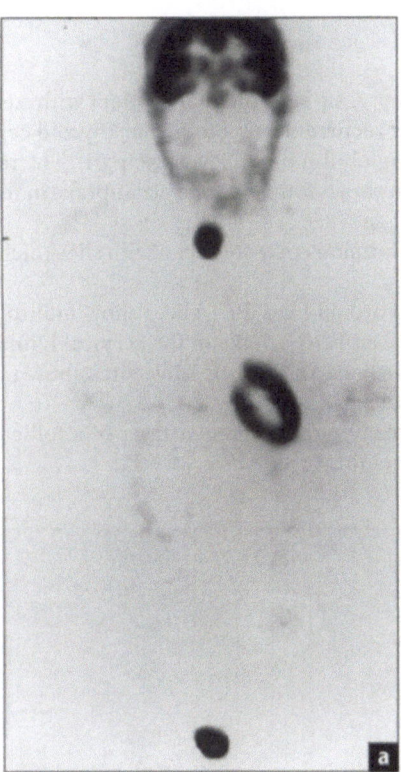

Figure 1 a–c

Patient and History: A 27-year-old male patient, scanned for staging of malignant melanoma.

Technique: Non-transmission corrected scan with slice thickness of 4 mm.

PET Results: The coronal FDG-PET slices show a large area of increased FDG uptake in the right lobe of the thyroid gland (**a**).

Further Clinical History: Clinical examination revealed a palpable mass in the right thyroid lobe. Ultrasound showed a 42 × 34 × 35-mm nodule in the right lobe (**b**), which was cold in the pertechnetate scintigraphy (**c**).

Histology: Papillary thyroid carcinoma pT2a N0 M0.

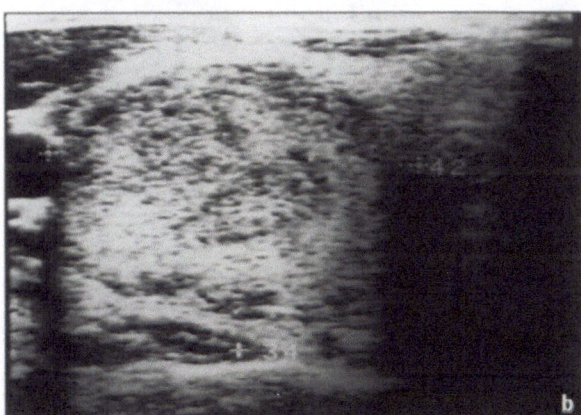

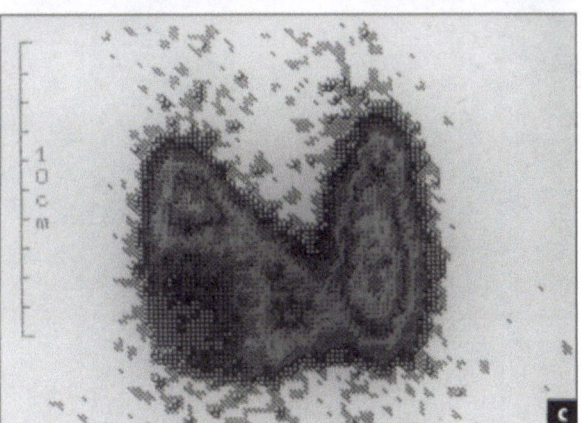

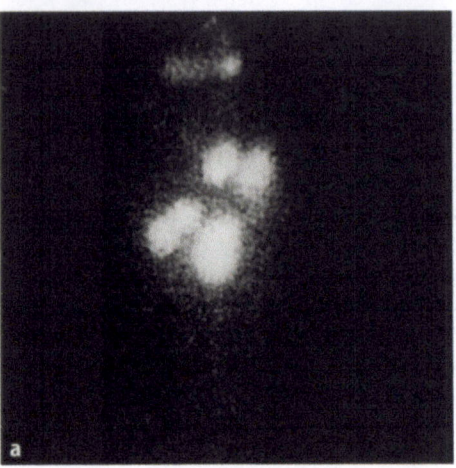

Figure 2 a, b

Patient and History: A 54-year-old male patient with suspicion of local recurrence of a follicular thyroid carcinoma (thyroglobulin blood level: 850 µg/l). The radioiodine scan shows four sites of tracer uptake in the neck (**a**).

Technique: Transmission corrected scan with slice thickness of 4 mm.

PET Results: The coronal FDG-PET slices show multiple areas of increased FDG uptake in the cervical lymph nodes (**b**). **Cave:** not all FDG-positive sites show radioiodine uptake.

Histology: Multiple lymph node metastases of a follicular thyroid carcinoma.

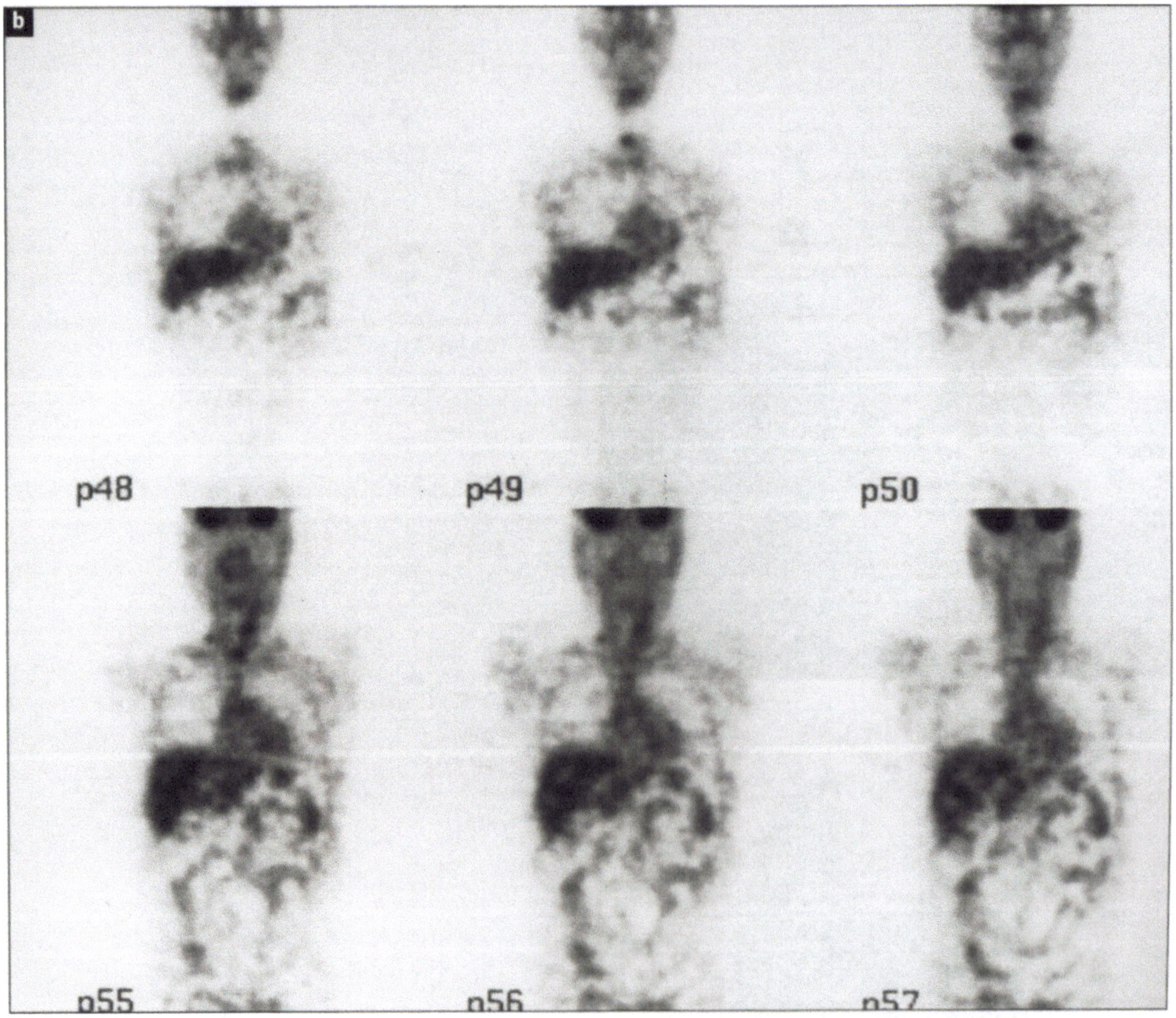

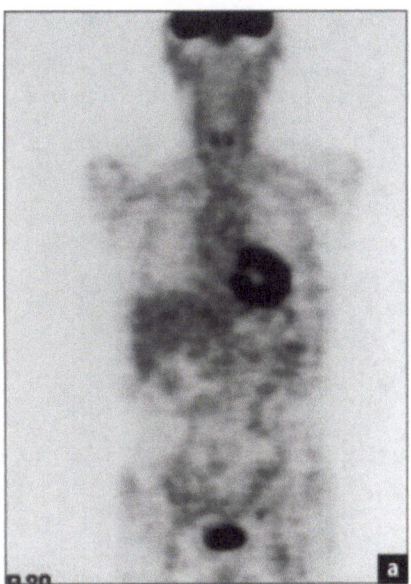

Figure 3 a, b

Patient and History: A 34-year-old female patient, studied for staging of a malignant melanoma.

Technique: Transmission corrected scan with slice thickness of 4 mm.

PET Results: The coronal (**a**) and transaxial (**b**) FDG-PET slices show an increased FDG uptake in the larynx. Cave: the larynx can show up with an increased FDG uptake, particularly if the patient is talking in the first minutes after tracer injection.

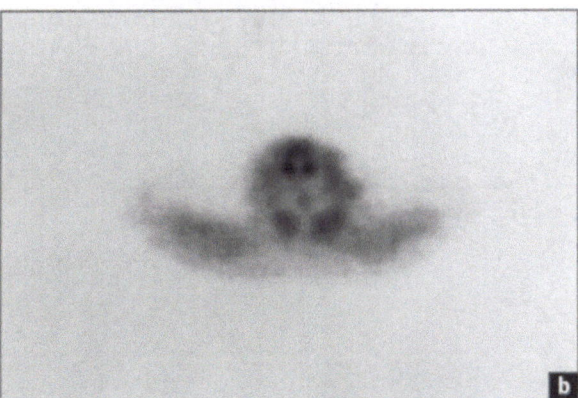

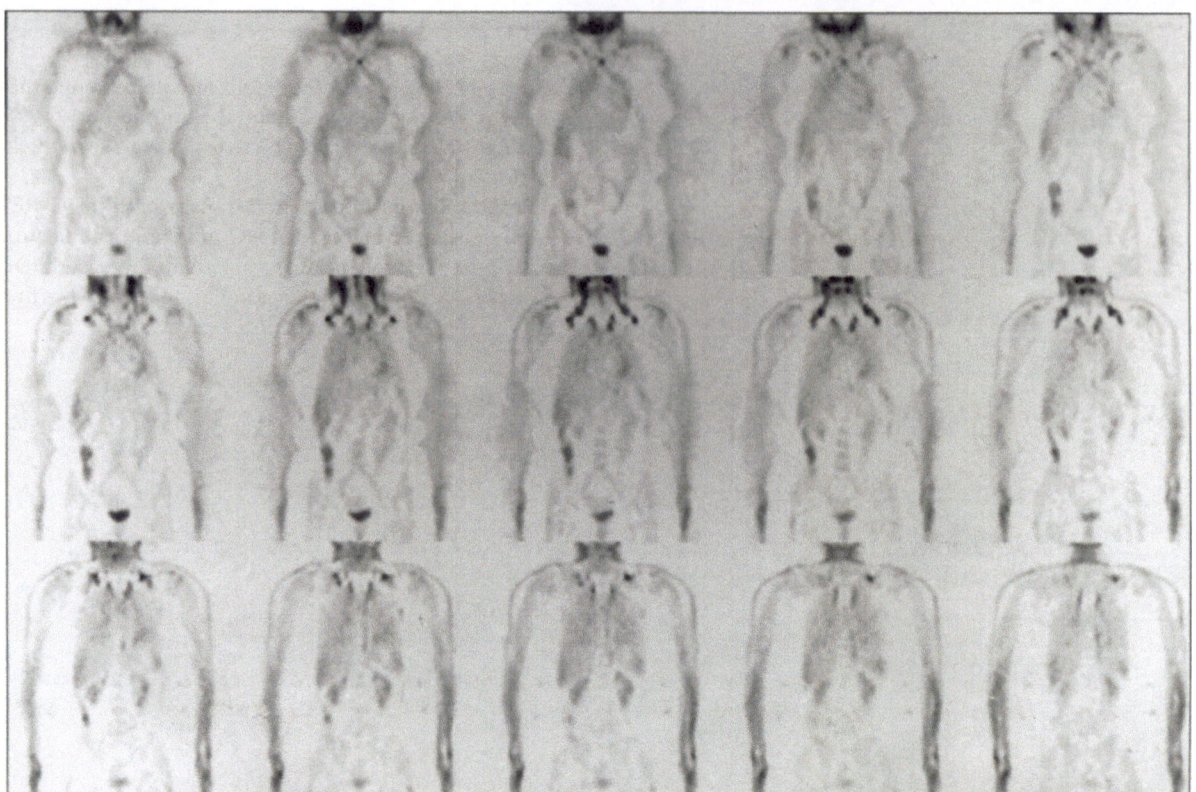

Figure 4

Patient and History: A 27-year-old female patient, studied because of suspected osteomyelitis.

Technique: Non-transmission corrected scan with slice thickness of 4 mm.

PET Results: The coronal FDG-PET slices show multiple areas of increased FDG uptake in the muscles and muscular insertions of the neck and upper thorax (predominantly symmetrical, **a**). **Cave:** the cervical muscles can have an intensively increased FDG uptake, particularly in young women with high muscle tension.

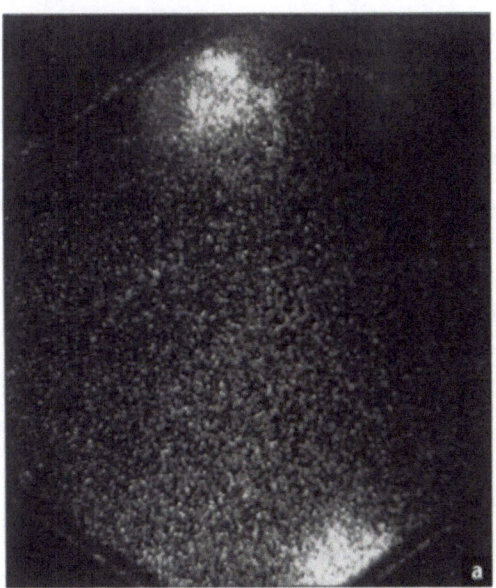

Figure 5 a–c

Patient and History: A 73-year-old female patient with suspicion of metastases of a papillary thyroid carcinoma (thyroglobulin blood level: 124 μg/l). The radioiodine scan shows no tracer uptake (**a**).

Technique: Non-transmission corrected scan with slice thickness of 4 mm.

PET Results: The coronal (**b**) and transaxial (**c**) FDG-PET slices show areas of increased FDG uptake in the mediastinum.

Further Clinical History: No surgery could be performed; the patient was treated with radiotherapy.

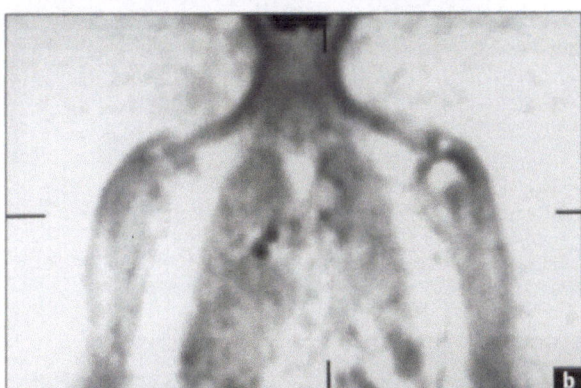

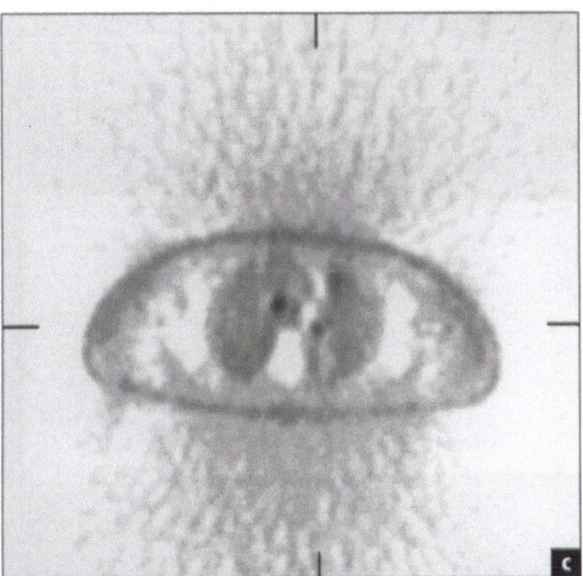

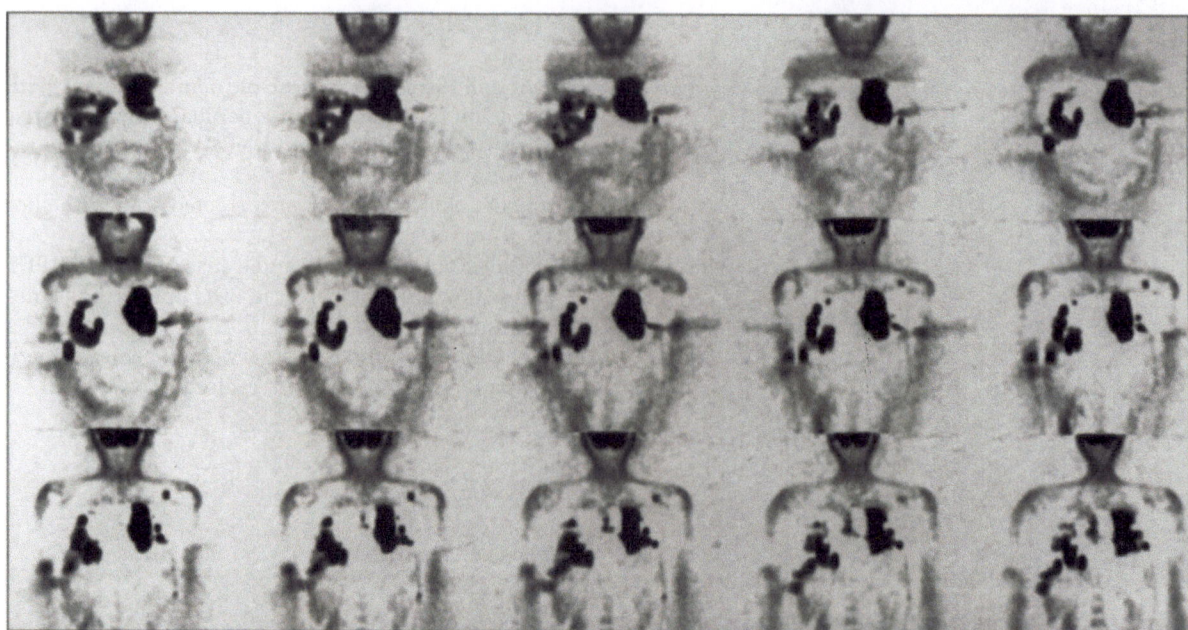

Figure 6

Patient and History: A 54-year-old male patient, suffering from dyspnea, treated with thyroidectomy and ablative radioiodine therapy because of a follicular thyroid cancer.

Technique: Non-transmission corrected scan with slice thickness of 4 mm.

PET Results: The coronal FDG-PET slices show multiple sites of intensively increased FDG uptake in both lungs and the left shoulder.

Further Clinical History: The patient was not operated. No radioiodine therapy could be performed since the metastases did not take up radioiodine. Redifferentiation therapy and subsequently chemotherapy were performed.

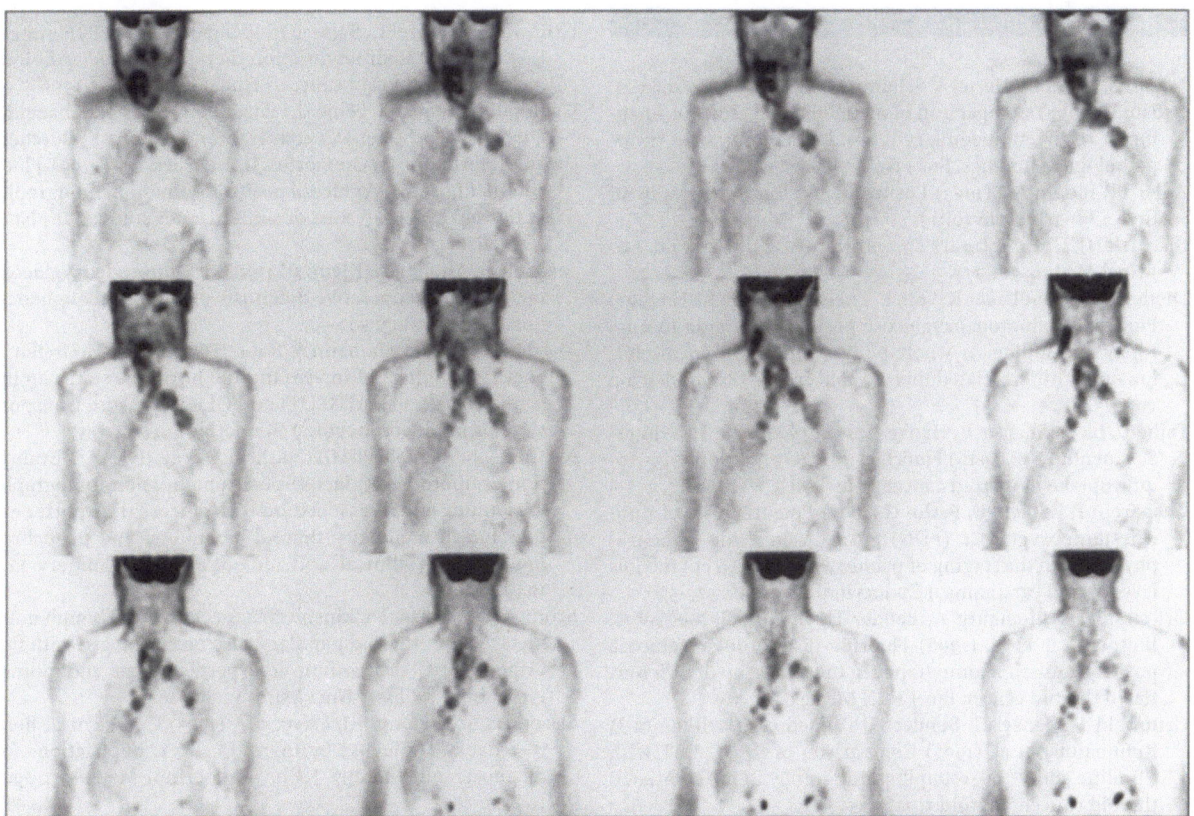

Figure 7

Patient and History: A 49-year-old male patient with a cervical tumor, suspected to be malignant (e.g., lymphoma or thyroid carcinoma).

Technique: Non-transmission corrected scan with slice thickness of 4 mm.

PET Results: The coronal FDG-PET slices show multiple areas of increased FDG uptake in the right thyroid lobe, in the cervical lymph nodes (predominantly on the right side) and in the thorax (**a**).

Histology: Medullary thyroid cancer with multiple cervical and mediastinal lymph node metastases.

References

Adams S, Baum RP, Hertel A, Schumm-Draeger PM, Usadel KH, Hör G (1998) Comparison of metabolic and receptor imaging in recurrent medullary thyroid carcinoma with histopathological findings. Eur J Nucl Med 25: 1277-1283

Adler LP, Bloom AD (1993) Positron emission tomography of thyroid masses. Thyroid 3: 195-200

Biersack HJ, Hotze A (1991) The clinician and the thyroid. Eur J Nucl Med 18: 761-778

Dietlein M, Scheidhauer K, Voth E, Theissen P, Schicha H (1997) Fluorine-18 fluorodeoxyglucose positron emission tomography and iodine-131 whole-body scintigraphy in the follow-up of differentiated thyroid cancer. Eur J Nucl Med 24: 1342-1348

Feine U, Lietzenmayer R, Hanke JP, Held J, Wöhrle H, Müller-Schauenburg W (1996) Fluorine-18-FDG and Iodine-131-Iodide uptake in thyroid cancer. J Nucl Med 37: 1468-1472

Gasparoni P, Rubello D, Ferlin G (1997) Potential role of fluorine-18-deoxyglucose (FDG) positron emission tomography (PET) in the staging of primitive and recurrent medullary thyroid carcinoma. J Endocrinol Invest 20: 527-530

Grünwald F, Schomburg A, Bender H, Klemm E, Menzel C, Bultmann T et al. (1996) Fluorine-18 fluorodeoxyglucose positron emission tomography in the follow-up of differentiated thyroid cancer. Eur J Nucl Med 23: 312-319

Grünwald F, Menzel C, Bender H, Palmedo H, Willkomm P, Ruhlmann J et al. (1997) Comparison of [18]FDG-PET with [131]Iodine and ^{99m}Tc-sestamibi scintigraphy in differentiated thyroid cancer. Thyroid 7: 327-335

Grünwald F, Menzel C, Bender H, Palmedo H, Otte R, Fimmers R et al. (1998) Redifferentiation therapy-induced radioiodine uptake in thyroid cancer. J Nucl Med 39: 1903-1906

Grünwald F, Kälicke T, Feine U, Lietzenmayer R, Scheidhauer K, Dietlein M, Schober O, Lerch H, Brandt-Mainz K, Burchert W, Hiltermann G, Cremerius U, Biersack HJ (1999) Fluorine-18 fluorodeoxyglucose positron-emission tomography in thyroid cancer: results of a multicenter study; Eur J Nucl Med 26: 1547–1552

Joensuu H, Ahonen A, Klemi PJ (1988) ^{18}F-fluorodeoxyglucose imaging in preoperative diagnosis of thyroid malignancy. Eur J Nucl Med 13: 502-506

Matthaei S, Trost B, Hamann A, Kausch C, Benecke H, Greten H et al. (1995) Effect of in vivo thyroid hormone status on insuline signalling and GLUT1 and GLUT4 glucose transport systems in rat adipocytes. J Endocrinol 144:347-357

Musholt TJ, Musholt PB, Dehdashti F, Moley JF (1997) Evaluation of fluorodeoxyglucose-positron emission tomographic scanning and its association with glucose transporter expression in medullary thyroid carcinoma and pheochromocytoma: a clinical and molecular study. Surgery 122: 1049-1060

Scott GC, Meier DA, Dickinson CZ (1995) Cervical lymph node metastasis of thyroid papillary carcinoma imaged with fluorine-18-FDG, technetium-99m-pertechnetate and iodine-131-sodium iodide. J Nucl Med 36: 1843-1845

Sisson JC, Ackermann RJ, Meyer MA (1993) Uptake of 18-fluoro-2-deoxy-D-glucose by thyroid cancer: implications for diagnosis and therapy. J Clin Endocrinol Metab 77:1090-1094

Non-Small Cell Lung Cancer

R. J. Hagge, A. Al-Sugair and R. E. Coleman

Lung cancer is the number one cause of cancer deaths worldwide. According to the World Health Organization, over 660,000 new cases are diagnosed each year. According to the American Cancer Society, almost 180,000 new cases are diagnosed annually within the United States. Overall 5-year survival in these patients is about 13%, and depends strongly on the stage of the disease at diagnosis. Five-year survival is greater than 60% in stage I disease, 30–50% in stage II, 10–30% in stage IIIa, and less than 5% in stages IIIb and IV. Accurate, noninvasive methods of staging are needed so that decisions for definitive versus palliative therapy can be made appropriately.

FDG PET imaging is a powerful tool in the initial diagnosis and staging of lung cancer, and in follow-up surveillance for recurrent and metastatic disease. Hypermetabolism within a solitary pulmonary nodule, i.e., a standardized uptake value (SUV) greater than 2.5, is suggestive of malignancy, and can be used as an indication for biopsy. PET is also useful for staging the mediastinum, for detecting distant metastases, and in selecting sites for biopsy when clinically indicated.

8.1 PET Imaging Protocols Used in This Chapter

- PET scanner: GE advance
- Patient preparation: NPO 4–6 h
- Radiopharmaceutical: 140 µCi/kg F-18 fluorodeoxyglucose (FDG), administered intravenously (maximum dose 20.0 mCi)
- Postinjection delay: 45–120 min
- Image acquisition
  - Chest with measured attenuation correction:
    2D emission scans (8 min per bed position)
    2D transmission scans (10 min per bed position)
  - Whole body survey without attenuation correction:
    2D emission scans (4 min per bed position)
- Image reconstruction:
  - 2D filtered backprojection
  - 7.0-mm Hann filter
  - 128×128 matrix
  - 4.25-mm transaxial slice thickness

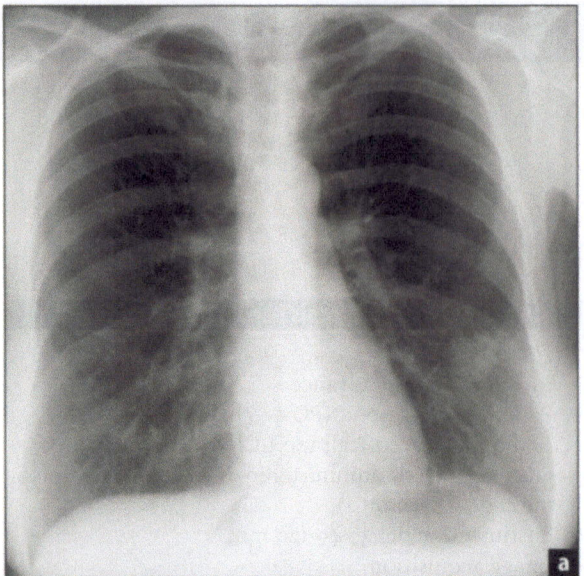

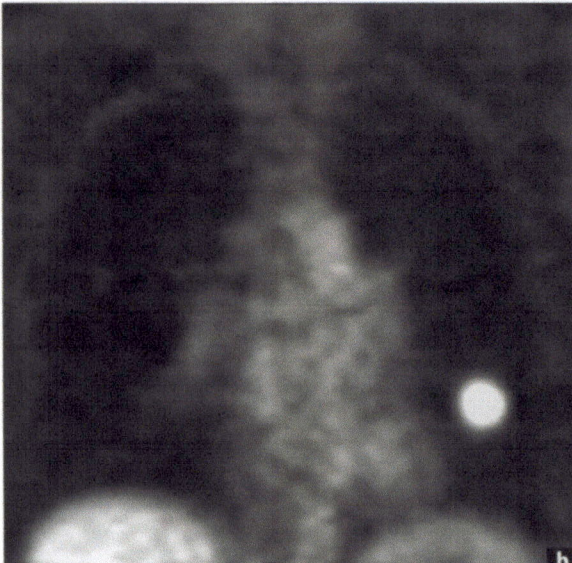

8.2 Primary Tumor

Figure 1 a, b

Patient and History: This 43-year-old woman presented with a seizure. A brain MRI showed an enhancing left frontal mass with surrounding edema (not shown). A chest radiograph revealed a left lung nodule (**a**).

PET Results: A coronal image of the chest demonstrates intense hypermetabolism within the left lung nodule, consistent with a primary malignancy (**b**). No hypermetabolic metastases were identified elsewhere within the chest, abdomen, or pelvis. The brain lesion was hypermetabolic, consistent with either a solitary metastasis or a primary high grade glioma (not shown).

Histology: Bronchoscopy revealed adenocarcinoma of the lung.

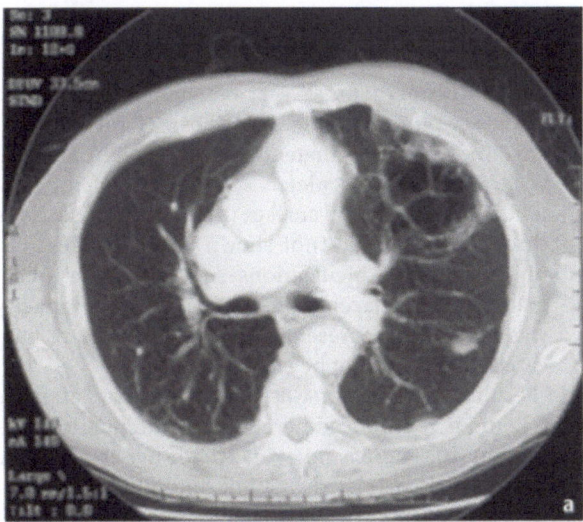

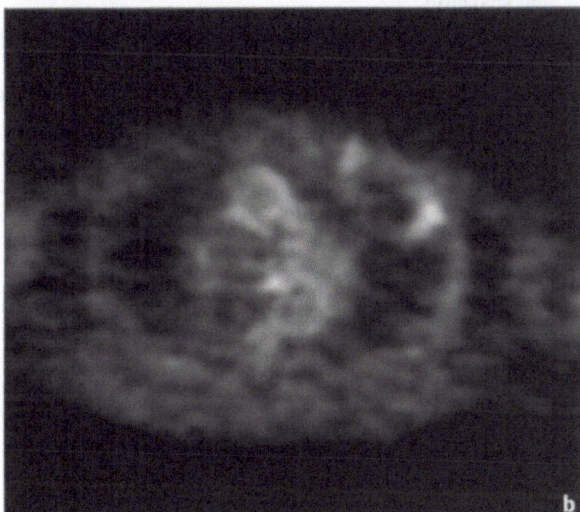

Figure 2 a, b

Patient and History: This 76-year-old man presented with 5 months of progressive hemoptysis. Bronchoscopy revealed non-small cell carcinoma in the lingula. CT showed a cavitary lesion in the lingula, and a 1.5 × 1.0-cm nodule separate from and posterior to the cavity (**a**).

PET Results: The PET scan was performed on the same day as the CT. Hypermetabolism is demonstrated along the rim of the lingular cavity, consistent with a primary pulmonary malignancy (**b**). The small left lung nodule is not seen, favoring a benign process.

Histology: The patient underwent a lingular wedge resection and completion lobectomy. Bronchioloalveolar cell carcinoma (BAC) was found to be surrounding the periphery of the large bullous cystic area. No other pulmonary malignancy was found at surgery.

Cave! BAC is a potential source of false negative FDG PET scans. According to Higashi et al., about 57% of BAC cases are hypometabolic, and the mean SUV in BAC is 1.4 ± 0.8. According to Kim et al., the mean peak SUV in BAC is 3.5 ± 2.2, which is much lower than in other non-small cell lung carcinomas.

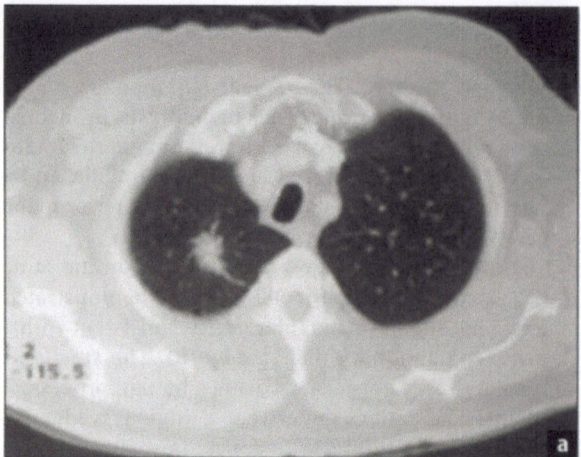

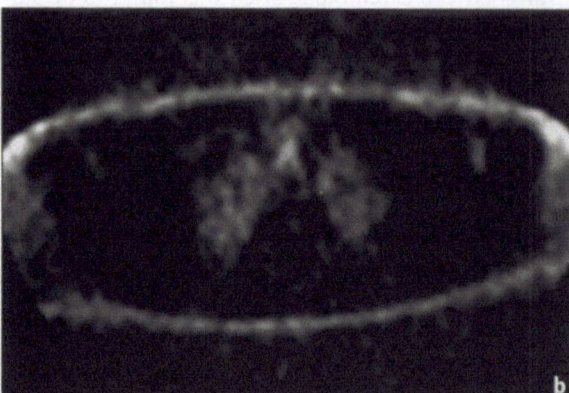

Figure 3 a, b

Patient and History: This 52-year-old man presented with a solitary pulmonary nodule. Chest CT revealed a 1-cm, smoothly marginated right upper lobe nodule, with associated spiculated soft tissue opacities extending to the pleural surface (**a**). Thin 1 mm sections through the nodule (not shown) demonstrated benign-appearing calcifications, suggestive of a tuberculoma. The adjacent spiculated soft tissue opacity was thought to represent scarring, but primary lung carcinoma could not be excluded.

PET Results: The PET scan was performed 5 days after the CT, and is reproduced here without attenuation correction (**b**). There is no evidence for hypermetabolic tumor. The correlated imaging findings are consistent with prior granulomatous disease and right apical scarring.

Cave! Without attenuation correction the lungs typically show increased activity compared to the chest wall and superior mediastinum, despite the fact that they contain less metabolically active tissue per unit volume. This is because air within the lungs is low in density, resulting in less photon attenuation. When measured attenuation correction is applied, the lungs appear hypometabolic relative to surrounding tissues.

8.3 Local Recurrence

Figure 4 a, b

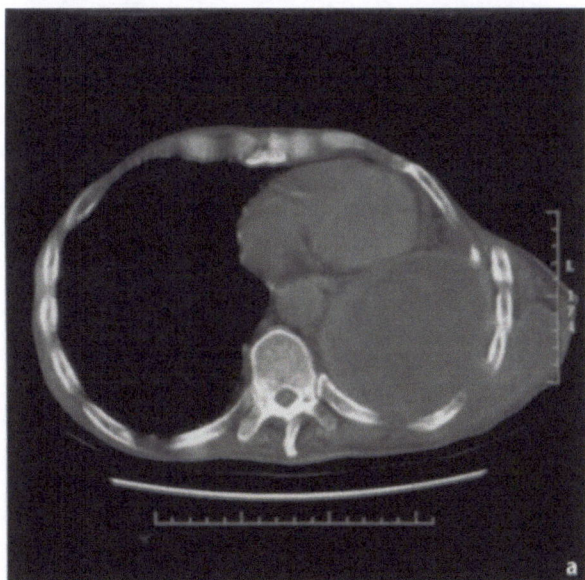

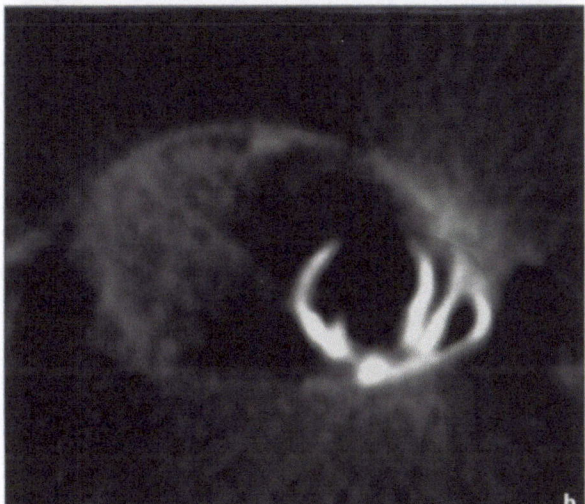

Patient and History: This 67-year-old man is 5 months status post left pneumonectomy for a well-differentiated squamous cell carcinoma, arising in the left lower lobe. The tumor was 10 cm in size, with extensive necrosis, and extended to the visceral pleura. There were no nodal or distant metastases. The postoperative course was complicated by a bronchopleural fistula and wound dehiscence, which were treated by repeat stapling of the left mainstem bronchus and placement of a left pectoralis flap. A pectoralis flap hematoma was later evacuated. He now presents with hypercalcemia, progressive weight loss, and left chest wall pain. A chest CT shows irregular soft tissue thickening surrounding the left pleural cavity (**a**). A soft tissue mass, with centrally decreased attenuation, extends into the left posterolateral chest wall.

PET Results: An intense rim of hypermetabolism surrounds the left pleural cavity and the left chest wall mass (**b**). The findings are highly suggestive of locally recurrent tumor.

Histology: A thin needle aspirate of the left chest wall revealed squamous cell carcinoma.

Cave! Healing postoperative wounds can also demonstrate hypermetabolism. Tissue diagnosis and/or close interval follow-up can be helpful in equivocal cases.

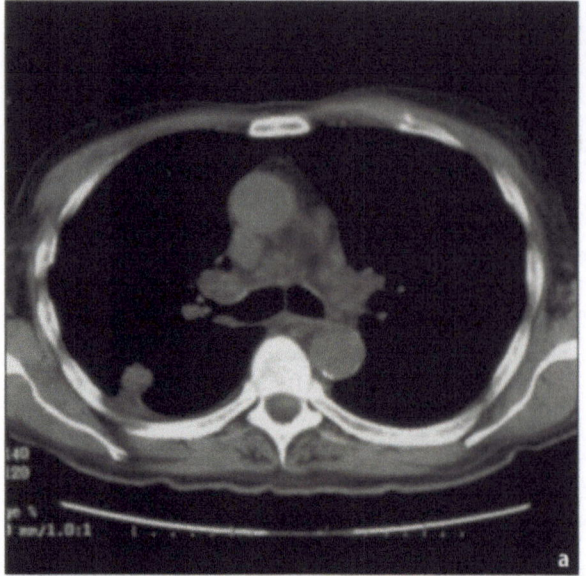

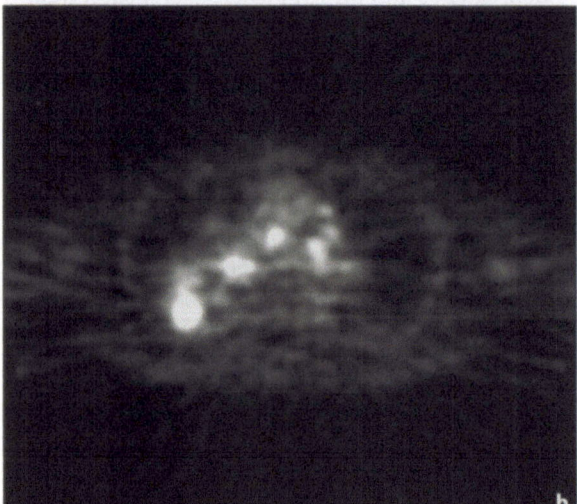

8.4 Lymph Node Metastases

Figure 5 a, b

Patient and History: This 78-year-old asymptomatic man has a 45 pack year smoking history. He presented with a right upper lung nodule on a screening chest radiograph. Chest CT showed a peripheral right lung mass, and adenopathy within the right hilum, precarinal space, and aortopulmonary window (**a**).

PET Results: The PET scan, performed 14 days after the CT, demonstrates hypermetabolism within both the lung mass and the hilar and mediastinal lymphadenopathy (**b**).

Histology: Bronchoscopy and mediastinoscopy revealed metastatic adenocarcinoma involving the right hilar and bilateral mediastinal lymph nodes.

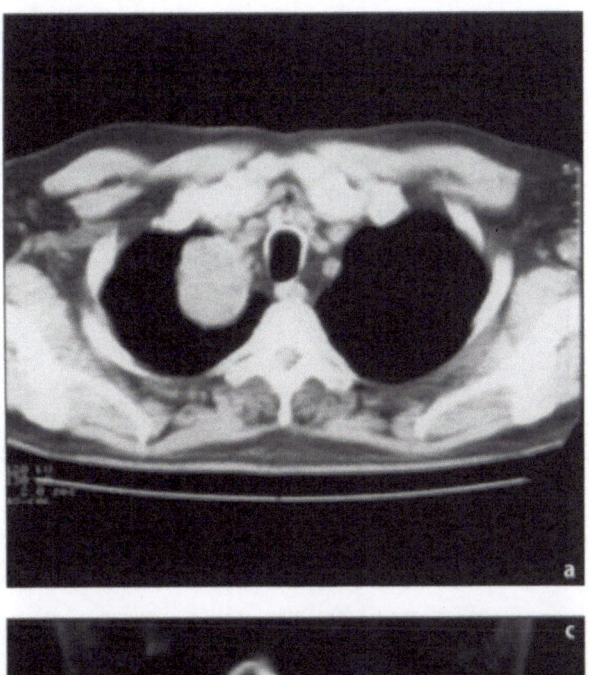
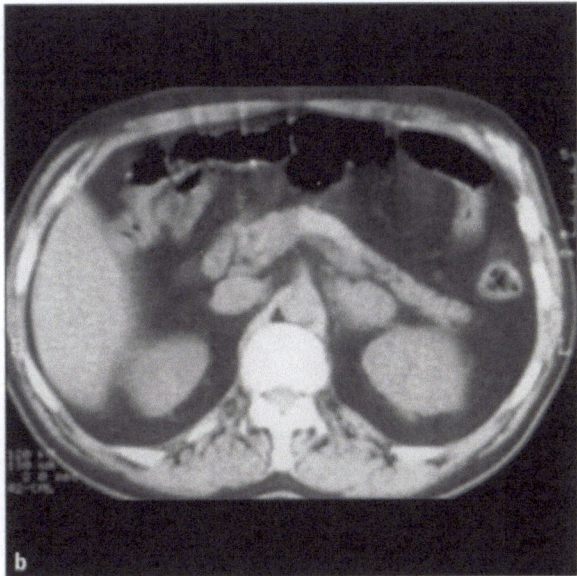
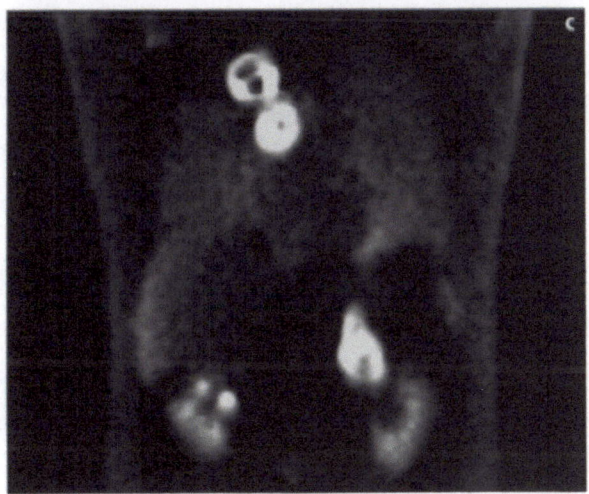
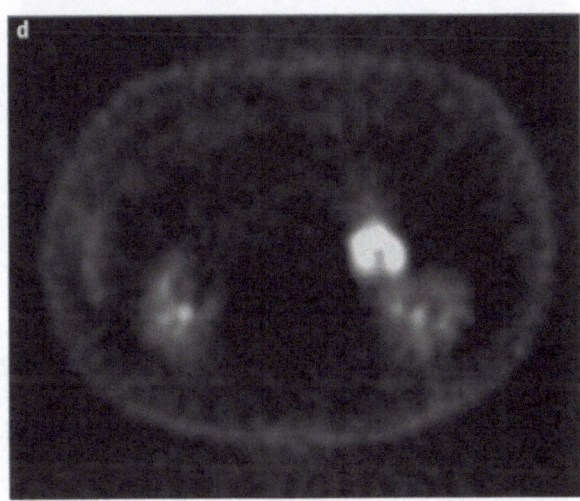

8.5 Distant Metastases

Figure 6 a–d

Patient and History: This 62-year-old man presented with a primary non-small cell carcinoma of the right upper lobe and right paratracheal lymphadenopathy, as seen by chest CT (**a**). The CT also revealed left adrenal enlargement concerning a metastasis (**b**).

PET Results: The coronal PET image demonstrates hypermetabolism within the right upper lobe mass and paratracheal adenopathy, consistent with malignant tumor (**c**). Hypermetabolism is also identified within the enlarged left adrenal gland (**c, d**). An unsuspected osseous metastasis was also discovered in the right ilium (not shown).

Follow-up: Despite chemotherapy, subsequent CT scans showed enlargement of the left adrenal metastasis, and progression of metastatic disease elsewhere.

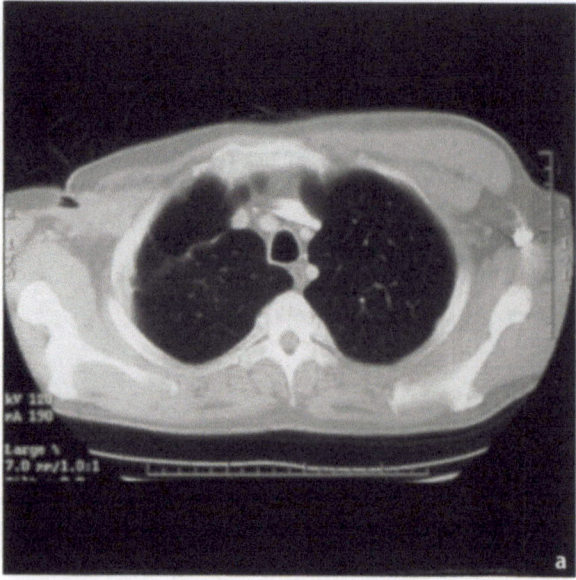
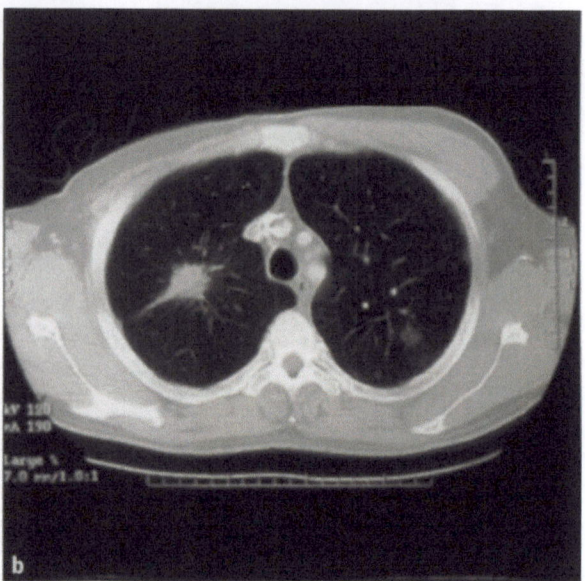
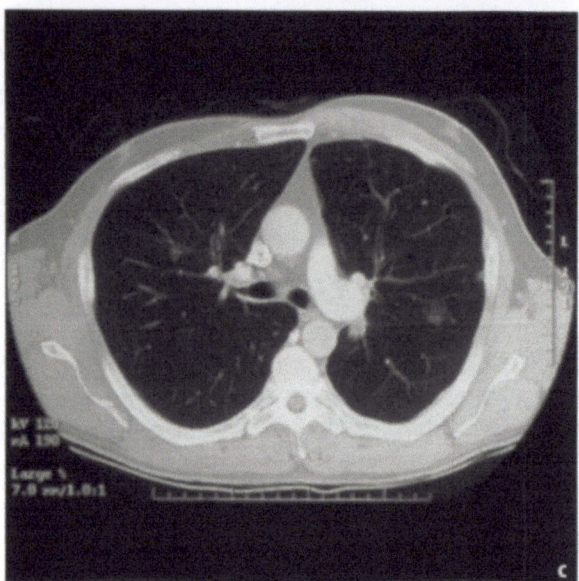
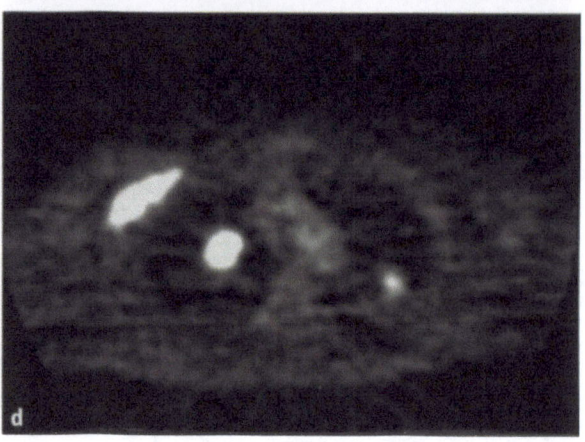
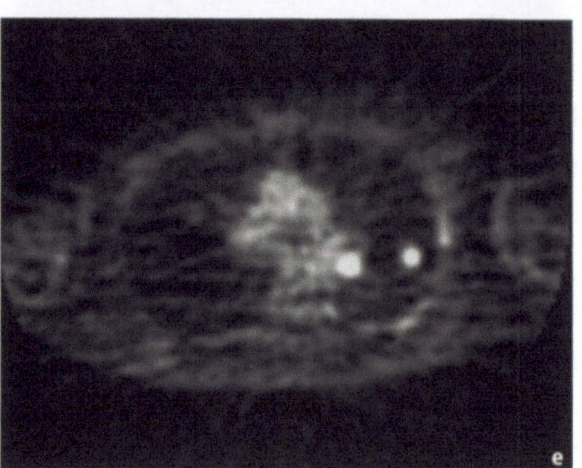

Figure 7 a–e

Patient and History: This 48-year-old man presented with 3 years of worsening pain in his right shoulder, chest wall, and axilla, and atrophy of the right pectoralis muscle. MRI showed a normal brachial plexus, but discovered an unsuspected right upper lobe mass (not shown). Chest CT (**a–c**) showed right pleural scarring, a primary right upper lobe tumor, and scattered left pulmonary nodules.

PET Results: Intense hypermetabolism is present in the right upper lobe tumor and in the left lung metastases (**d, e**). The right anterior chest wall also shows intense hypermetabolism suspicious for a metastasis, but the only CT correlate is mild pleural reaction.

Histology: Transthoracic needle aspiration revealed squamous cell carcinoma of the lung.

Follow-up: A subsequent chest CT confirmed a metastasis to the right anterior chest wall.

Figure 8 a–h

Patient and History: This 60-year-old man presented with sinus congestion and an abnormal chest radiograph. A noncontrast chest CT demonstrated a cavitary right upper lung mass, but no other suspicious lesions (**a**). A bone scan showed foci of increased activity suspicious for metastases in the left parietal bone, the anterior aspect of the right 4th rib, and the posterior aspect of the right 9th rib (**b**). A head CT demonstrated an osseous metastasis to the greater wing of the right sphenoid bone, with mass effect upon the right temporal lobe, invasion through the lateral wall of the right orbit, and impingement upon the right lateral rectus muscle (**c**). The head CT also showed a metastasis to the posterior aspect of the left parietal bone, with epidural mass effect upon the left parietal lobe (**d**).

Brain PET Technique: 3D emission scan for 6 min, with calculated attenuation correction.

PET Results: Intense hypermetabolism is seen within the cavitary right upper lobe tumor, and within unsuspected lymph node metastases to the right hilum, mediastinum, and right supraclavicular region (**e, f**). Numerous hypermetabolic liver metastases were also not shown by CT. Hypermetabolic osseous metastases are seen in several ribs, the right ilium, the right sphenoid bone (**g**) and the left parietal bone (**h**). The osseous metastases to the right ilium, the right sphenoid bone, and all but two ribs were not seen on the bone scan.

Histology: Fine-needle aspiration of a cervical lymph node demonstrated metastatic squamous cell carcinoma.

Cave! In patients who present with widespread metastases, PET can be used to identify an easily accessible biopsy site so that risks of the procedure can be minimized.

Figures 8 c–h see pages 86, 87

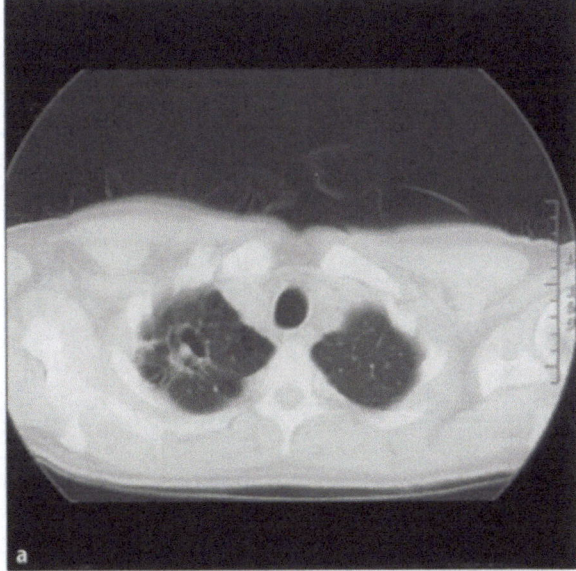

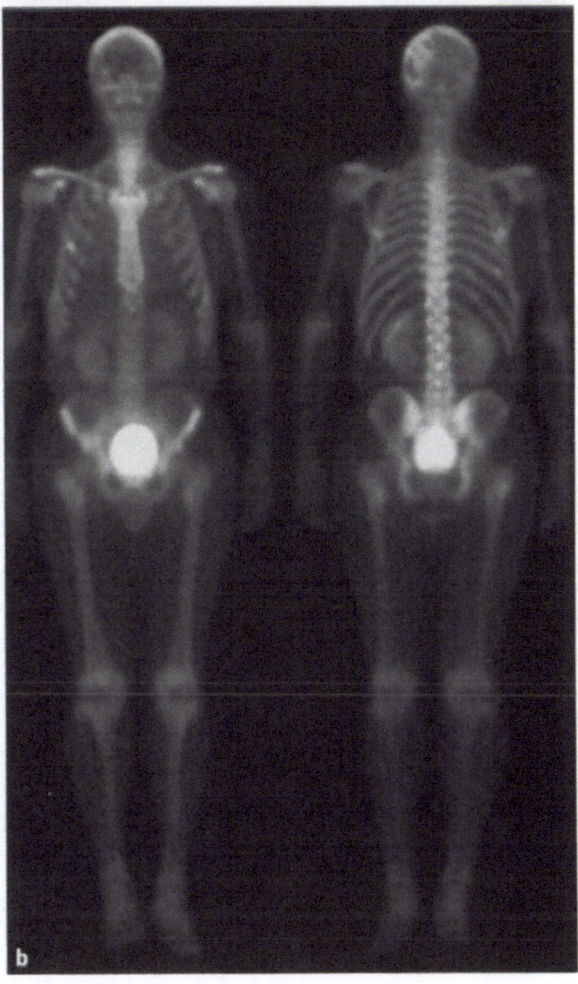

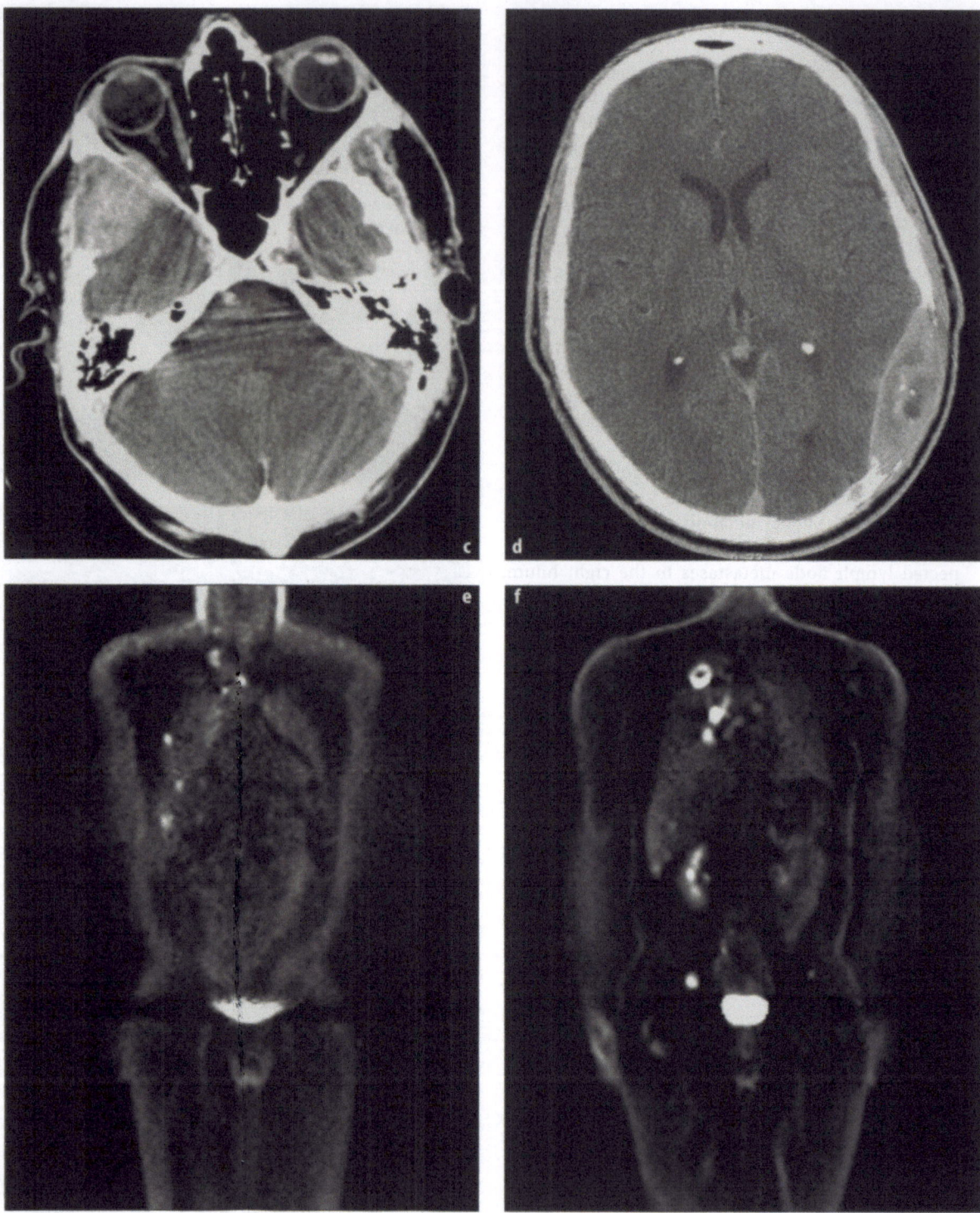

Figure 8 c–f

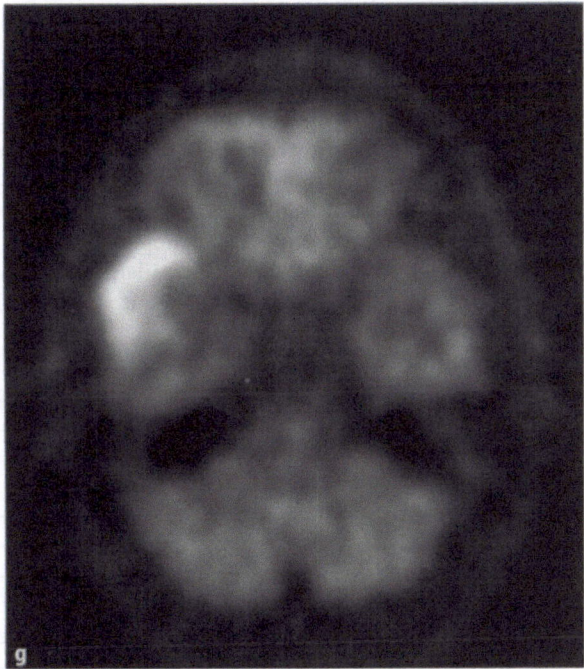

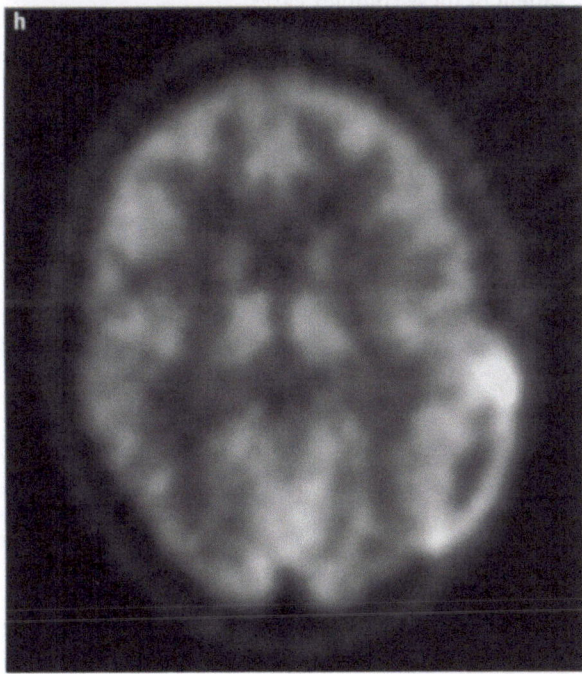

Figure 8 g, h

8.6 Variants and Pitfalls

There are many causes of false positive FDG PET scans. Active inflammatory processes can be hypermetabolic, particularly those which are granulomatous in nature and/or those which contain significant macrophage infiltration. Hypermetabolism can also be seen in benign entities such as healing thoracotomy wounds, postoperative inflammation of the pleura, healing post-traumatic and insufficiency fractures, and radiation fibrosis.

False negative studies are uncommon because nearly all lung cancers are intensely hypermetabolic. Small lesions that are below the limiting spatial resolution of the PET scanner (less than 6 mm) may be missed. Also, about half of all bronchioloalveolar cell carcinomas and primary pulmonary carcinoid tumors are hypometabolic.

Figure 9 a–d ▶

Patient and History: This 67-year-old woman underwent wedge resection of the right upper lobe and the superior segment of the right lower lobe 9 months ago for squamous cell carcinoma. She has a history of sarcoidosis, with serial CT scans demonstrating stable hilar, mediastinal, and periportal adenopathy (**a, b**).

PET Results: Intense hypermetabolism is identified within the bilateral hilar, mediastinal, and periportal lymph nodes (**c, d**).

Histology: Numerous biopsies of hilar and mediastinal lymph nodes have all demonstrated non-necrotizing granulomatous inflammation, consistent with the clinical history of sarcoidoisis. No metastatic adenopathy has been demonstrated.

Pitfall: Active granulomatous disease and nodal metastases are both hypermetabolic, and are thus indistinguishable by FDG PET imaging. This can be problematic in patients who carry both diagnoses. Close clinical and imaging follow-up, combined with tissue diagnosis as indicated, are important to the management of these complex cases.

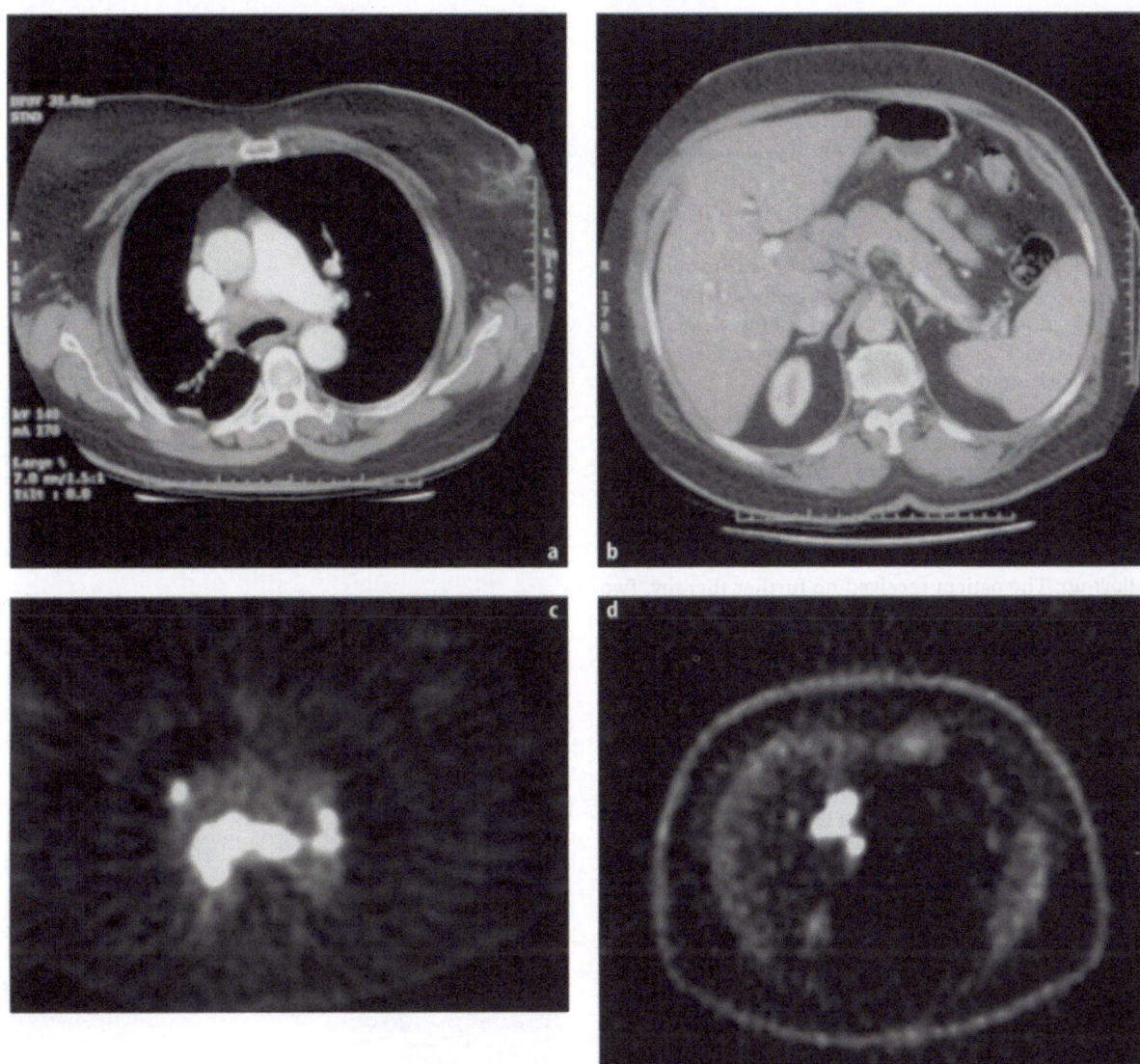

Figure 10 a–f

Patient and History: This 68-year-old man underwent left upper lobectomy for stage IIIA large cell undifferentiated carcinoma. Pleural and lymphovascular invasion were noted at the time of surgery, and there was metastatic involvement in 1 of 20 mediastinal lymph nodes. He received postoperative chemotherapy, followed by 6000 cGy external beam radiation therapy. Chest radiographs performed 1 month (**a**) and 3 months (**b**) after therapy showed increasing density in the aortopulmonary window, suspicious for recurrent disease.

PET Results: Increased metabolism is identified within the mediastinum and paramediastinal portions of the lungs, corresponding to the known anatomic distribution of the radiation port (**c–e**). A correlative chest CT confirms fibrosis related to the radiation port, but shows no definite mass lesion (**f**).

Follow-up: The patient received no further therapy. Two years later he is active and doing well, with no clinical evidence of recurrent tumor.

Cave! Although most fibrosis is hypometabolic on FDG imaging, hypermetabolism has been reported within fibrosis following therapeutic doses of radiation. Biopsy of these FDG-avid areas typically shows significant macrophage infiltration, which is thought to be the etiology of the increased FDG uptake. The expected time course of the FDG accumulation within radiation-therapy-induced fibrosis of the lung and mediastinum has not been determined.

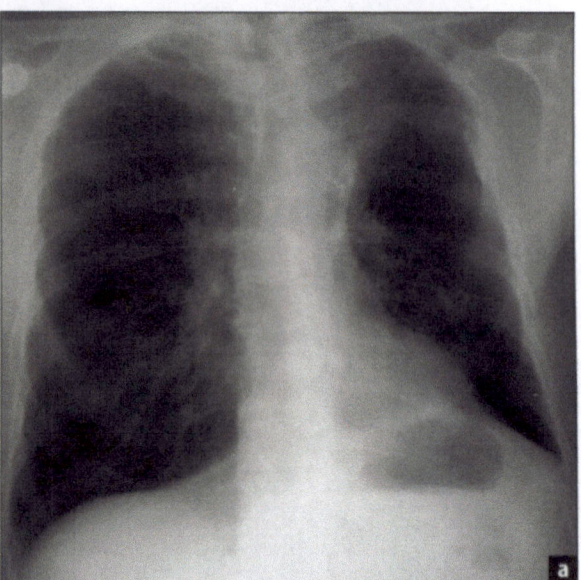

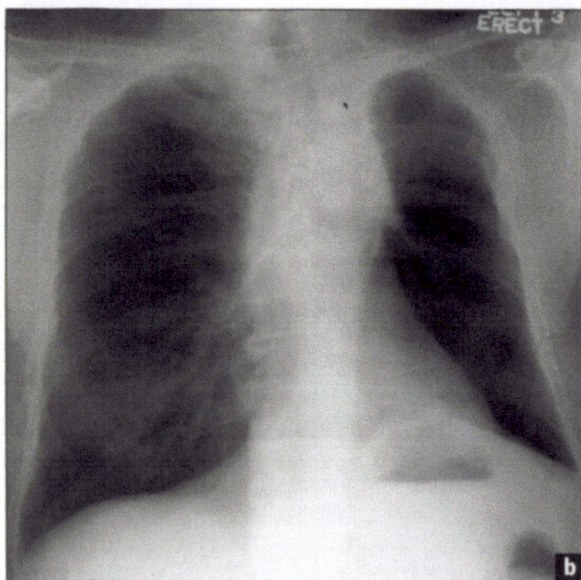

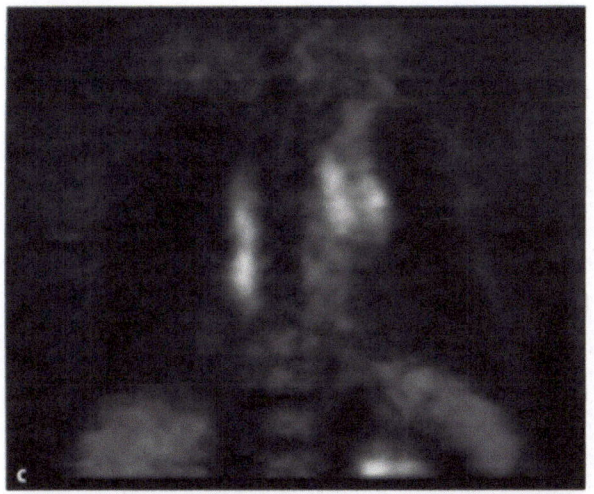

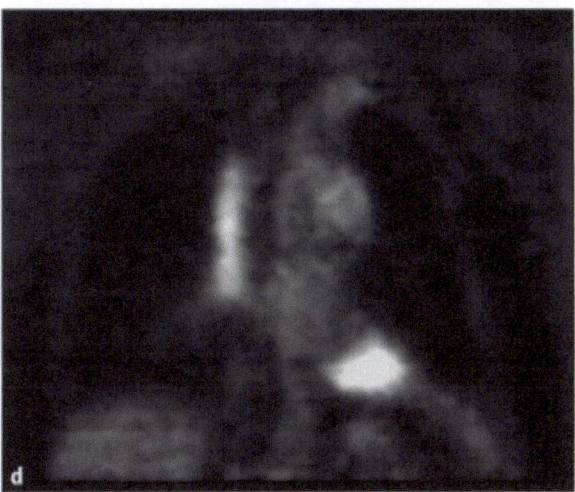

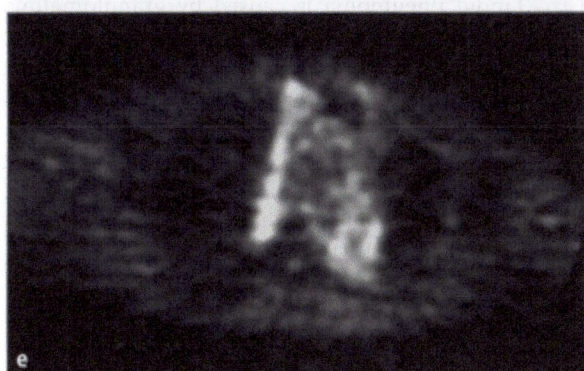

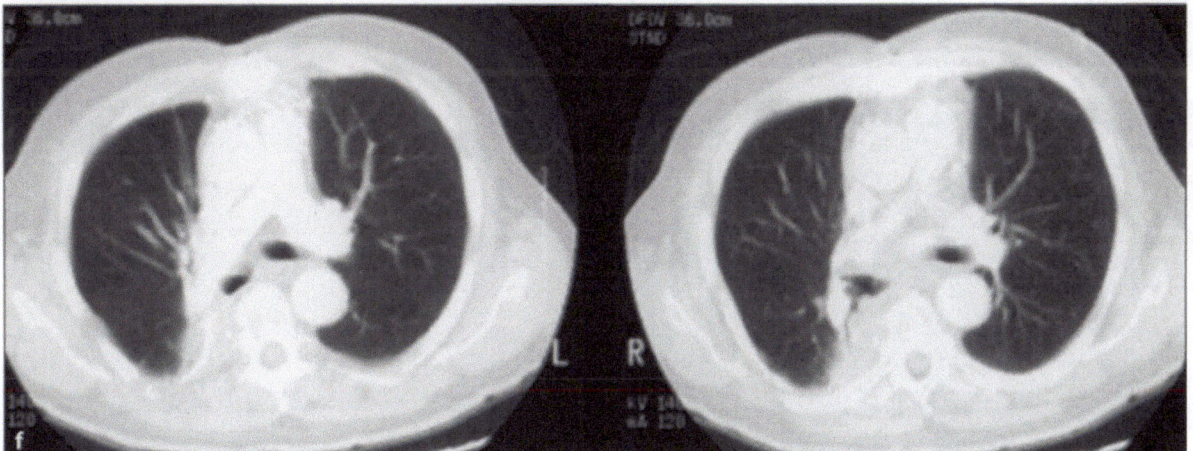

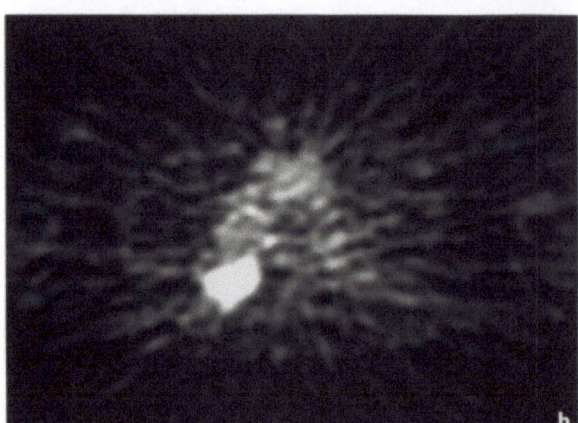

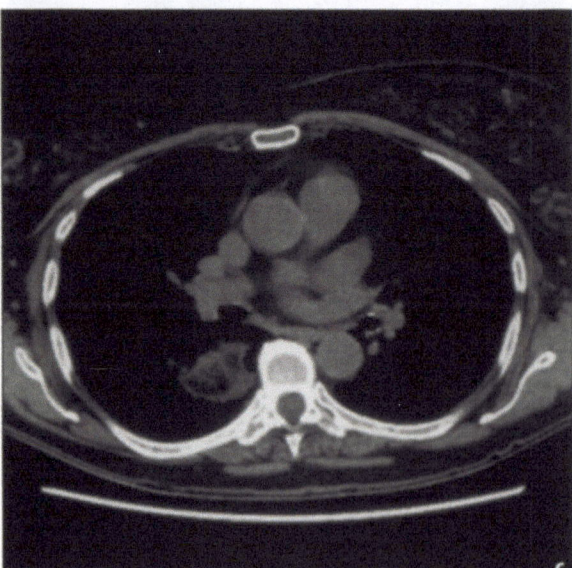

Figure 11 a–c

Patient and History: This 80-year-old woman had adenocarcinoma of the colon resected 8 years ago. She recently presented with malaise and mild shortness of breath. A chest radiograph demonstrated a large, heterogeneous opacity within the right middle and lower lobes (**a**). Needle biopsy of the right lower lobe was inconclusive.

PET Results: Intense hypermetabolism is identified within the right lung mass, suspicious for a primary malignancy (**b**).

Follow-up: A chest CT demonstrated fatty density within the mass, consistent with lipoid pneumonia (**c**). On further questioning, the patient gave a history of habitual mineral oil ingestion.

Cave! Lipoid pneumonia is caused by granulomatous reaction and fibrosis due to aspiration of mineral, vegetable, or animal oil. It typically occurs in elderly or debilitated people with swallowing problems, and most commonly presents in the right middle and lower lobes. A characteristic CT finding due to mineral oil aspiration is the "paraffinoma," a circumscribed peripheral mass lesion containing areas of fat density. As with other granulomatous inflammation, lipoid pneumonia can demonstrate increased FDG uptake.

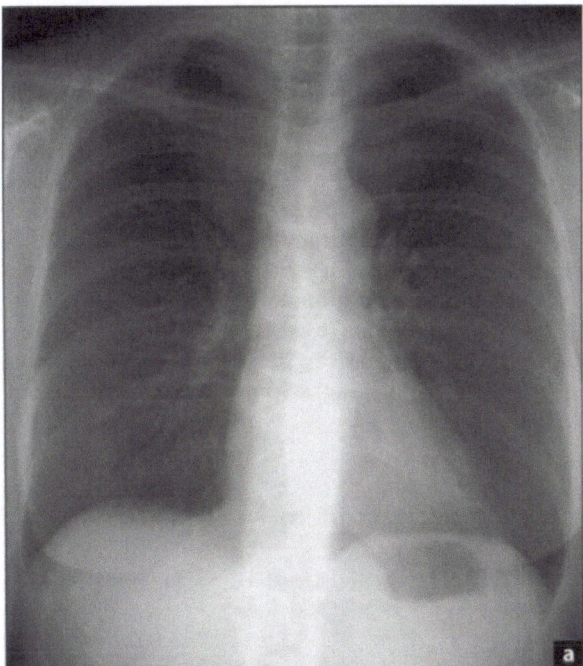

Figure 12 a–c

Patient and History: This 53-year-old woman presented with a carcinoid tumor of the appendix and metastases to the liver, peritoneal cavity, and retroperitoneum. She was treated for 5 years with alpha-interferon. A follow-up chest radiograph revealed a new, ill-defined opacity in the right middle lobe (**a, b**). I-131 MIBG imaging confirmed her abdominal metastases, but there was no MIBG-avid disease in the chest (not shown).

PET Results: FDG imaging of the chest shows hypermetabolism within the right middle lobe lesion (**c**). The abdominal carcinoid metastases were also hypermetabolic (not shown).

Histology: Thoracoscopic biopsy demonstrated granulomatous disease.

Cave! Active granulomatous disease can be hypermetabolic on FDG imaging.

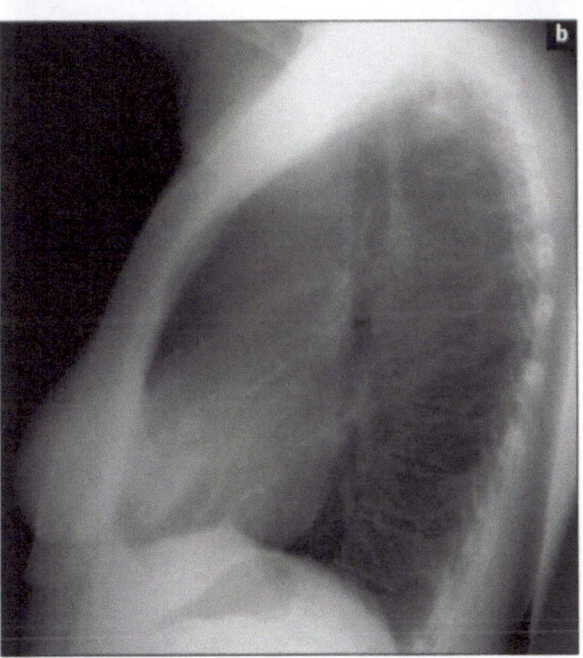

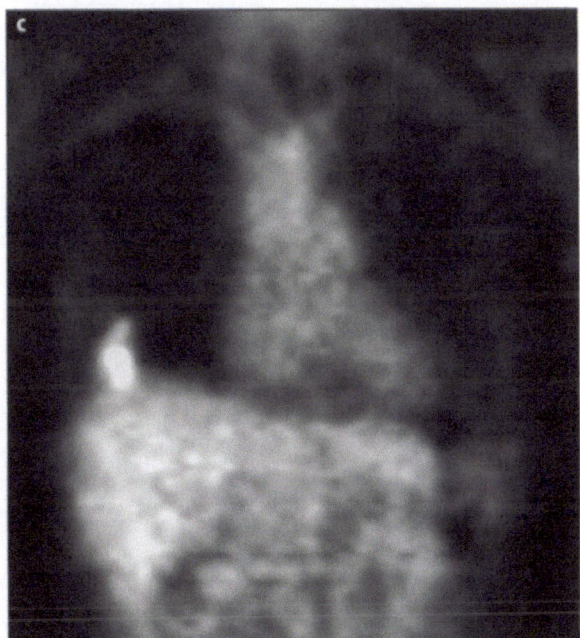

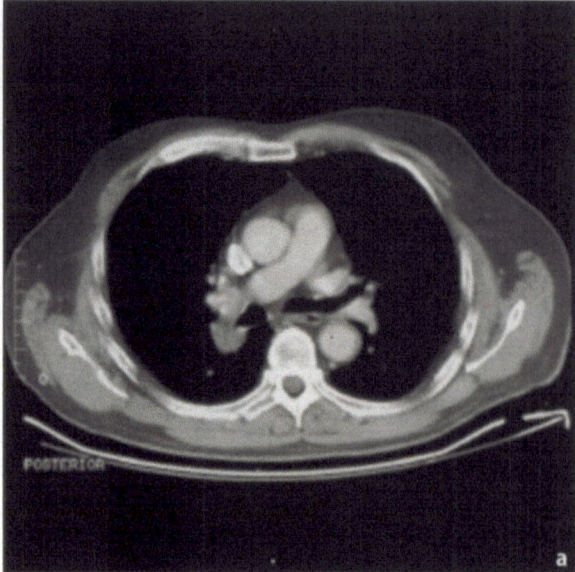

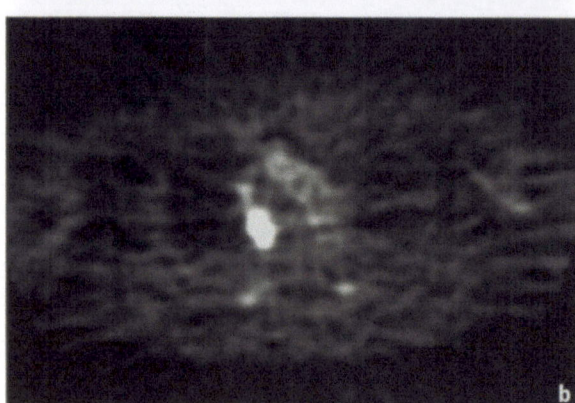

Figure 13 a, b

Patient and History: This 76-year-old man is status post-resection of a benign right lung hamartoma, followed by talc pleurodesis. A follow-up chest CT demonstrated numerous pleural-based nodules, several of which contained radiodense material. The CT findings were consistent with talc granulomata (**a**).

PET Results: FDG imaging shows intense hypermetabolism within a talc granuloma adjacent to the right mainstem bronchus (**b**).

Cave! Talc granulomas can demonstrate hypermetabolism on FDG imaging, as can any active granulomatous disease.

References

Kim et al. (1998) AJR 170: 935
Higashi et al.(1998) J Nucl Med 39: 1016

Breast Cancer

H. Palmedo

9.1 Primary Tumor

With worldwide more than 700,000 new cases, breast cancer presents the most frequent disease of women. The earlier the malignant tumor is detected the better the survival rate of patients. It has been shown that detection of smaller tumors (<1 cm) by mammography has resulted in an increase of overall survival.

Figure 1 a–d

Patient and History: 84-year-old patient with a big palpable mass in the upper part of the left breast.

Technique: Transmission-corrected scans with slice thickness of 4 mm.

PET Results: On the transversal slice (**a**) at the level of the lower mediastinum, focal FDG accumulation is demonstrated in the left breast near to the chest wall. On the sagittal view (**b**), focal accumulation is obvious and parts of the lower mediastinum, the liver and the renal pelvis can be identified. No axillary, mediastinal or lung disease can be noted. Additionally, an aneurysm of the aortic arc which was detected on the chest X-ray image (**c**) can also be seen on the coronal view of the PET images (**d**) as a filiform accumulation in the upper mediastinum.

Histology: Invasive combined ductal and lobular carcinoma pT4 without axillary lymph node metastases.

Figures 1 c, d see page 96

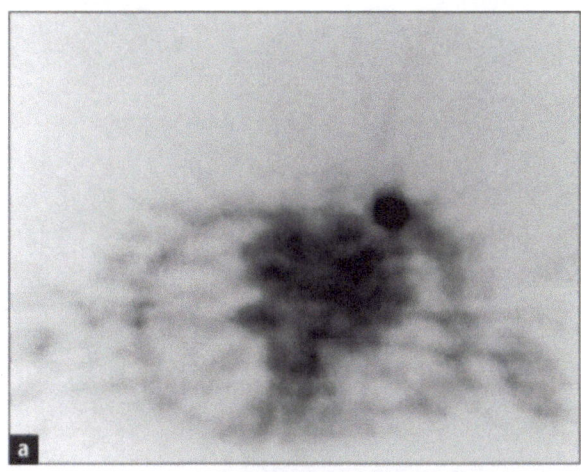

a

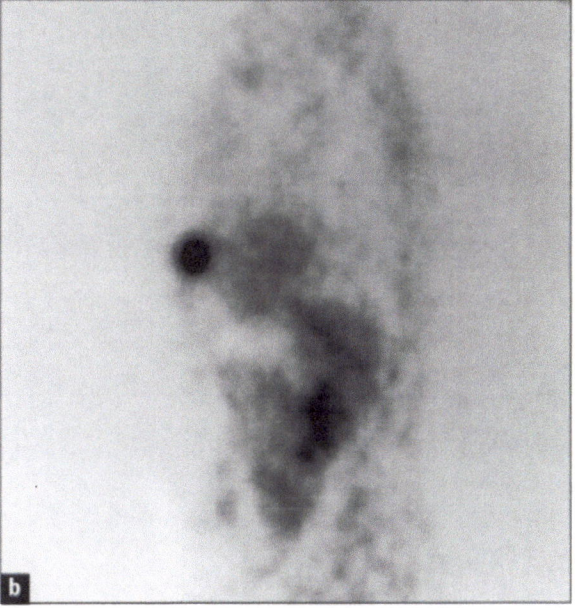

b

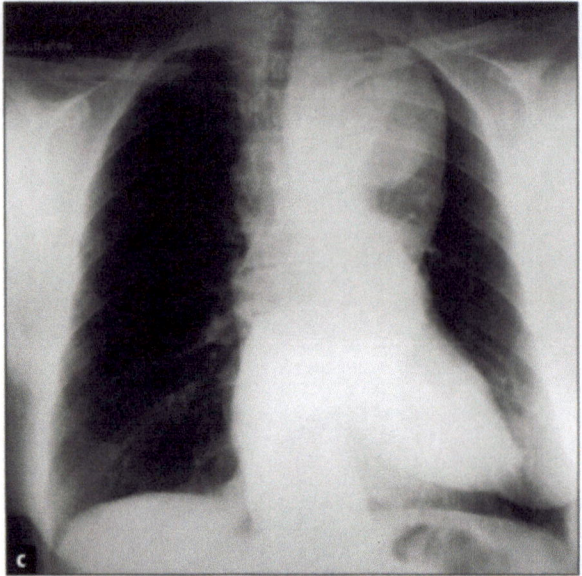

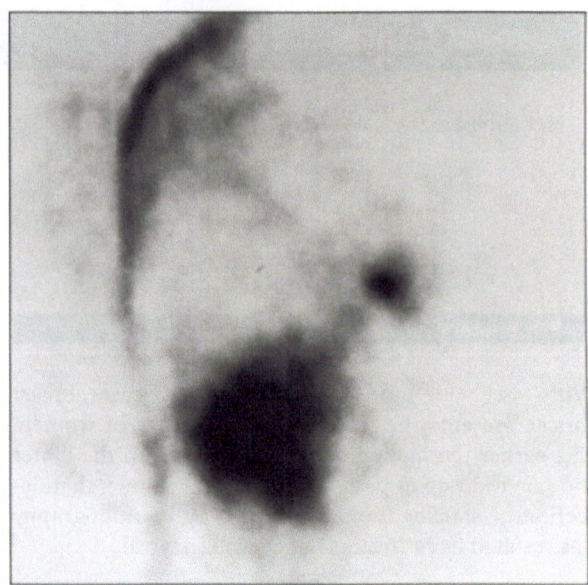

Figure 1 c, d

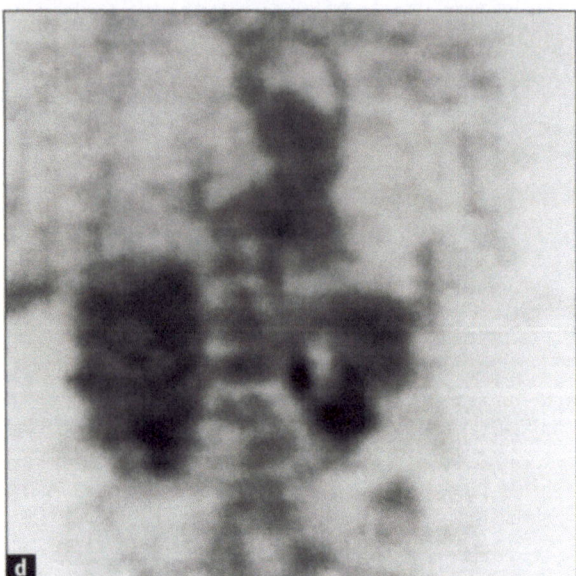

Figure 2 ▲

Patient and History: a 43-year-old patient who had detected a nodule in the right breast during self palpation.

Technique: Transmission-corrected scans with slice thickness of 4 mm.

PET Results: Sagittal view of FDG-PET scan demonstrates focal accumulation of high intensity which is typical for malignancy (FDG accumulation in the carcinoma of the breast equals the accumulation of the cerebrum). Furthermore, tracer uptake of the liver is demonstrated.

Histology: Invasive ductal carcinoma which was staged pT2 N0.

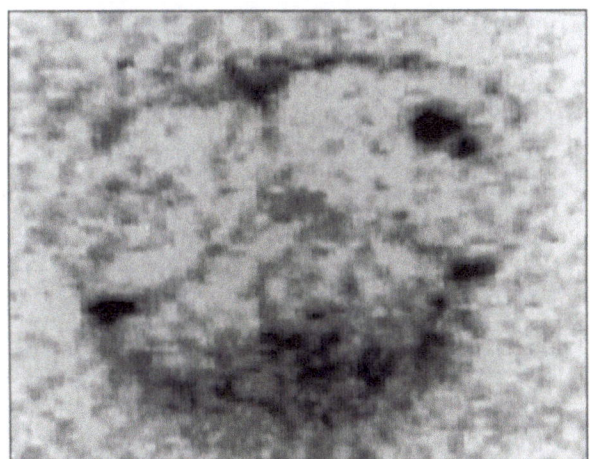

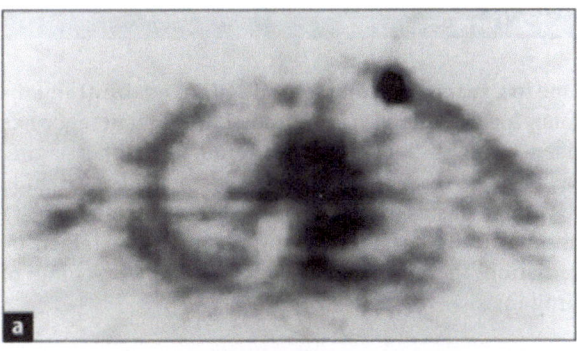

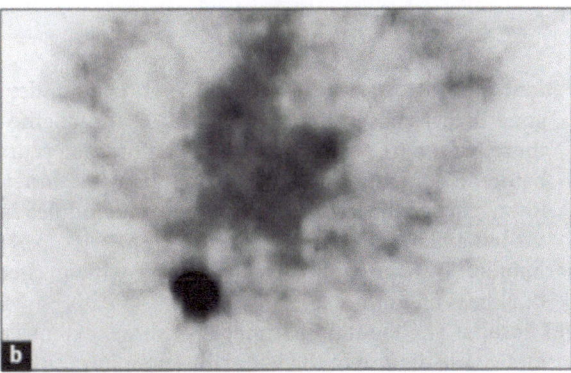

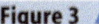
Figure 3 ▲

Patient and History: Patient with suspicion of multifocal breast cancer.
Technique: Non-transmission corrected scans with slice thickness of 4 mm.
PET Results: Coronal view of the breasts showing two foci of intense tracer uptake in the upper part of the right breast. The breasts are outlined by a filiform tracer accumulation which is typical for non-transmission attenuated PET images. At the lower part of the breasts symmetrical focal tracer uptake can be detected as a result of soft tissue superposition. Below the breasts, there is diffuse uptake in the abdominal wall.
Histology: Multifocal breast cancer pT2 N0.

Figure 4 a, b

Patient and History: Patient who had detected a nodule in the left breast.
Technique: Transmission-corrected scans with slice thickness of 4 mm.
PET Results: Transversal FDG-PET slices. The transversal view at the level of the upper mediastinum in the supine position (**a**) demonstrates a focus which is at the niveau of the chest wall. The same PET study with the patient examined in the prone position (**b**) showed focal tumor accumulation which is more distant from the chest wall.
Histology: Invasive ductal carcinoma which was staged pT2 N0 and poorly differentiated.
Cave! Examination of the breast should ideally be performed in the prone position to differentiate breast lesions from lesions of the chest wall.

9.2 Local Recurrence

One to 2 years after complete tumor removal, intramammary local recurrence may occur. If local recurrence has been diagnosed by clinical examination or imaging techniques, restaging should be performed to exclude distant metastases of disease. If distant metastases are absent locally, surgical therapy eventually sustained by radiation therapy is sufficient without worsening of prognosis.

Figure 5 a–d ▶

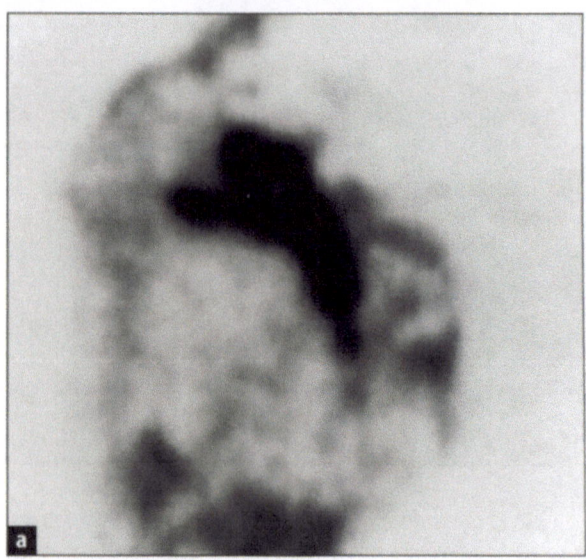

Patient and History: 66-year-old patient who had undergone breast conserving surgery, radio- and chemotherapy for a pT4 carcinoma of the left breast 2 years before. Examination revealed a nodule in the inner, lower part of the left breast and multiple nodules in the left axilla.

Technique: Transmission-corrected scans with a slice thickness of 4 mm.

PET Results: The sagittal PET image (**a**) shows extensive metastatic disease in the left axilla (note intensity of accumulation is much higher than in the spleen visualized in the lower part of the image). As bone scintigraphy (**b**) could exclude osseous involvement, the axillary FDG accumulation is due to soft tissue and lymph node disease. The transversal image (**c**) at the level of the middle mediastinum shows the lower part of FDG accumulation visualized on the sagittal view. This demonstrates that soft tissue uptake near to the chest wall cannot be differentiated from bone uptake. The transverse slice (**d**) at the level of the lower left breast shows focal uptake in the axilla and in two lesions in the inner part of the breast corresponding to two local tumor recurrences.

Cave! Bone scintigraphy is necessary to exclude or confirm osseous metastases if FDG uptake near to the chest wall occurs.

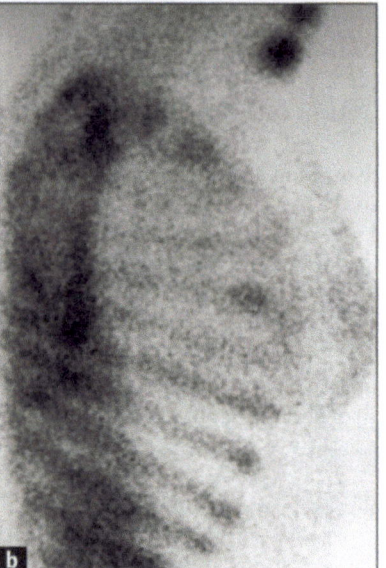

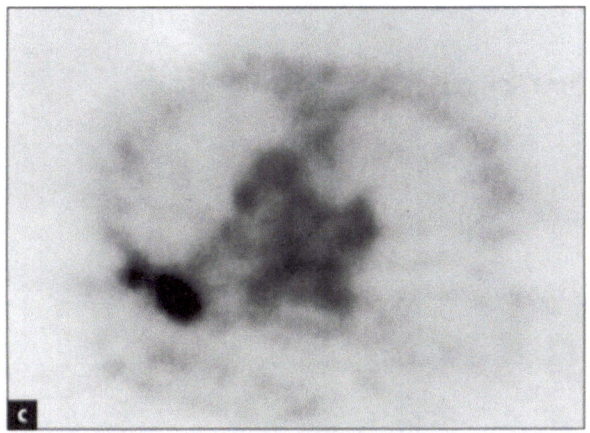

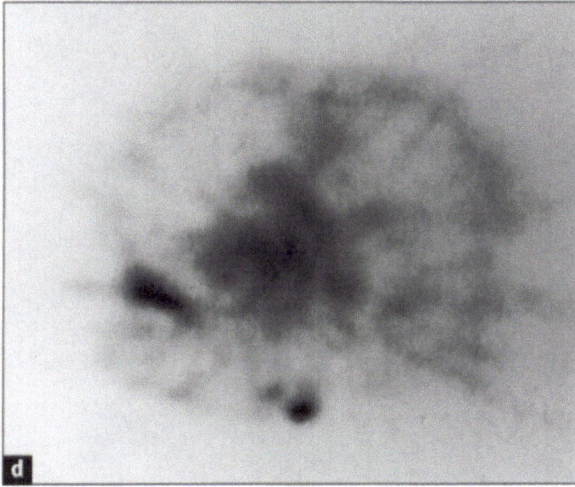

Figure 5 c, d

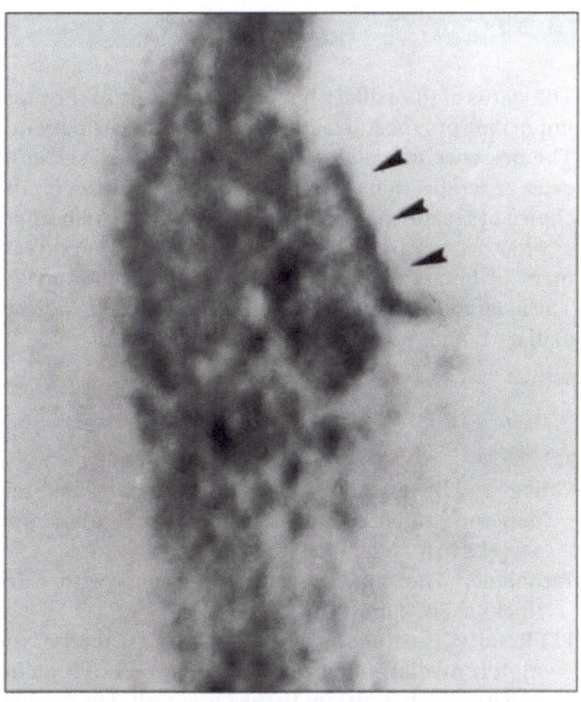

Figure 6 ▲

Patient and History: 32-year-old patient. She had mastectomy and axillary dissection 2 years before because of invasive ductal breast cancer staged pT2 N1 M0. She underwent restaging because of cutaneous infiltration at the scar.

Technique: Transmission-corrected scans with slice thickness of 4 mm.

PET Results and Histology: Sagittal image shows long filiform accumulation (arrows) of moderate intensity at the left chest wall. This was due to diffuse dermal infiltration with carcinoma cells.

9.3 Axillary Lymph Node Metastases

The status of the axillary lymph nodes is one of the most important prognostic factors in breast cancer patients. The presence of axillary lymph node metastases indicates generalization of disease and has an impact on the choice of treatment after surgery. Adjuvant chemotherapy has been proven to be effective in the primary treatment of breast cancer patients with metastatic axilla. The likelihood of a positive axillary PET scan to indicate axillary lymph node metastases is very high.

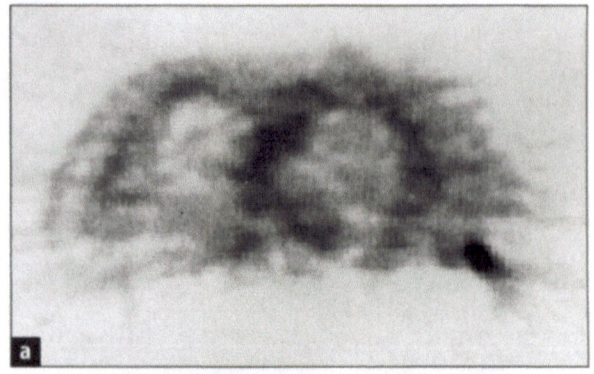

Figure 7 a, b

Patient and History: a 60-year-old patient who had undergone tumorectomy and axillary dissection 3 weeks before the PET studies.

Technique: Transmission-corrected scans with slice thickness of 4 mm.

PET Results: The transversal image (**a**) at the level of the middle mediastinum shows tracer uptake of high intensity which is distant to the chest wall. The coronal cut through this accumulation (**b**) demonstrates clearly this axillary uptake on the right side (see liver accumulation, patient studied in prone position).

Histology: Histopathology had revealed a poorly differentiated carcinoma of the right breast and lymph node metastases. Due to the poor differentiation of the tumor, staging was initiated. Axillary uptake was due to three histopathologically proven lymph node metastases in the right axilla.

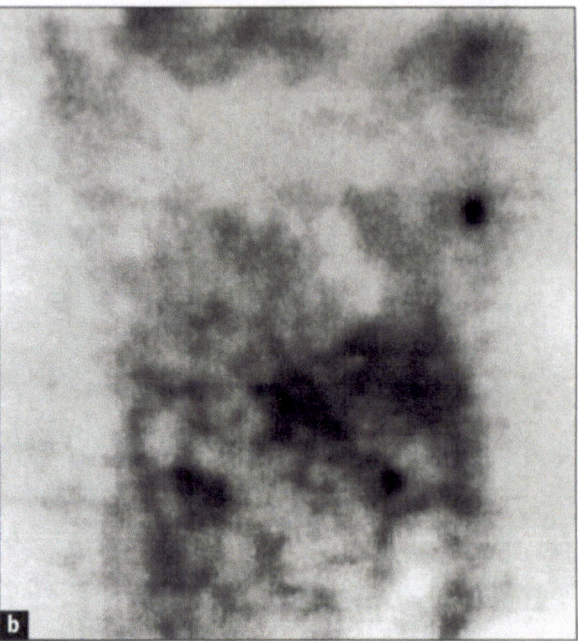

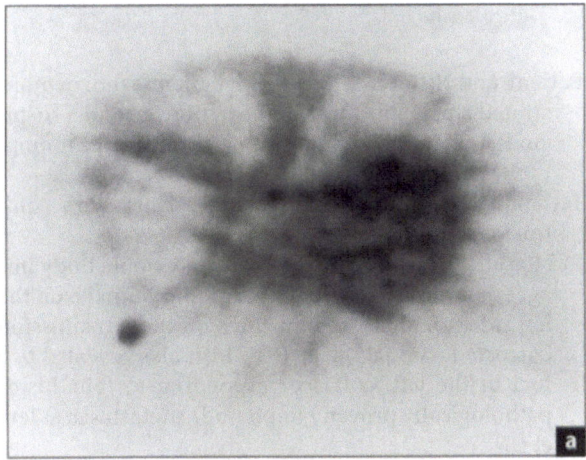

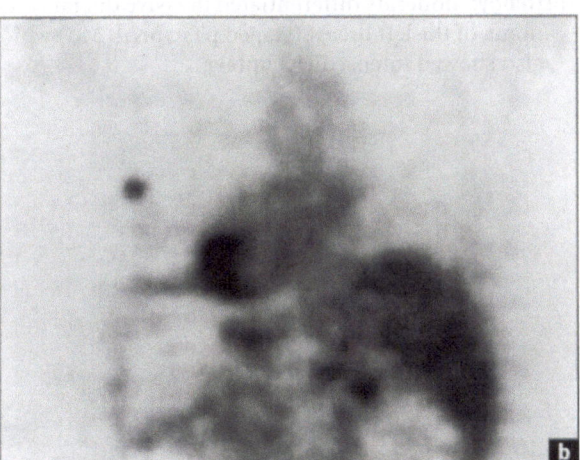

Figure 8 a, b

Patient and History: 52-year-old patient presented with a suspicious, palpable nodule in the left breast but negative axillary palpation.

Technique: Transmission-corrected scans with slice thickness of 4 mm.

PET Results: PET studies demonstrated focal tracer accumulation in the lower, outer part of the left breast on the transversal image (**a**) and also left axillary uptake at the level of the middle mediastinum in the coronal section (**b**) (note tracer uptake in the heart and the liver, patient studies in prone position).

Histology: Invasive, ductal carcinoma of the left breast (diameter 1.7 cm) which was moderately differentiated and one single, axillary lymph node metastases (from 14 dissected lymph nodes).

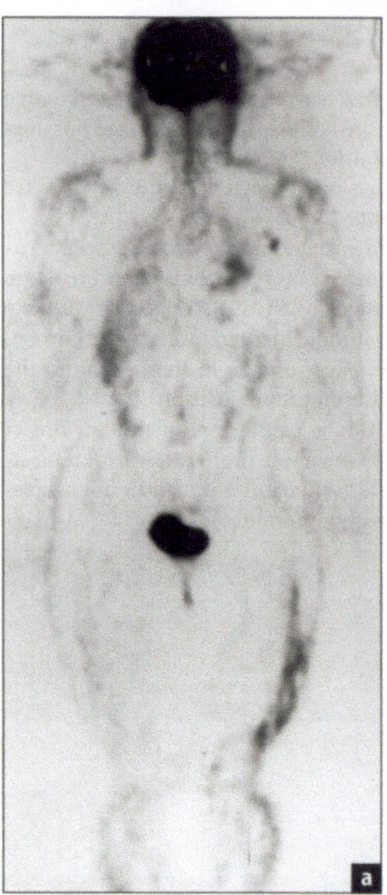

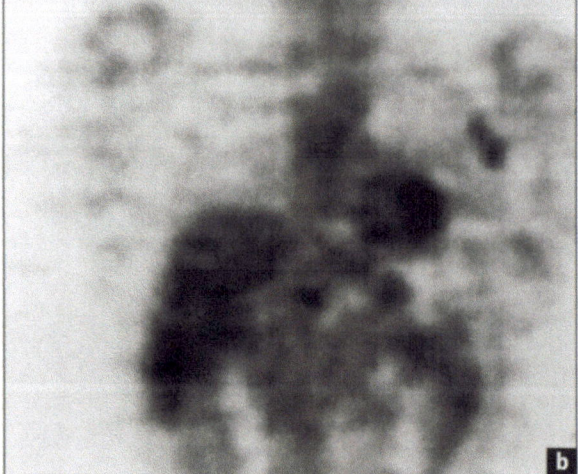

Figure 9 a, b

Patient and History: 50-year-old patient who demonstrated a palpable mass in the left breast and a suspicious axillary palpation. Magnetic resonance tomography showed one axillary lymph node.

Technique: Transmission-corrected scans with slice thickness of 4 mm.

PET Results: Non-attenuation corrected whole body images demonstrated two foci of axillary uptake on the left side (**a**). This was confirmed on the transmission corrected coronal image (**b**) which also revealed two foci in the left axilla corresponding to four histopathologically proven lymph node metastases at level 1.

Histology: Moderate differentiated invasive ductal carcinoma of the left breast (staged pT1c pN1b M0) which also showed intense FDG uptake.

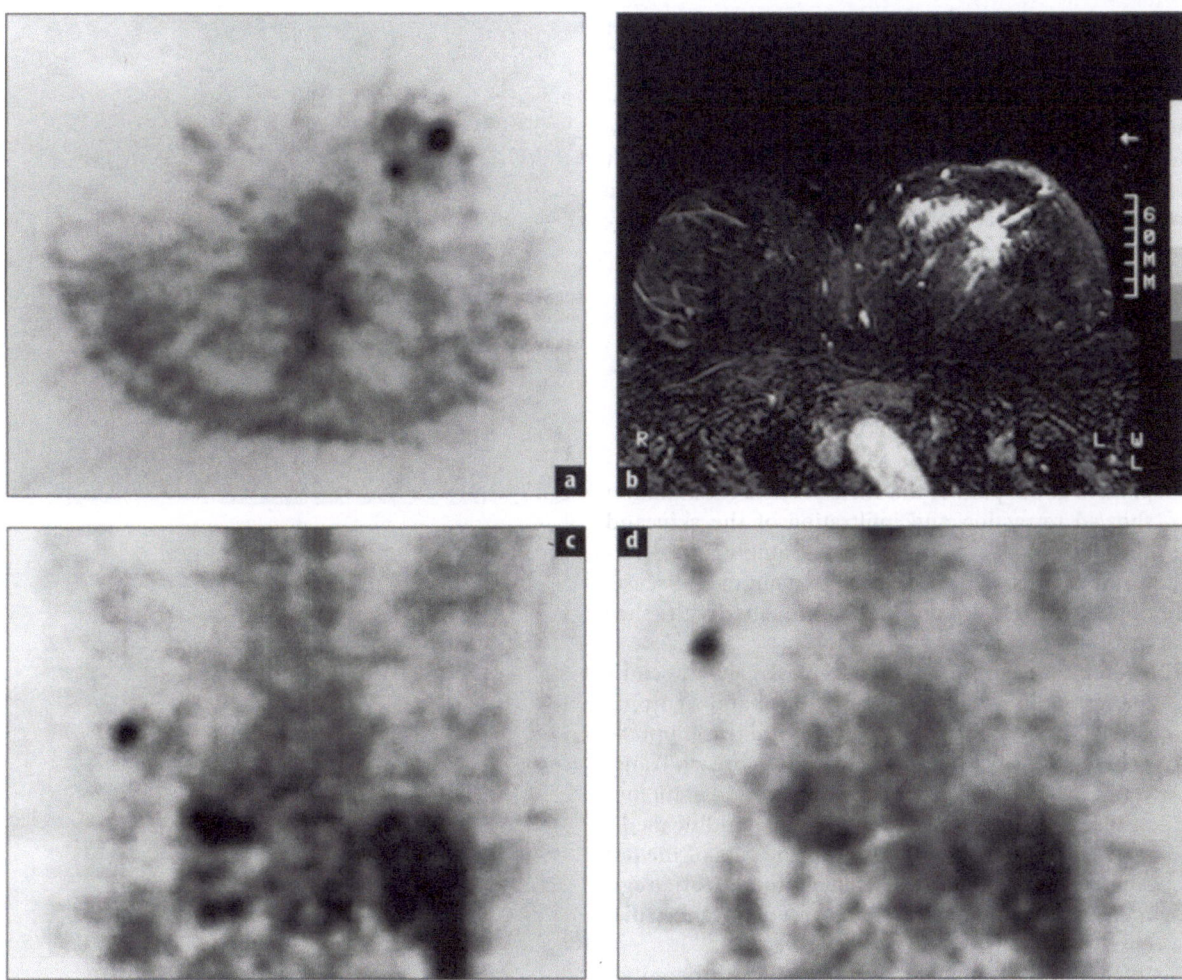

Figure 10 a–d

Patient and History: 54-year-old patient who had detected a nodule in the left breast. Mammography showed an irregular opacity and palpation was also suspicious for malignancy.

Technique: Transmission corrected scans with slice thickness of 4 mm.

PET Results: Transverse PET image (**a**) demonstrated three foci of FDG accumulation in the left breast. Also MRI (**b**) of the breasts showed gadolineum enhancement in several regions. These findings correspond to multifocal carcinoma of the left breast. The first coronal image (**c**) demonstrates intense focal accumulation in the left axilla which was in the axial view at the level of the suspicious tumor in the left breast. This corresponded to one single lower axillary lymph node metastasis. The second coronal image (**d**) shows a more ventral section with another focal tracer uptake of high intensity in the left axilla which is situated cranially in comparison to the first focus (compare distance between upper liver pole and a horizontal line through the focus). This corresponded to three metastatic lymph nodes each of which measured 3 mm.

Histology: Poorly differentiated, multifocal invasive lobular and ductal carcinoma staged pT3 pN1 MO G3.

9.4 Distant Metastases

If distant metastases are present, the disease has become incurable. The median of suspected overall survival is less than 2 years. Quality of life is the most important factor for the patient and aggressive chemotherapeutic regimens are not acceptable. If patients show local recurrence of breast cancer, it is important to exclude distant metastases to make further therapeutic decisions.

Figure 11 a–c

Patient and History: 70-year-old patient who had detected a mass in the left breast. Additionally, she complained about pain of the back. Clinical examination showed retraction and infiltration of the skin and suspicious axillary lymph nodes. Staging was performed to define the extension of malignant disease.

Technique: Transmission-corrected scans with slice thickness of 4 mm.

PET Results: Images of a planar ventral view of scintimammography with Tc-99m MIBI (**a**) and a coronal slice of FDG-PET (**b**) demonstrate focal tracer uptake of high intensity in the tumor of the left breast. Transversal slice (**c**) of PET additionally proves distant metastases by intense tracer uptake in the middle mediastinum, in the thoracic vertebra, the ribs of the left side and the left axilla. The chemotherapeutic regimen was modified due to this aspect of advanced disease.

Histology: Invasive ductal carcinoma of low differentiation which was pT4 pN2 M1 G3.

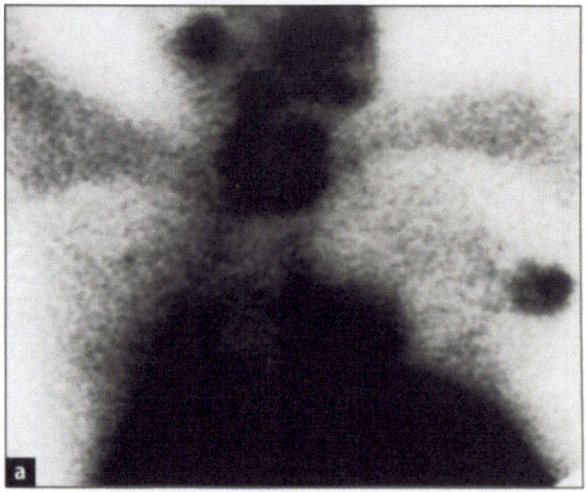

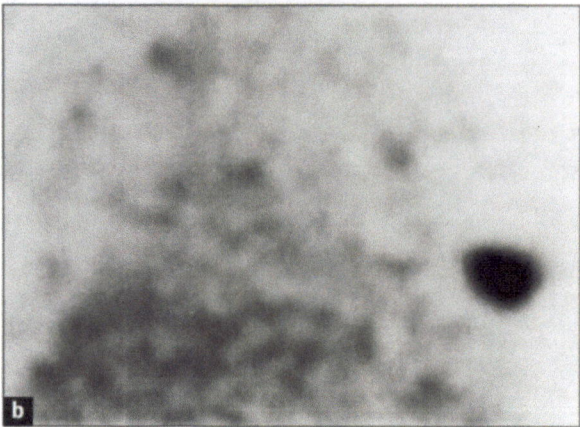

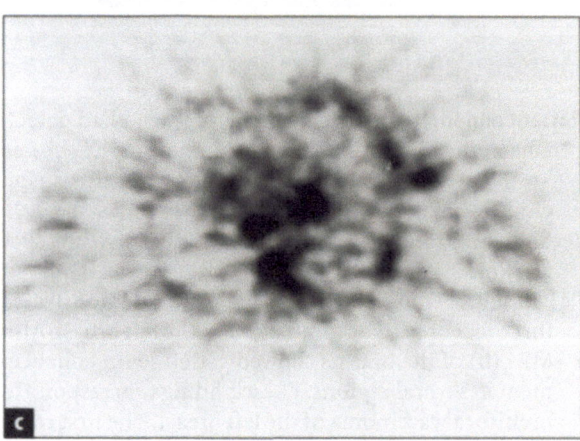

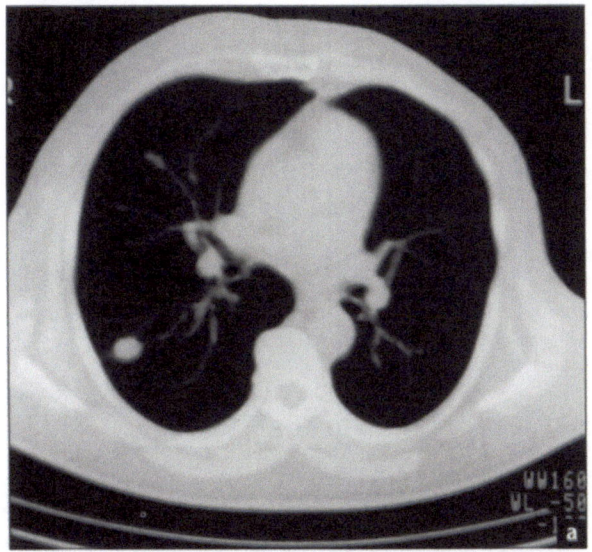

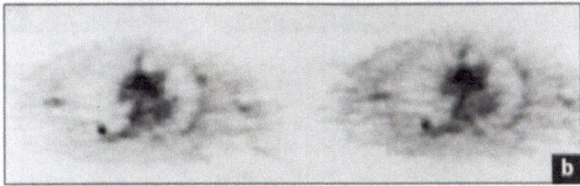

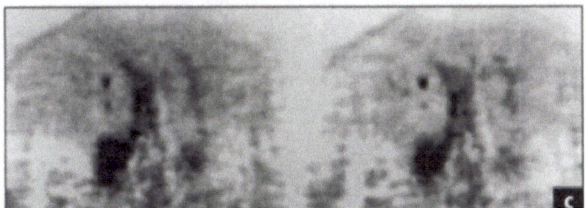

Figure 12 a–c

Patient and History: 68-year-old patient who had been operated on because of bilateral breast cancer 5 years ago was examined as local recurrence was suspected. After histology had confirmed cancer cells at the site of the old scar, restaging was initiated.

Technique: Transmission-corrected scans with slice thickness of 4 mm.

PET Results: Computed tomography of the thorax demonstrated two single lesions in segment 6 (**a**) and 9 of the right lung which had a size of about 11 mm and 8 mm. To confirm lung metastases and to look for further metastatic disease FDG-PET was performed in the supine position. Transversal slices of PET (**b**) which correspond to the CT image show focal tracer uptake of high intensity in segment 6 of the right lung. Coronal PET images (**c**) demonstrate the second focus in segment 9, which was smaller than the first one but shows intense tracer uptake (note tracer uptake in the liver and the spleen).

Histology: Biopsy confirmed lung metastases of breast carcinoma.

Figure 13 a–d

Patient and History: 31-year-old patient who had been operated on because of an invasive ductal carcinoma of the right breast 5 years ago. She presented with a local recurrence in the form of cutaneous and axillary lymph node metastases. A first PET revealed metastatic disease in the axillary, mediastinal and paraaortal lymph nodes and in the bones. After a conventional chemotherapy, PET-restaging was performed.

Technique: Transmission-corrected scans with slice thickness of 4 mm.

PET Results: Coronal slices demonstrate multiple focal uptake in the middle and lower mediastinum (**a**) and in the 2nd lumbar vertebra and the 12th thoracic vertebra (**b**) corresponding to lymph node and bone metastases. Note the diffuse increase of tracer uptake in the lumbar vertebrae due to bone marrow activation after chemotherapy. Because of this persisting metastatic disease, high dose chemotherapy had been initiated and a third PET study was performed 1 week after high dose chemotherapy. The corresponding coronal images show a significant decrease of tracer uptake in mediastinal lymph node metastases (**c**) and also in bone metastases (**d**). However, high intensity uptake in bone marrow and spleen demonstrating chemotherapy induced activation may mask residual disease. Quantification of PET images confirmed a significant decrease of FDG uptake in soft tissue metastases indicating a positive response to high dose chemotherapy.

Cave! Activation of bone marrow after chemotherapy can enhance diffuse FDG uptake throughout the bone marrow which may mask osseous metastases.

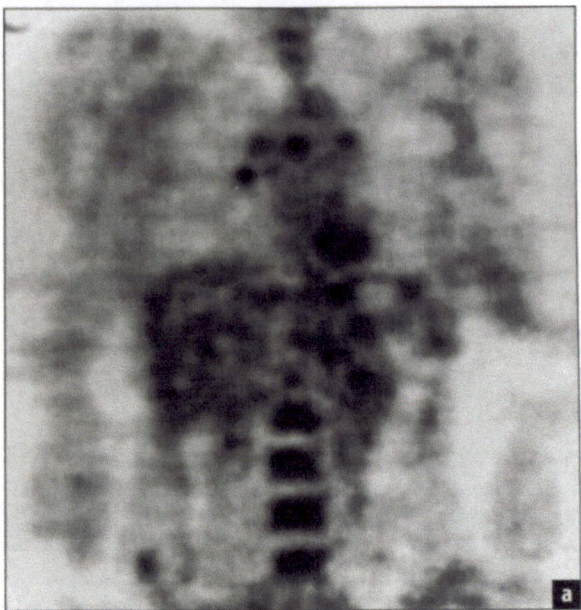

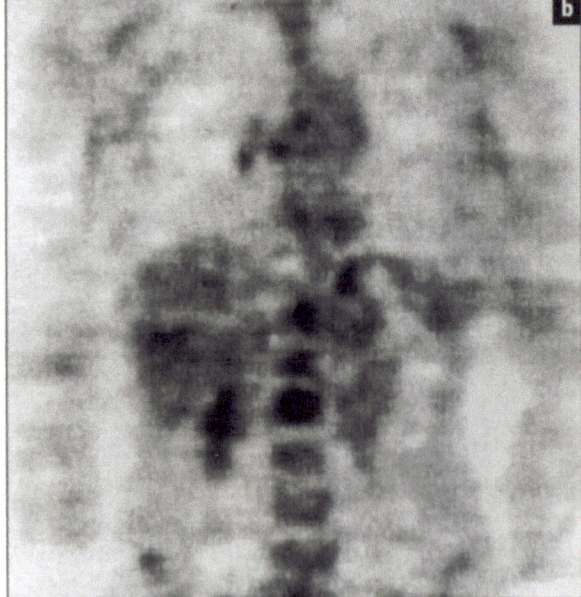

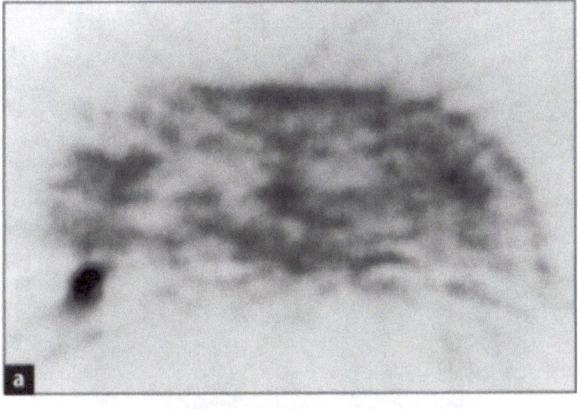

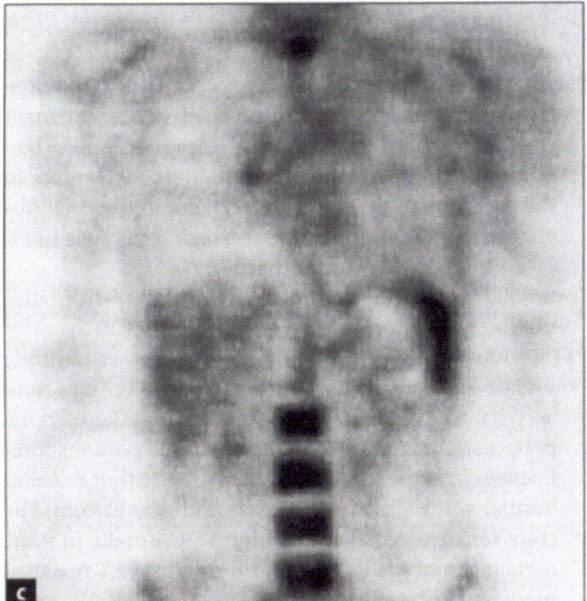

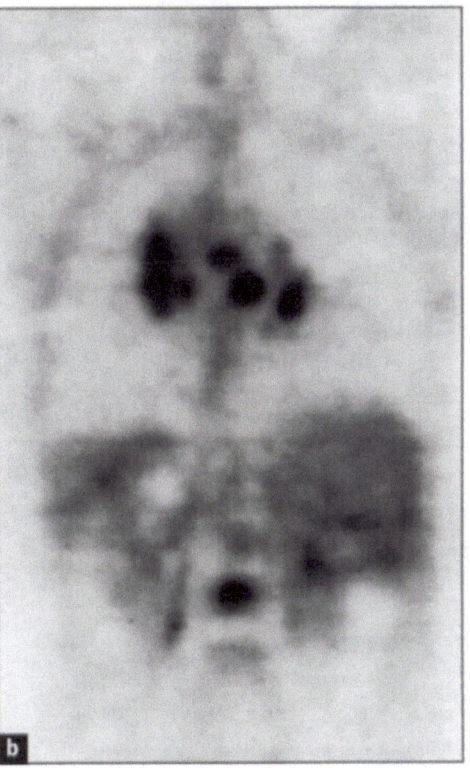

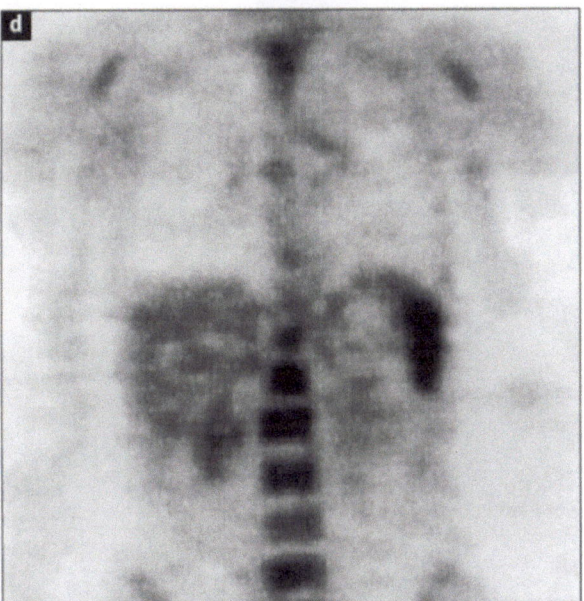

Figure 13 c, d

Figure 14 a, b ▲

Patient and History: 43-year-old patient who had undergone breast conserving surgery 4 years ago because of an invasive ductal carcinoma of the left breast. She was presented with suspicious, palpable lymph nodes in the left axilla. For restaging PET was performed.

Technique: Transmission-corrected scans with slice thickness of 4 mm.

PET Results: The transverse image (**a**) shows focal tracer uptake in the left axilla corresponding to three histopathologically proven lymph node metastases. Additionally, PET could reveal distant metastases. The coronal image (**b**) demonstrates several foci of intense tracer uptake in the posterior mediastinum and one focus in the second lumbar vertebra. With regard to the PET findings, the patient received a stage-of-disease adapted chemotherapy regimen.

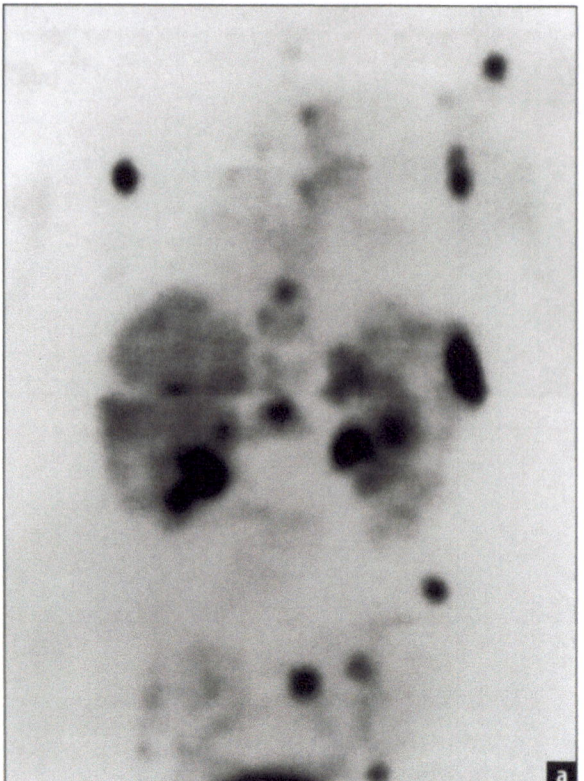

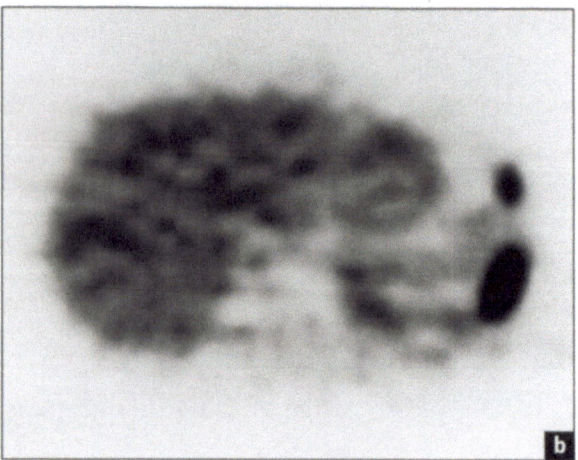

Figure 15 a, b

Patient and History: 55-year-old patient with tamoxifen treatment because of receptor positive breast cancer which had been diagnosed 5 years ago. There had been radiation therapy of single bone metastases in the sternum and the lumbar vertebra in the previous year. The patient underwent restaging because of elevation of Ca 15–3 tumor marker.

Technique: Transmission corrected scans with slice thickness of 4 mm.

PET Results: The coronal PET image (**a**) shows multiple foci of extremely intense tracer uptake (compare to activity of liver and to the bilateral uptake of renal pelvices!) corresponding to multiple osseous metastases in the left shoulder, the ribs, the thoracic and lumbar spine, the os ilium and the iliosacral joint. The transversal slice (**b**) shows high FDG uptake in bone metastases of the left ribs. Additionally, PET revealed mediastinal lymph node metastases.

Testicular Germ Cell Tumors

P. Albers and H. Bender

Testicular cancer is a rare disease and represents 1% of all cancers in males. In the age groups between 20 and 40 years it is the most common cancer. Histologically 40–50% are seminoma and 50% are non-seminomatous cancers. Testicular cancer has become a model for a curable neoplasm.

Figure 1 a–d

Diagnosis: NSGCT, clinical stage II.

Patient and History: The 25-year-old patient underwent an orchidectomy having a right-sided non-seminomatous testicular germ cell tumor (embryonal carcinoma, seminoma and mature teratoma). AFP and b-HCG were negative. His CT scan showed two suspicious lesions interaortocaval in the region of the lower poles of the kidneys (**d**).

Technique: Transmission-corrected scans with a slice thickness of 4 mm; image reconstruction by filtered backprojection.

PET Results: PET scan was positive in the same area and the direct comparison between PET and CT scan confirmed a suspicion of a lymph node metastasis of the right-sided testicular tumor. The lesion is less than 2 cm in maximal transverse diameter. The retroperitoneal lymph node dissection (RPLND) (left-sided nerve sparing) confirmed a lymph node metastasis. The patient received two adjuvant cycles of PEB chemotherapy and has been recurrence free for more than 3 years.

Histology: Non-seminomatous testicular germ cell tumor (embryonal carcinoma, seminoma and mature teratoma).

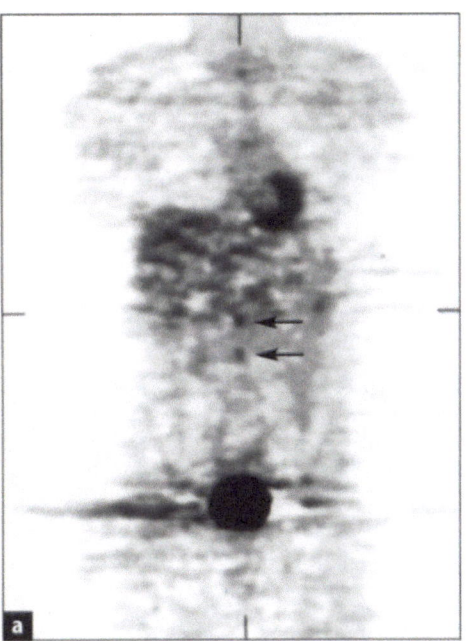

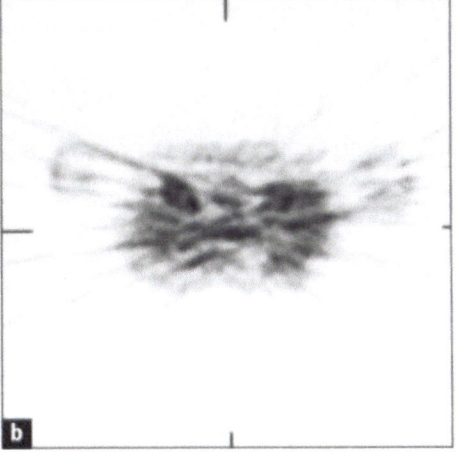

Figures 1 c, d see page 110

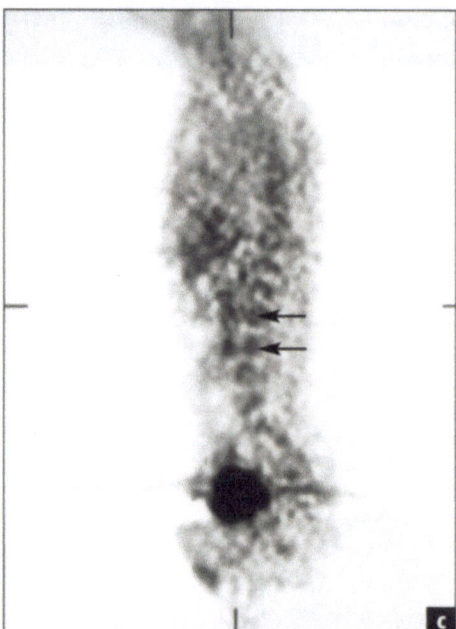

Figure 2 a–d ▶

Diagnosis: Contralateral retroperitoneal recurrence after pathological stage I non-seminoma.

Patient and History: This 26-year-old patient was diagnosed with a right-sided non-seminomatous germ cell tumor (pure embryonal carcinoma with vascular invasion). He underwent nerve sparing RPLND on the right side with 27 tumor negative lymph nodes of the right template. Three months postoperatively he showed rising markers (AFP) and a CT scan was performed that showed the rare case of a contralateral retroperitoneal tumor recurrence.

Technique: Transmission-corrected scans with a slice thickness of 4 mm; image reconstruction by filtered backprojection.

PET Results: The lesion was less than 2 cm in the left paraaortic region at the lower pole of the left kidney. PET scan confirmed a positive focus in this area and the patient was treated with three cycles of PEB chemotherapy. The residual tumor after chemotherapy, which was less than 1 cm, was resected and showed complete necrosis of this recurrent germ cell tumor.

Histology: Non-seminomatous germ cell tumor (pure embryonal carcinoma with vascular invasion).

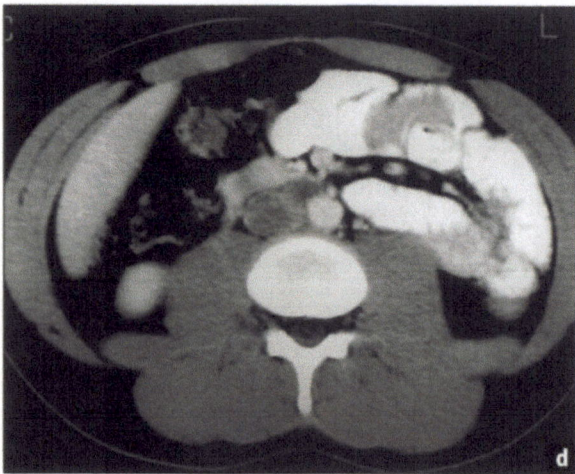

Figure 1 c, d

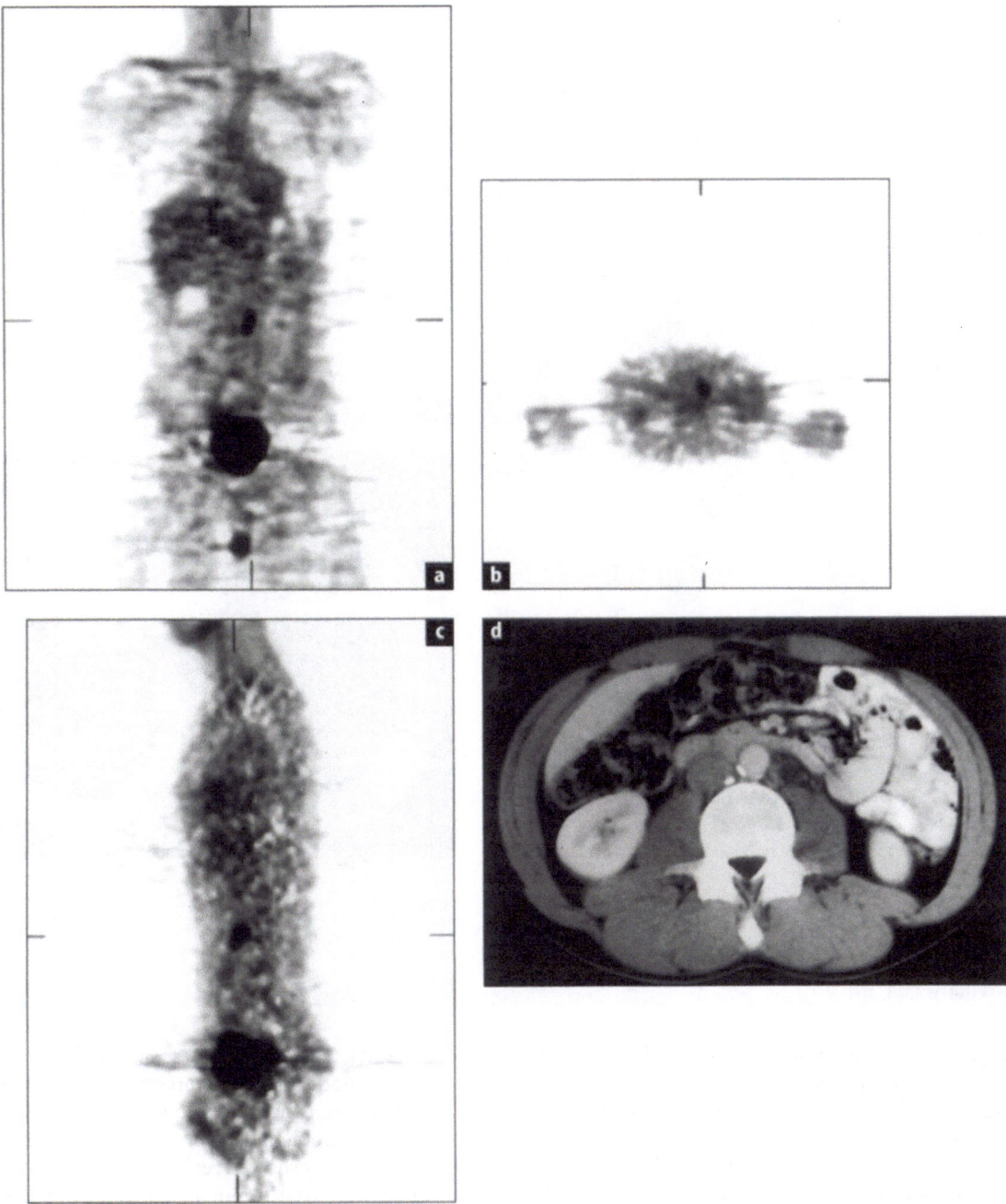

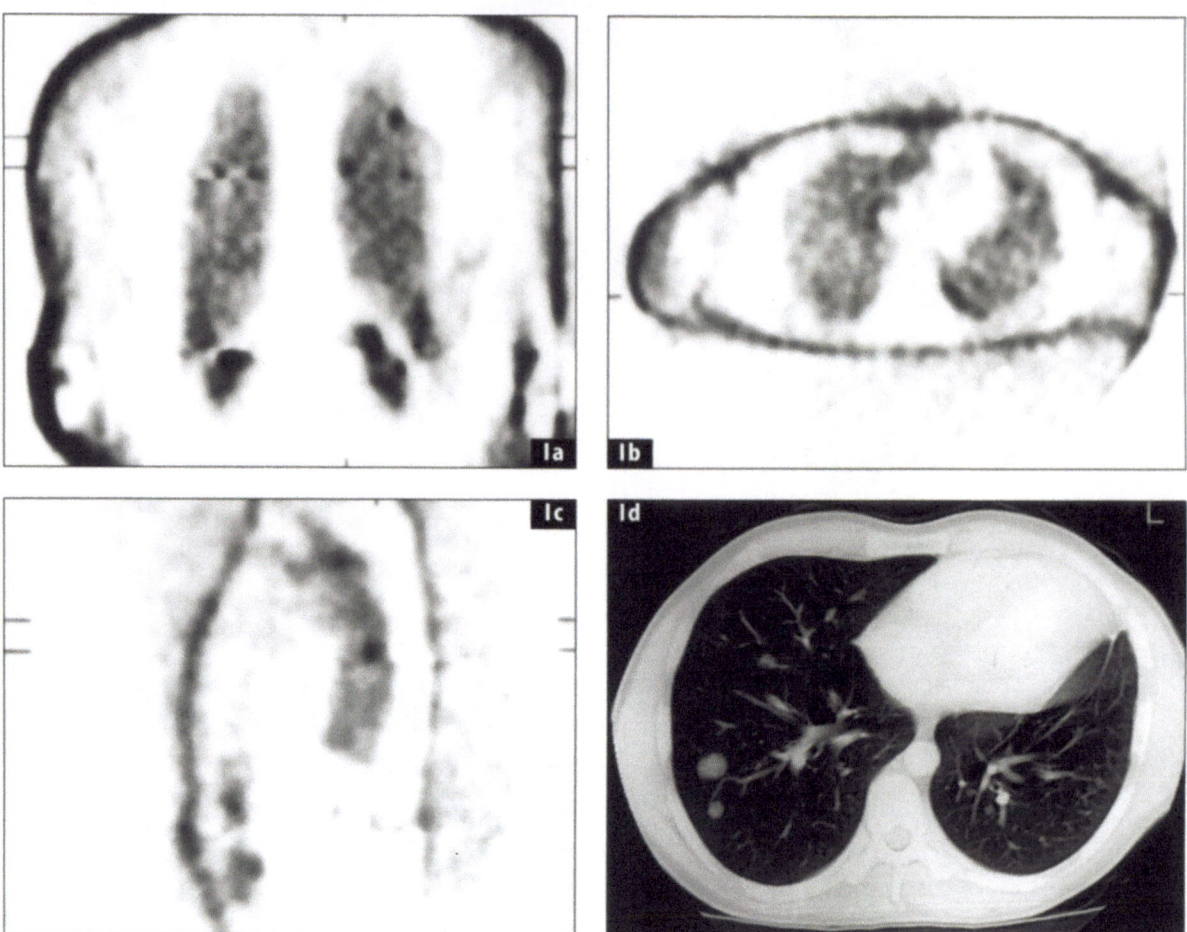

Figure 3/Ia–d/IIa–c

Diagnosis: Non-seminomatous germ cell tumor with retroperitoneal and pulmonary metastasis.

Patient and History: The 32-year-old patient had a non-seminomatous germ cell tumor (mainly chorion carcinoma) with retroperitoneal and pulmonary metastasis (see chest CT scan). A PET scan confirmed the pulmonary lesions. The patient underwent four cycles of PEB chemotherapy. The CT scan was repeated and showed a decrease of the pulmonary metastasis in size and number. A residual tumor was seen also in the left upper lung (CT scan not shown).

Technique: Transmission-corrected scans with a slice thickness of 4 mm; image reconstruction by filtered backprojection.

PET Results: The initial PET scans (Ia–c) show multiple foci in both lungs. A representative CT view (Id) is shown. After chemotherapy, the activity in various lesions (example in IIa–c) was markedly reduced. The thoracotomy showed residual tumor with mainly necrosis but vital tumor in the center of the residual pulmonary mass. The patient was repeatedly treated with high dose chemotherapy and died in tumor progress.

Histology: Non-seminomatous germ cell tumor (mainly chorion carcinoma).

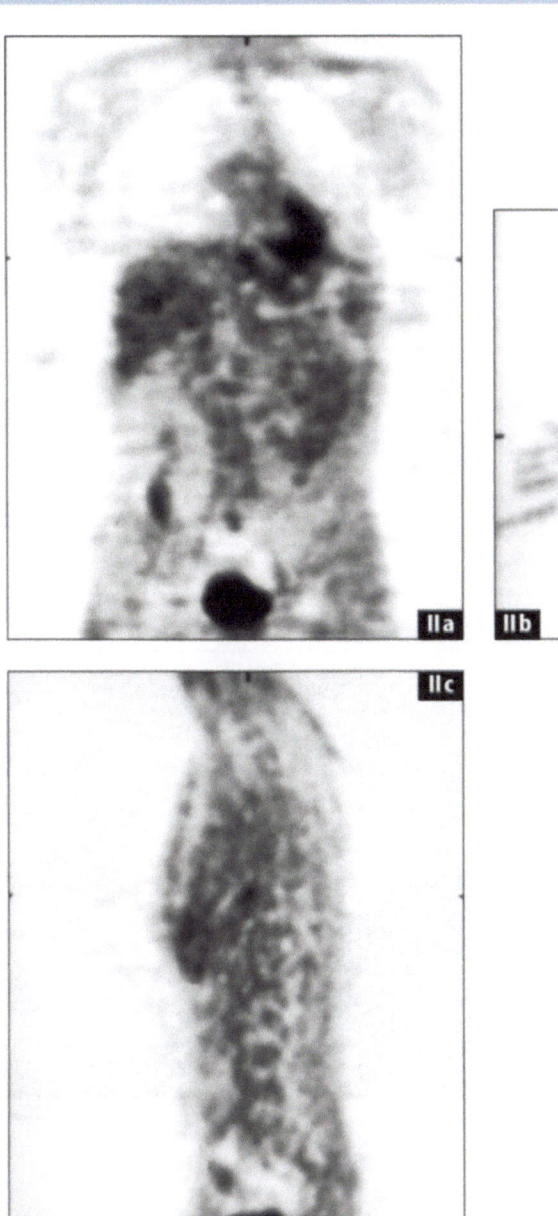

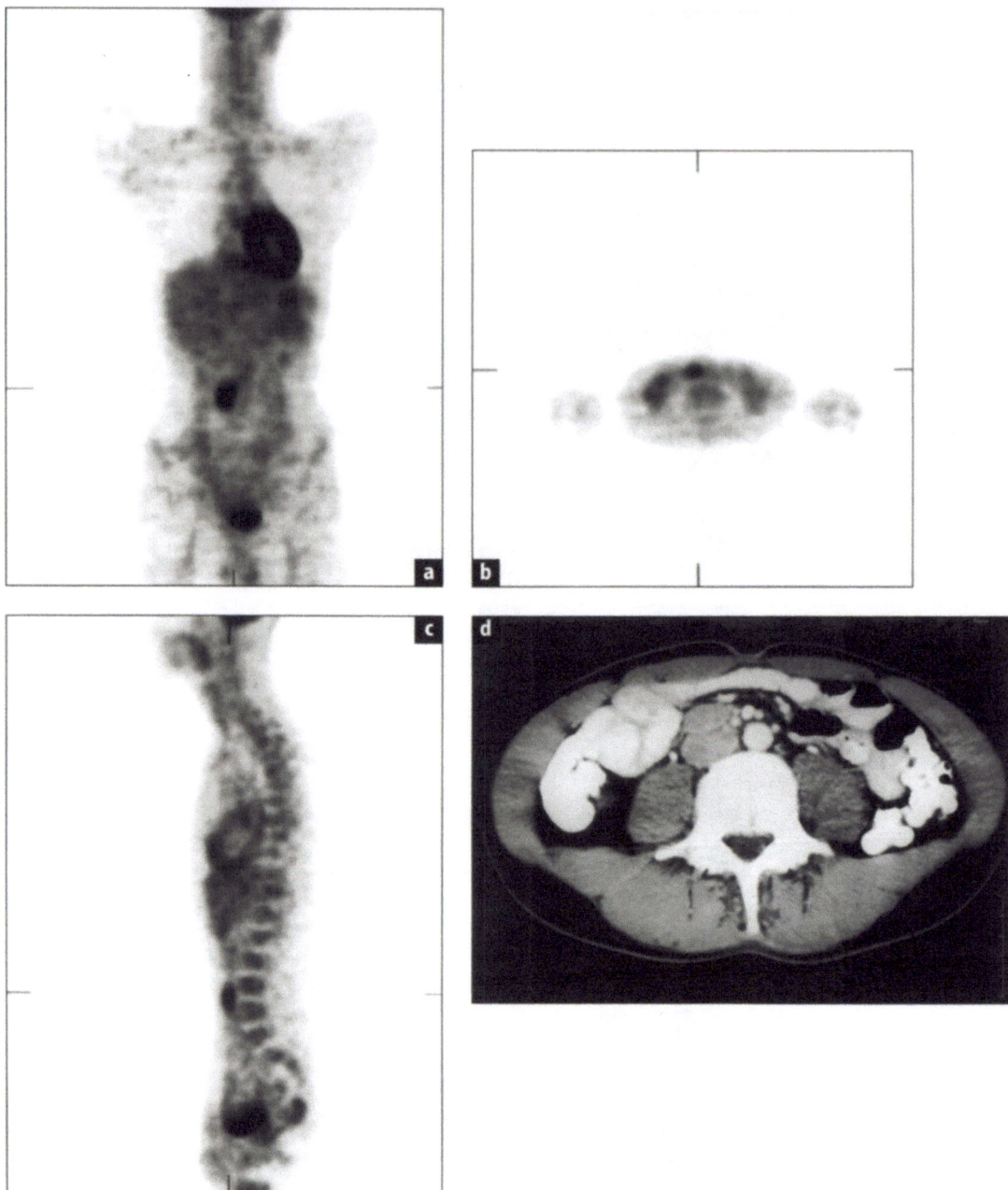

Figure 4 a–d

Diagnosis: Seminoma.

Patient and History: The 27-year-old patient was diagnosed with a right-sided pure seminoma. The tumor did not express any markers (AFP, b-HCG, or PLAP). His staging CT was primarily rated unsuspicious. Due to low oral contrast a non-enhancing mass in front of the v. cava remained unclear. The repeated spiral CT scan with sufficient contrasting of the duodenum revealed a 3-cm lesion in maximal transverse diameter suspicious of a lymph node metastasis.

Technique: Transmission-corrected scans with a slice thickness of 4 mm; iterative image reconstruction.

PET Results: The PET scan verified this lesion to be a malignancy (metastases). The patient was treated with chemotherapy.

Histology: Seminoma.

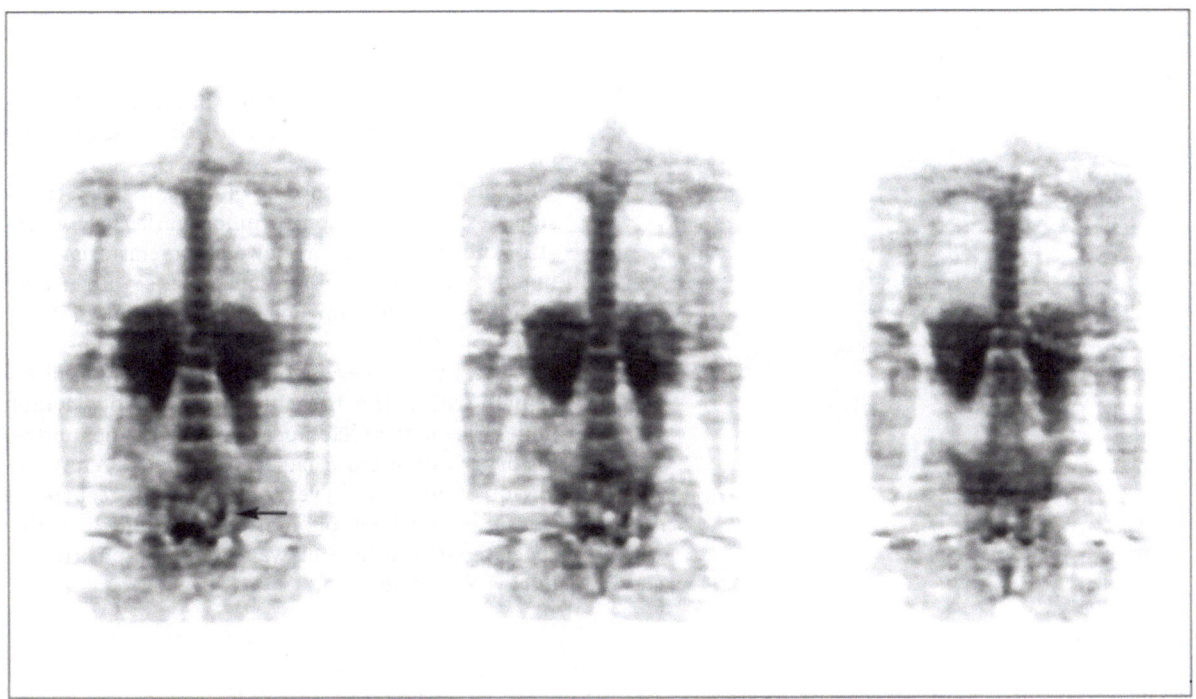

Figure 5

Diagnosis: Germ cell tumor (no metastases); misinterpretation of ureter activity as lymph node metastasis.

Patient and History: This 35-year-old patient had a left-sided testicular germ cell tumor (embryonal carcinoma, mature teratoma and yolk sac tumor). His tumor markers normalized within the usual half-time and his spiral CT scan was unsuspicious of lymph node metastases.

Technique: Transmission-corrected scans with a slice thickness of 4 mm; image reconstruction by filtered backprojection.

PET Results: Positron-emission tomography showed a left-sided focus in the area of the left common iliac artery. This lesion was initially graded as tumor suspicious. Staging retroperitoneal lymph node dissection (RPLND) had been performed in ipsilateral nerve sparing technique. The patient is recurrence free with a follow-up of more than 3 years. Retrospectively, the PET signal was interpreted as temporary urinary stasis in the distal ureter.

Histology: No evidence of cancer cells.

Cave! Ureter activity may be misinterpreted as malignoma.

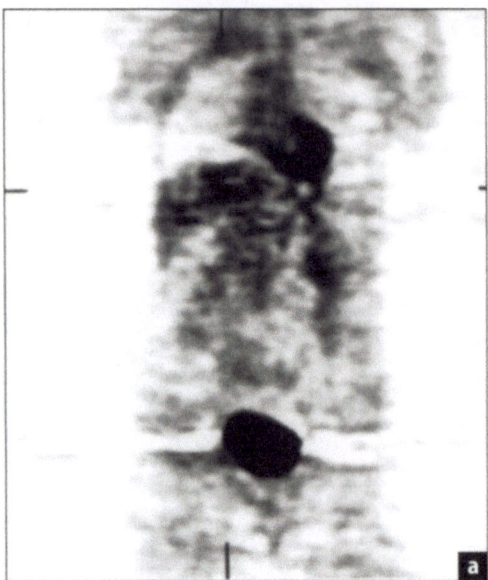

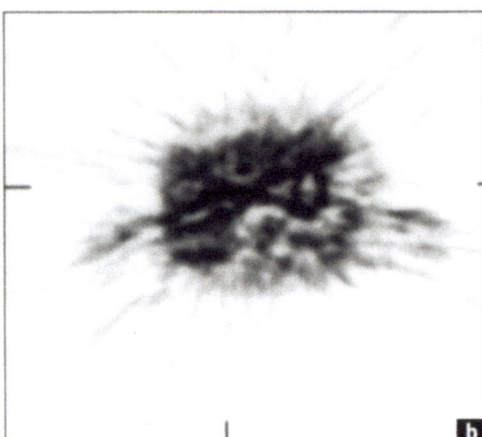

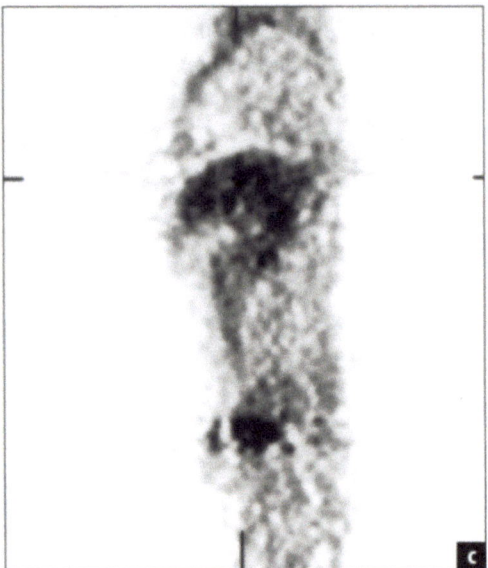

Figure 6 a–c

Diagnosis: Seminoma (no evidence of metastasis); misinterpretation of reconstruction artifacts as liver metastasis.

Patient and History: The 36-year-old patient had a right-sided testicular seminoma. Tumor markers were negative and spiral CT scan showed no metastasis.

Technique: Transmission-corrected scans with a slice thickness of 4 mm; image reconstruction by filtered backprojection.

PET Results: PET scan evaluation demonstrated multiple signals within the liver but no suspicious lymph nodes. The patient had normal liver enzymes and no history of liver disease had been evaluated. With a follow-up of more than 3 years the patient is recurrence free after adjuvant paraaortic radiation. In retrospect, the PET evaluation was rated false-positive.

Histology: Not performed.

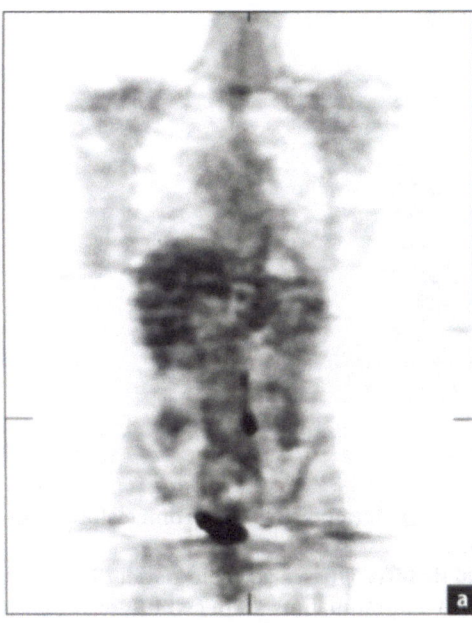

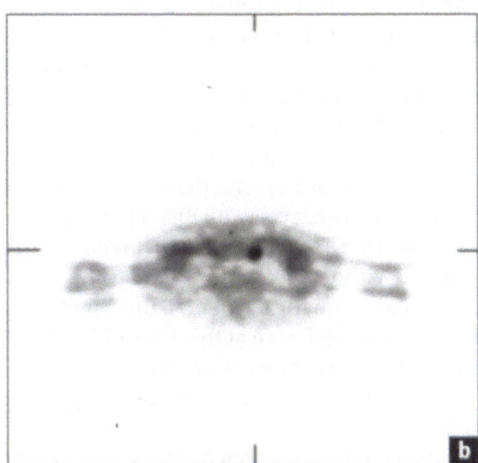

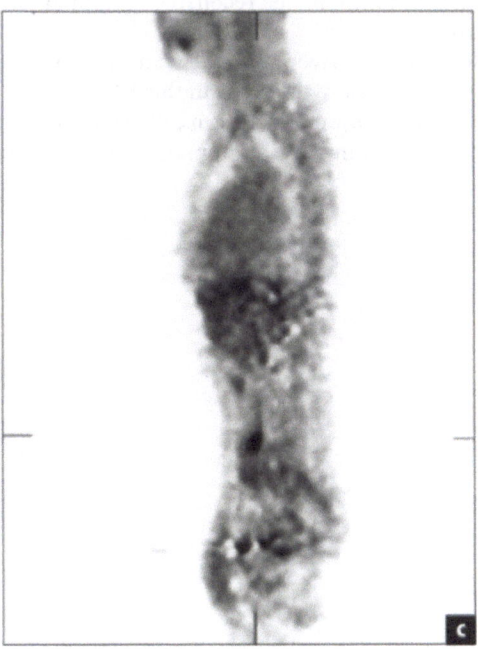

Figure 7 a–c

Diagnosis: Seminoma (no evidence of metastases); misinterpretation of renal activity as metastases.

Patient and History: This 32-year-old patient was diagnosed with a left-sided seminoma. Tumor markers were negative and spiral CT was unsuspicious.

Technique: Transmission-corrected scans with a slice thickness of 4 mm; image reconstruction by filtered backprojection.

PET Results: PET views showed a tumor-suspicious activity uptake in projection on both distal ureters. After adjuvant radiation the patient is more than 2 years recurrence free. In retrospect, the PET scan evaluation with positive signals in the renal area was caused by low hydration and trapping of the tracer.

Histology: Not performed.

Cave! Renal or pelvic activity may be misinterpreted as metastases.

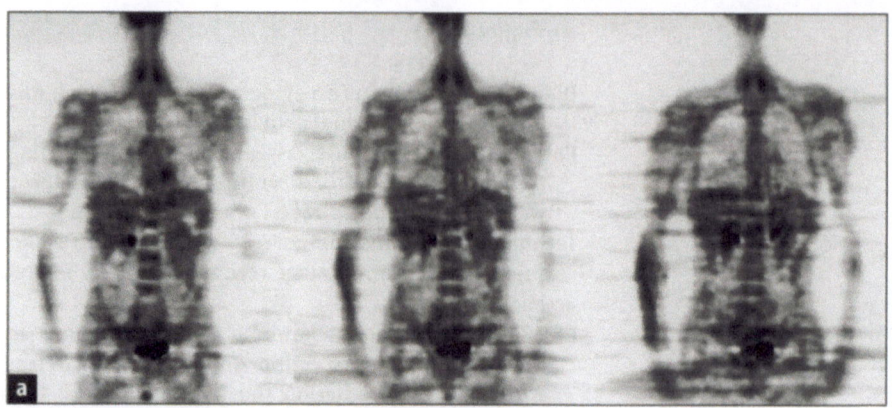

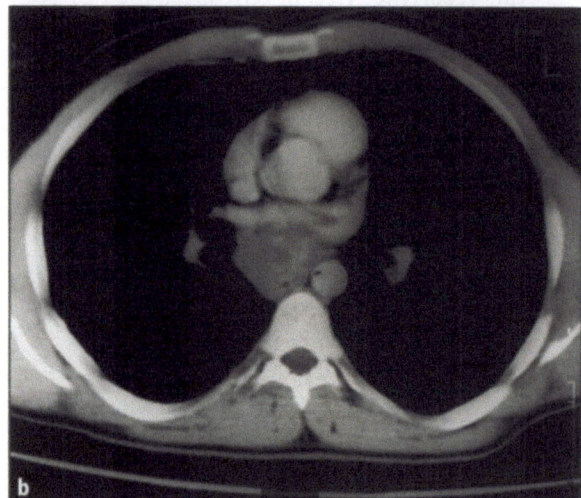

Figure 8 a, b

Diagnosis: Mature teratoma with micrometastatic lymph node metastases.

Patient and History: This 27-year-old patient had a left-sided non-seminomatous germ cell tumor (embryonal carcinoma, mature teratoma and yolk sac tumor). He had a history of drug abuse with a consecutive hepatitis A. The spiral CT scan was unsuspicious and an initial PET scan was negative. In RPLND he showed micrometastasis and was classified as having pathological stage IIa tumor. A left-sided nerve sparing RPLND was performed and the patient was treated with adjuvant two cycles of PEB chemotherapy. One year later he showed a chest recurrence in the mediastinum without rising tumor markers. Additionally he had a small peripheral lung metastasis (see CT scan). The PET scan at this time did not show any signal in the chest. The patient underwent thoracotomy and tumor resection in the lung which showed mature teratoma.

Technique: Transmission-corrected scans with a slice thickness of 4 mm; image reconstruction by filtered backprojection.

PET Results: Retrospectively, the PET scan was false-negative because of pure teratoma in the lung.

Histology: Non-seminomatous germ cell tumor (embryonal carcinoma, mature teratoma and yolk sac tumor)

Malignant Lymphoma

U. Cremerius

The two major variants of malignant lymphoma are non-Hodgkin's lymphoma and Hodgkin's disease. About 40,000 new cases of non-Hodgkin's lymphoma and 7500 new cases of Hodgkin's disease occur each year in the United States. The incidence of non-Hodgkin's lymphoma has increased rapidly in the last few years. Malignant lymphomas are the most common neoplasm in patients between the ages of 20 and 40 years. Thus, although the total number of patients is relatively small, malignant lymphomas rank fourth in the total number of person-years of life lost to cancer.

11.1 Nodal Disease

Most patients present with persistent peripheral lymphadenopathy. Hodgkin's disease is located exclusively in the supradiaphragmatic lymph nodes in 54%, exclusively in the infradiaphragmatic lymph nodes in 6%, and on both sides of the diaphragm in 40% of cases. Non-Hodgkin's lymphomas tend to be more generalized with nodal spread on both sides of the diaphragm in 70%. The modified Ann Arbor staging system is used to describe the stage of malignant lymphomas. In stages I and II, sites of disease are on the same side of the diaphragm. Stage III disease involves both sides of the diaphragm, and stage IV is defined as disseminated involvement of one or more extralymphatic organs. CT scans and chest X-ray are the major imaging techniques for clinical staging while lymphangiography has been abandoned for the most part. PET has been shown to be more sensitive than CT imaging in the detection of nodal disease, as it can detect malignancy also in normal-sized lymph nodes.

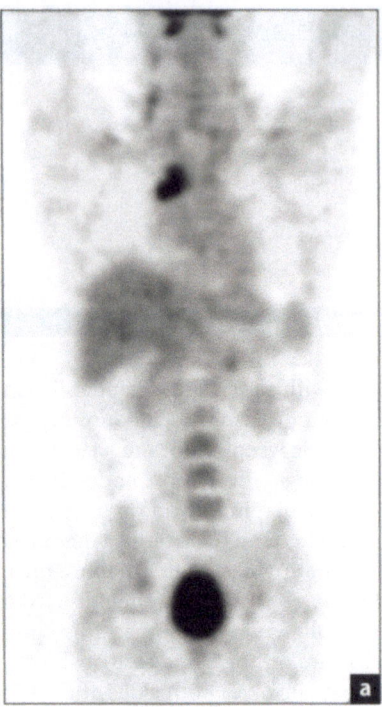

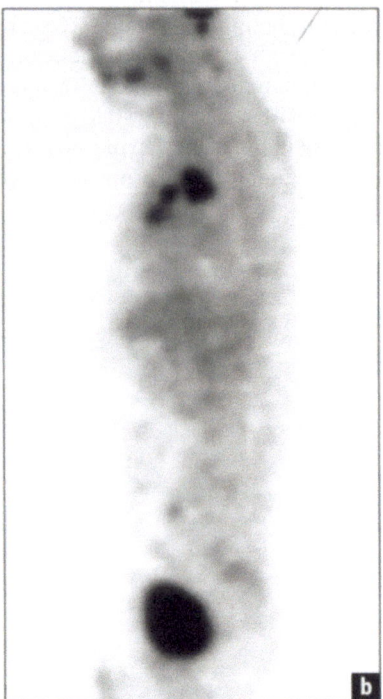

Figure 1 a, b

Patient and History: 27-year-old male with mediastinal lymphadenopathy, accidentally diagnosed on chest X-ray done for chronic bronchitis.

Technique: Attenuation-corrected whole-body scan after injection of 300 MBq FDG. Hydration and administration of 20 mg furosemide. Documentation in coronal and sagittal slices of 7 mm thickness. Iterative reconstruction.

PET Results: Increased focal uptake in three lesions of the anterior and superior mediastinum. Regular uptake in all other lymph node stations and homogeneous uptake in liver, spleen and bone marrow. **Note** faint non-specific uptake in neck muscles and radioactivity-filled bladder.

Histology: Hodgkin's lymphoma of nodular sclerosing subtype. Clinical stage IIA.

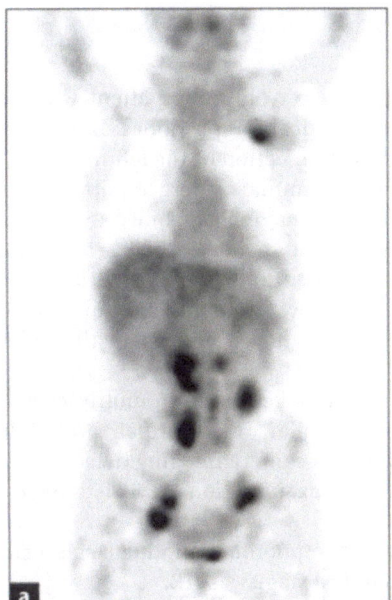
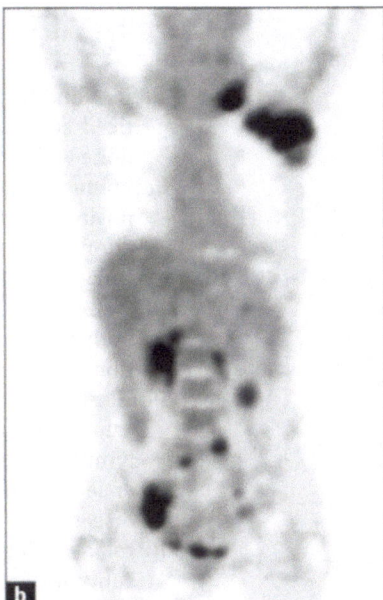
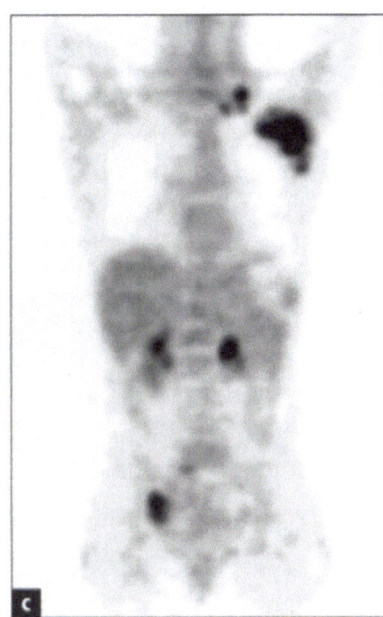

Figure 2 a–c

Patient and History: 44-year-old female patient who noted growth of a left supraclavicular node. Physical examination revealed enlarged lymph nodes in the left axilla and in both inguinal regions.

Technique: Transmission-corrected whole-body PET scan after injection of 190 MBq FDG. Application of furosemide, hydration and bladder catheterization. Iterative reconstruction from ventral (**a**) to dorsal (**b**) of the coronal view.

PET Results: Increased focal uptake in left axillary, left supraclavicular, paraaortic, iliac and inguinal lymph nodes. Regular uptake in liver, spleen and bone marrow.

Histology: Diffuse large B-cell non-Hodgkin's lymphoma. Stage IV due to small-volume (<5%) bone marrow infiltration with grade I follicular lymphoma. Discordant histology is explained by secondary transformation into a high-grade lymphoma.

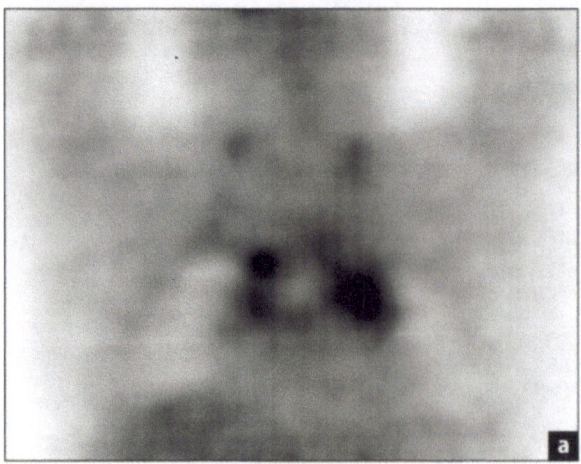

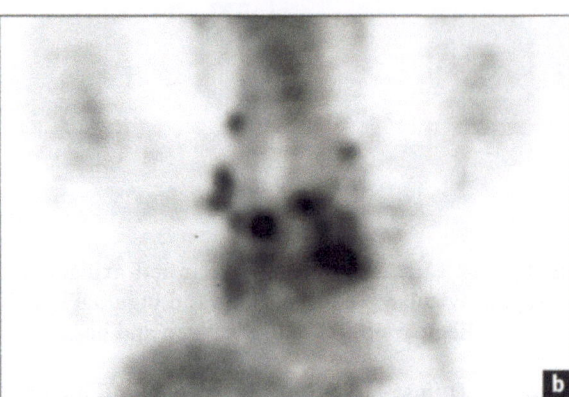

Figure 3 a, b

Patient and History: 45-year-old male patient who noticed swelling of cervical lymph nodes. Biopsy was done with modified dissection of the left neck.

Technique: Dual-head gamma camera equipped with positron coincidence imaging capability and attenuation correction (**a**) and dedicated PET scanner (**b**). Imaging was performed first on the dedicated PET system (the image shows a detail of a coronal whole body slice), then on the dual-head camera after injection of 270 MBq FDG.

PET Results: Increased uptake is seen in multiple cervical, supra/infraclavicular, mediastinal and hilar lymph nodes. Gamma camera imaging detected fewer lesions, but both examinations revealed stage II disease.

Histology: Hodgkin's lymphoma of nodular sclerosing subtype. Final clinical stage was IIB.

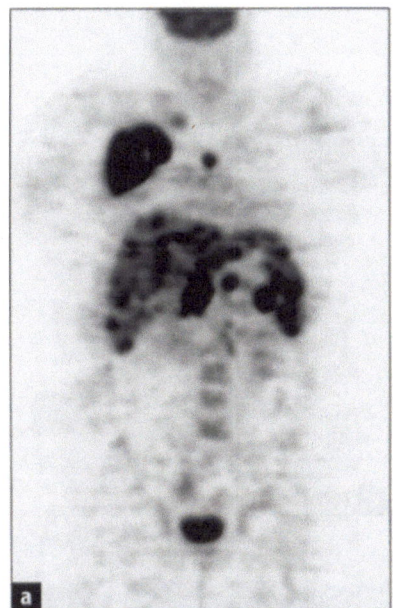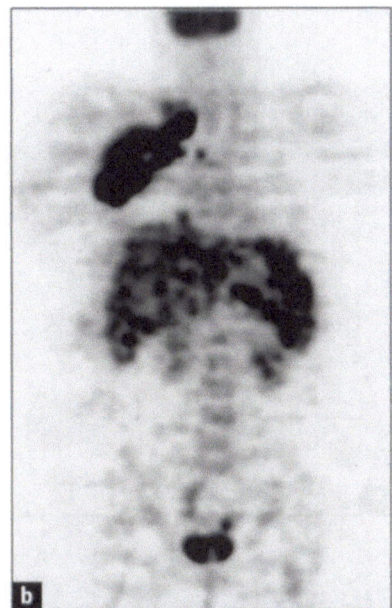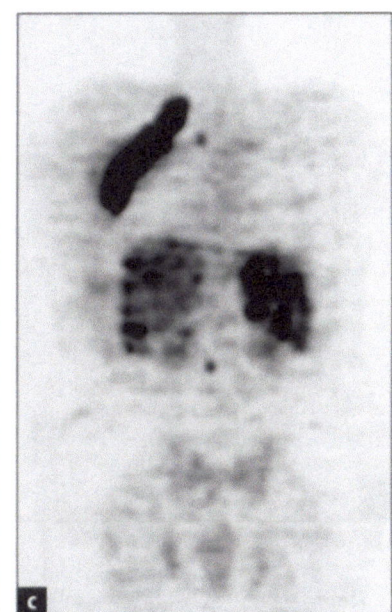

11.2 Extranodal Disease

Figure 4 a–c

While most malignant lymphomas originate from lymph nodes, non-Hodgkin's lymphoma may also originate from extralymphatic organs in up to 30%. Extranodal disease has been found in Hodgkin's disease in about 35% affecting the spleen, and in 4% for liver or bone marrow. In non-Hodgkin's lymphoma, extralymphatic involvement is far more common and may occur in up to 60%. A wide variety of diagnostic procedures is used to verify extranodal disease, including CT scans, bone marrow biopsy, bone scan, magnetic resonance imaging of the spine, endoscopic examinations, lumbar puncture, barium studies of the GI tract, liver biopsy, and staging laparatomy. Staging laparatomy is now rarely performed because of relevant morbidity. PET whole-body imaging has been shown to be a very sensitive method for detection of extralymphatic disease in almost every organ (with the exception of the brain).

Patient and History: Female 26-year-old patient, weight 106 kg, with complaints of pain and swelling in the right arm.

Technique: Transmission-corrected scan after injection of 380 MBq FDG, application of furosemide, hydration and bladder catheterization. Documentation in coronal planes of 7 mm slice thickness. Iterative reconstruction.

PET Results: Increased focal FDG uptake is shown in the right axillary mass, right supraclavicular lymph nodes, a single mediastinal lymph node and paraaortic lymph nodes (**a–c**). Increased multifocal uptake is also seen in liver and spleen. PET findings are compatible with nodal and extranodal involvement. Interestingly, liver involvement was not suspected from the CT scan.

Histology: T-cell-rich B-cell lymphoma, a rare entity of high-grade non-Hodgkin's lymphoma. Final clinical staging was stage IVB.

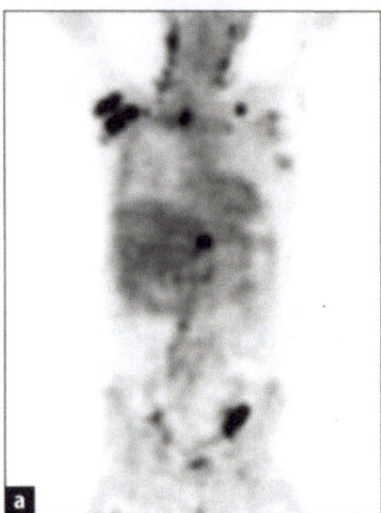
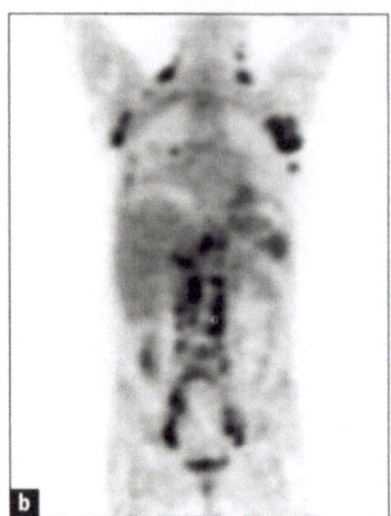
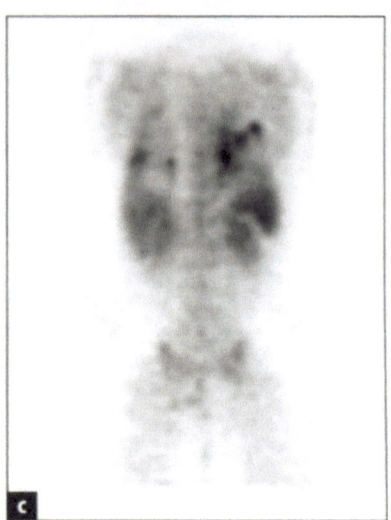

Figure 5 a–c

Patient and History: A 62-year-old female patient complained of persistent cough. Chest X-ray showed multiple pulmonary nodules. Enlarged lymph nodes were palpable cervical and inguinal. Cervical lymph node biopsy was done.

Technique: Attenuation-corrected whole body scan after injection of 200 MBq FDG, application of furosemide, hydration and bladder catheterization. Documentation in coronal planes of 7 mm slice thickness. Iterative reconstruction.

PET Results: Increased focal uptake in multiple lymph nodes (cervical, supra/infraclavicular, axillary, para-aortic, iliac and inguinal) (**a, b**) and in multiple pulmonary lesions (**c**). Diffuse enhanced uptake of the spleen (in comparison to liver uptake).

Histology: Follicular non-Hodgkin's lymphoma. Clinical staging was IVA due to suspected pulmonary involvement.

11.3 Lymphoma Relapse

The prognosis of patients who experience a relapse after systemic treatment for Hodgkin's disease or high-grade non-Hodgkin's lymphoma is significantly worse. Some of these patients are now regarded as candidates for high-dose chemotherapy with stem cell transplantation or bone marrow transplantation, and may still achieve long-standing progression-free survival. The curative chance is improved if relapse can be detected with small tumor volumes.

Figure 6 a, b

Patient and History: 60-year-old male after 13 courses of polychemotherapy for high-grade non-Hodgkin's lymphoma. The patient complains of persistent dyspnea. X-rays show compression fracture of the vertebral body, Th9.

Technique: Non-corrected (**a**) and attenuation-corrected (**b**) PET scan after injection of 230 MBq FDG. Hydration and application of furosemide. Shown are selected coronal whole-body (**a**) and sagittal thoracic (**b**) images with 7 mm slice thickness.

PET Results: On the whole-body study (**a**) increased focal uptake is seen in the right supraclavicular region, mediastinum, lung hili, spleen and pelvis. Bone marrow involvement was suspected in thoracic vertebrae and in the pelvis. Note that differentiation between involvement of the posterior mediastinum or thoracic vertebrae is difficult in coronal view (**a**), but much easier in the sagittal view (**b**). The sagittal slice shows lymphomas of the anterior and posterior mediastinum and increased uptake in several vertebrae. Note myocardial uptake and missing glucose consumption corresponding to the known compression fracture.

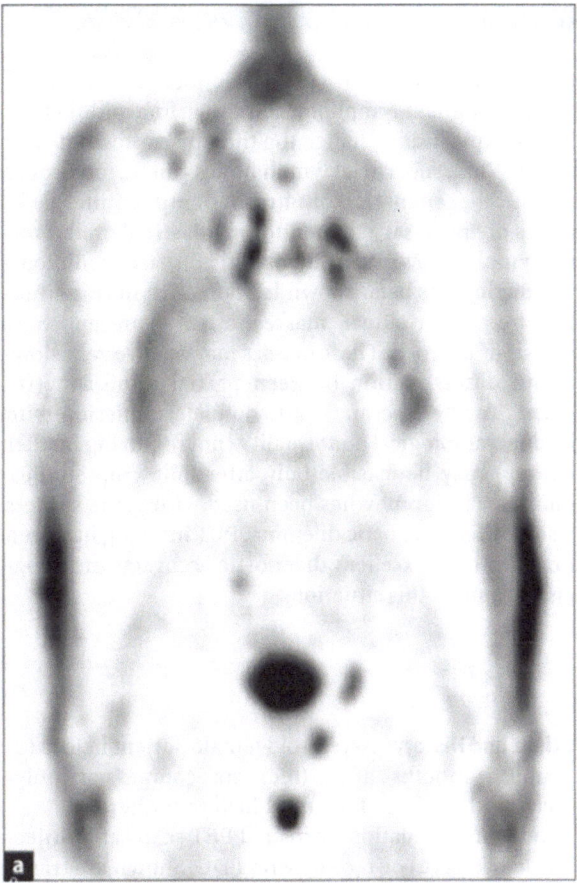

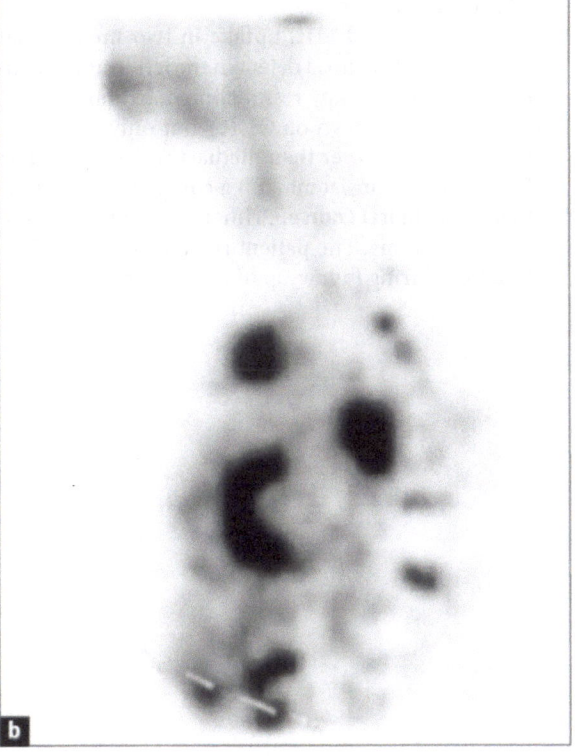

11.4 Therapy Control

It is mandatory to control the efficacy of aggressive therapy in malignant lymphomas in order to avoid ineffective therapy and to change the therapy protocol if necessary. While superficial lymph nodes can be monitored by clinical examination or ultrasonography, other techniques are necessary to monitor mediastinal or abdominal lymph nodes or extralymphatic disease. Radiological imaging has been shown less effective in this situation because residual masses often represent only fibrosis or necrosis. These masses may resolve very slowly, and differentiation between partial remission (requiring further therapy) and complete remission with residual radiological abnormality (not requiring further therapy) may be feasible only after follow-up studies. Gallium scintigraphy has been used with some success to solve this diagnostic dilemma. PET imaging has been shown to have excellent diagnostic accuracy and prognostic value in this situation.

Figure 7 a–c

Patient and History: 35-year-old female patient before (**a**) and 3 months after (**b,c**) six courses of polychemotherapy and involved field radiotherapy.

Technique: Attenuation-corrected PET scans after injection of 285 (**a**) or 140 (**b**) MBq FDG. Shown are transversal slices of 7 mm thickness. Native chest CT scan of 8 mm slice thickness.

PET Results: Increased FDG uptake in two mediastinal lesions (**a**). Note central defect in the left lesion due to necrosis. After therapy residual mediastinal mass of 4×2 cm size is shown on CT (**c**), but only very faint uptake on PET (lower than mediastinal uptake). The PET finding is consistent with a complete remission.

Histology and Clinical Course: Primary mediastinal large B-cell lymphoma. The patient remained in complete remission during follow-up of more than 3 years.

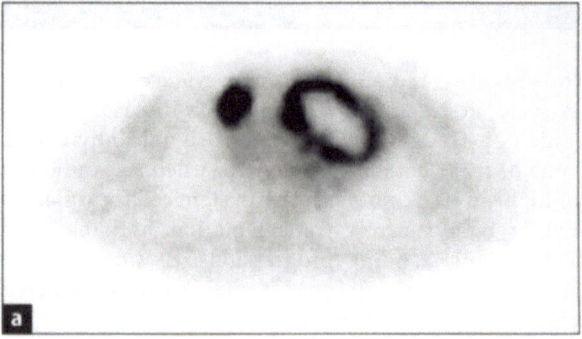

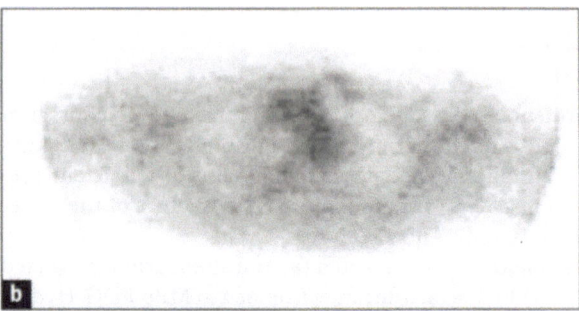

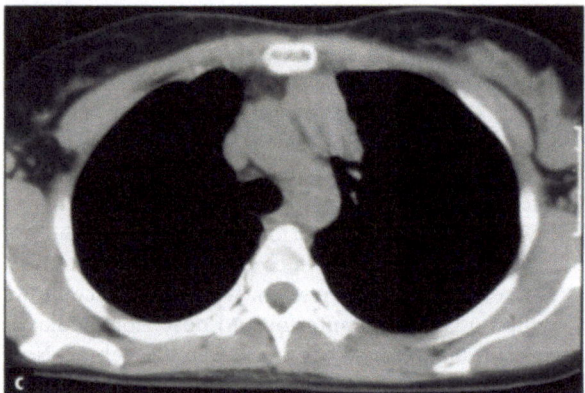

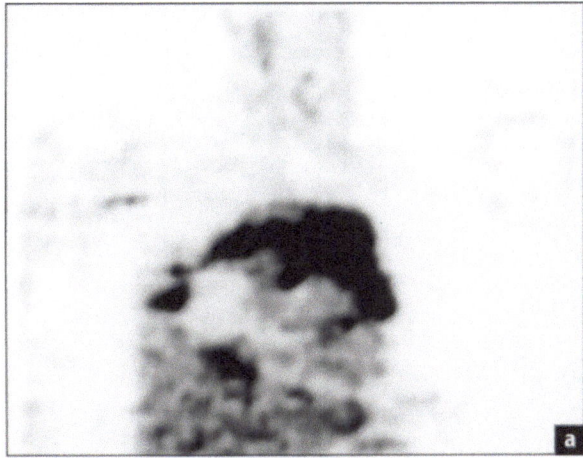

Figure 8 a–c

Patient and History: 34-year-old male patient at diagnosis (**a**), after eight courses of polychemotherapy (**b**) and 2 months after additional radiotherapy (**c**).

Technique: Attenuation-corrected PET scans after injection of 210–305 MBq FDG. Coronal slices of the chest (7 mm slice thickness). Reduced image quality in (**a**) due to shorter acquisition time per bed position using a scanner with a small field of view.

PET Results: Increased FDG uptake in a large mediastinal mass (bulky disease) at the time of diagnosis (**a**). Focal pathological uptake in the upper mediastinum after chemotherapy (**b**) indicating residual disease. Local disease progression on PET despite additional radiotherapy (**c**).

Histology and Clinical Course: Hodgkin's lymphoma of nodular sclerosing subtype. Lymphoma relapse became clinically apparent with development of pulmonal lesions 2 months after PET imaging in (**c**).

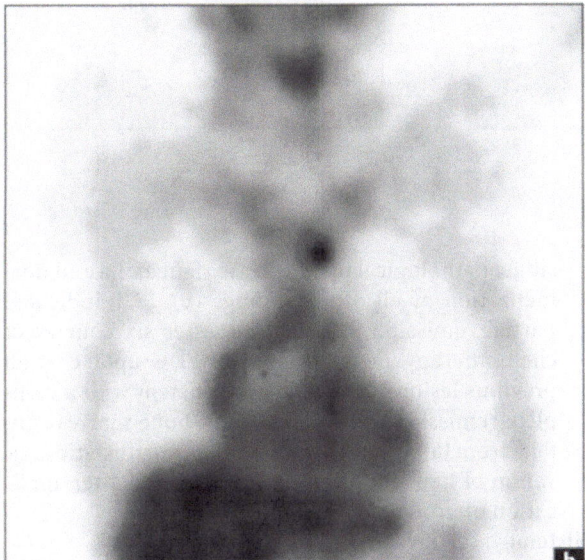

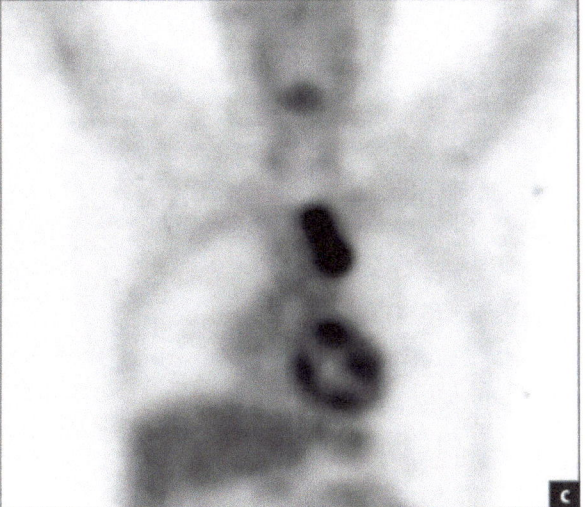

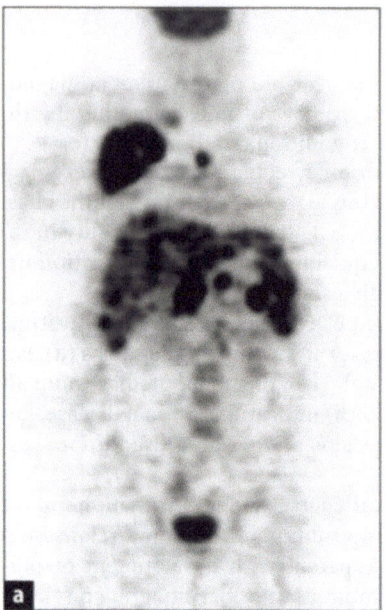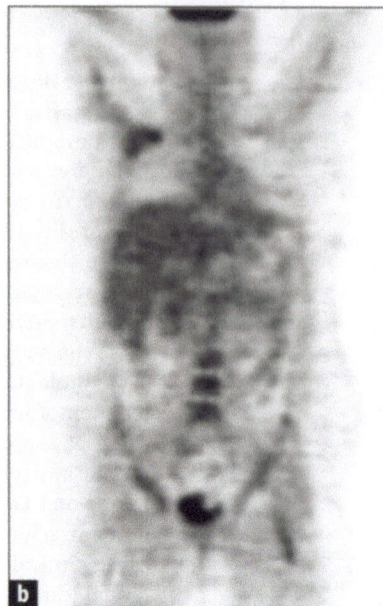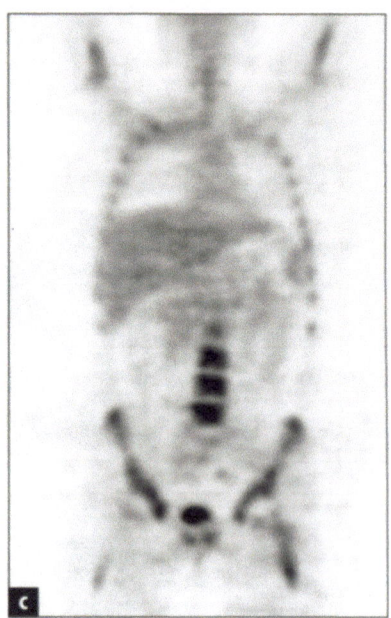

Figure 9 a–c

Patient and History: see Fig. 4.

Technique: Attenuation-corrected whole body scans after injection of 200–385 MBq FDG. 7-mm coronal slices. PET imaging was done before therapy (**a**), at mid-treatment (**b**) and after six courses of polychemotherapy (**c**).

PET Results: At the time of diagnosis, increased uptake in right axillary, mediastinal and paraaortal lymph nodes. PET also indicated multifocal involvement of spleen and liver (**a**). After three courses of therapy, residual pathological uptake in the right axilla and normalization of all other findings (**b**). PET indicated partial remission at that time. After six courses of chemotherapy, normalization of FDG uptake in all previous lesions (**c**). PET was consistent with a complete remission. Note elevation of bone marrow uptake from (**a**) to (**c**). This is due to postcytostatic activation of hematopoiesis, in (**c**) enhanced after application of growth factors (G-CSF).

Histology: see Fig. 4.

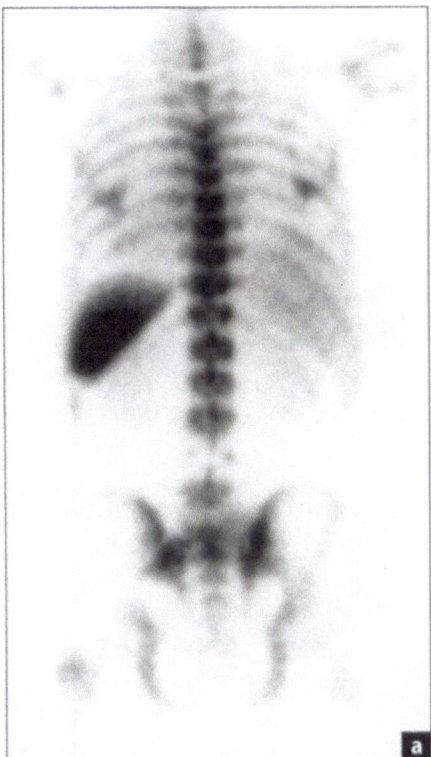

Figure 10 a, b

Patient and History: 30-year-old male patient who was treated with polychemotherapy for high-grade B-cell lymphoma stage IV with osseous involvement.

Technique: Posterior view of a planar bone marrow scintigraphy performed 3 h after injection of 300 MBq ^{99m}Tc-anti-NCA-95 (**a**). Coronal 7-mm slice of a corresponding PET scan 1 h after injection of 200 MBq FDG (**b**). The patient was hydrated and 20 mg furosemide administered. Iterative reconstruction.

PET Results: Corresponding defect in L3 both on bone marrow scintigraphy and on PET. While bone marrow scintigraphy cannot differentiate marrow infiltration and marrow fibrosis, a lack of glucose metabolism in L3 is in favor of marrow fibrosis. Concordant defects were also found in the left hip bone and in the upper thoracic vertebrae (PET not shown).

Clinical Course: The patient remained relapse-free during a follow-up of 3 years after treatment.

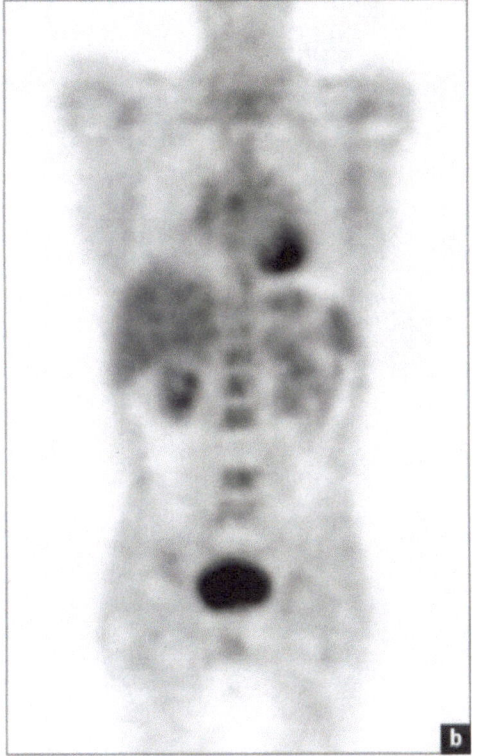

11.5 Variants and Pitfalls

Figure 11 a, b

Patient and History: 20-year-old female patient who received polychemotherapy for Hodgkin's lymphoma (stage III) with involvement of cervical, paraaortal and iliac lymph nodes. Five months after treatment, a retrosternal mass was evident on CT. She was clinically well.

Technique: Whole-body scan with (**a**) and without (**b**) transmission scan after injection of 175 MBq FDG. Documentation in coronal slices of 7 mm thickness.

PET Results: Moderately increased uptake (standardized uptake value 4.4) in the anterior mediastinum corresponding to the mass seen on CT. No pathological uptake in regions of initial involvement. In this clinical context the finding suggests rebound thymic hyperplasia after chemotherapy. **Cave!** Rebound thymic hyperplasia is sometimes seen in children and young adults recovering from severe illness or intensive chemotherapy.

Clinical Course: Three months later the finding was unchanged on a follow-up PET scan. The patient was clinically well.

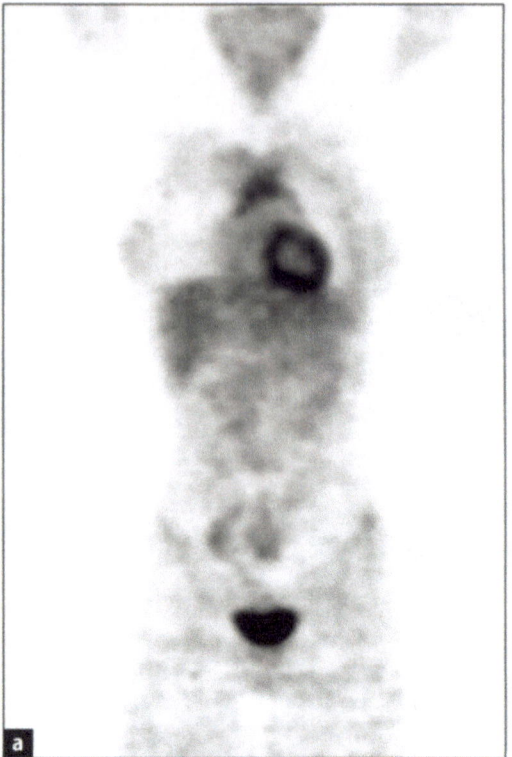

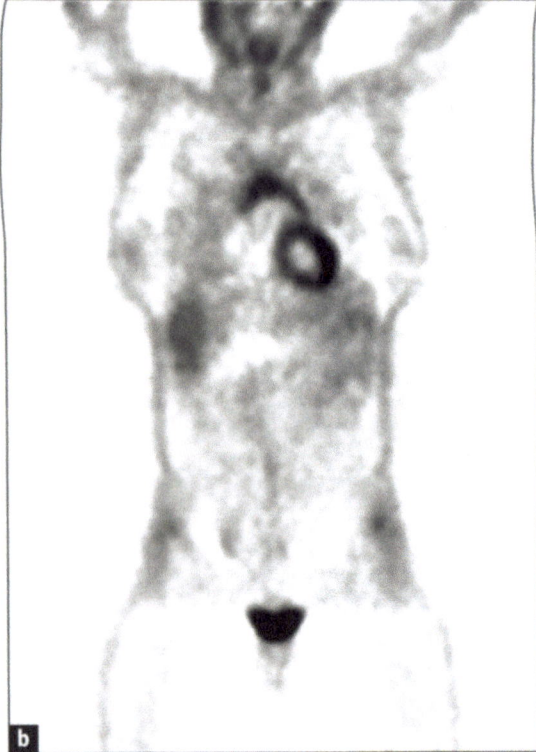

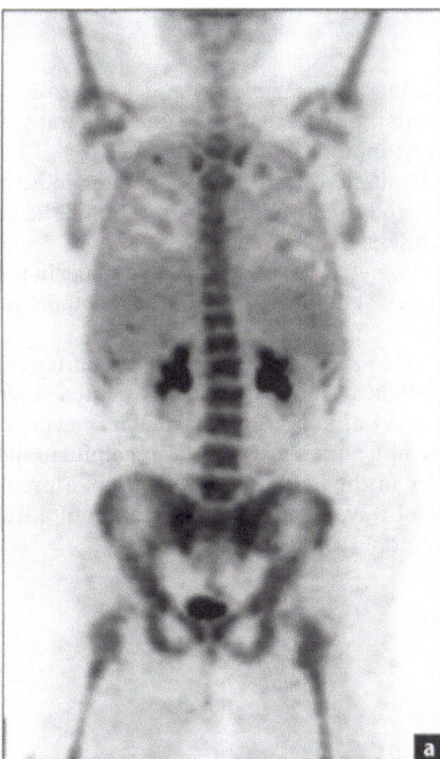

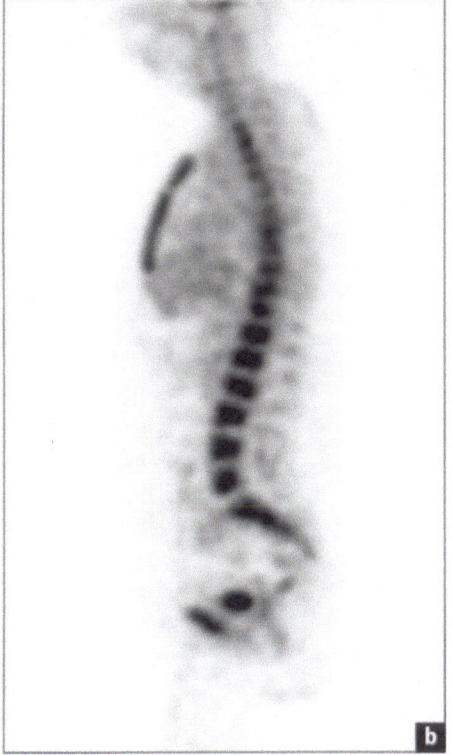

Figure 12 a, b

Patient and History: 26-year-old female patient after six courses of polychemotherapy for T-cell-rich B-cell lymphoma (see Figs. 4, 9). Bone marrow was stimulated with G-CSF in the last days before PET imaging.

Technique: Attenuation-corrected PET scan after injection of 200 MBq FDG. Shown are an anterioposterior maximum intensity projection (**a**) and a sagittal slice of 7 mm thickness (**b**).

PET Results: Homogeneous intense bone marrow uptake throughout the hematopoietic active marrow (higher than liver and spleen FDG uptake). Cave! This finding is typical after bone marrow stimulation with growth factors (to some extent also after endogenous stimulation following chemotherapy). However, diffuse lymphoma involvement cannot be excluded.

Histology: Bone marrow biopsy was not performed.

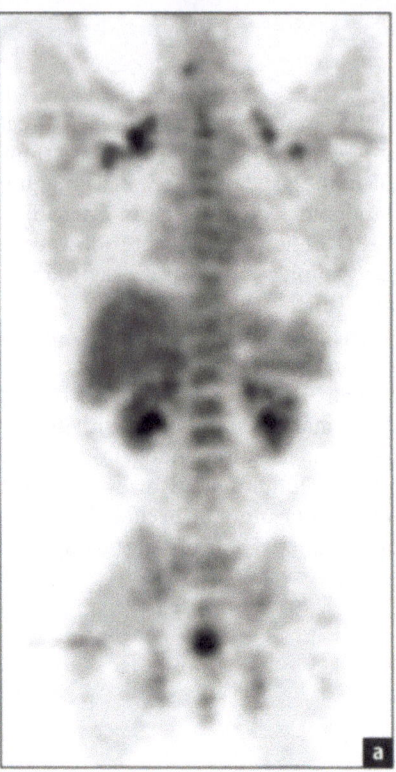

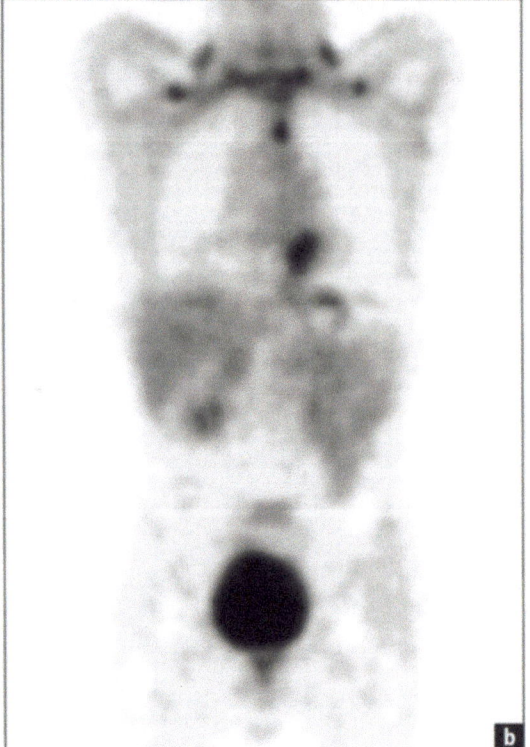

Figure 13 a, b

Patient and History: 28-year-old (**a**) and 34-year-old (**b**) male patients both treated with chemotherapy for Hodgkin's lymphoma and clinically well.

Technique: Attenuation-corrected scans after injection of 300 and 270 MBq FDG. Shown are coronal slices of 7 mm thickness. Iterative reconstruction

PET Results: Symmetric focally enhanced uptake in neck and shoulders, sometimes reaching to the upper mediastinum.

Cave! This is often seen in the musculature of tense or anxious patients. This may be easily confused with uptake of cervical, supra/infraclavicular or even mediastinal lymph nodes. A 3D display is helpful to show the muscles in the longitudinal direction. Muscular tension can be avoided by the application of a tranquilizer before FDG injection.

Pancreatic Lesions

C. G. Diederichs

12.1 Ductal Adenocarcinoma

About one-fifth of all gastrointestinal cancers are of pancreatic origin. More than 97% of these patients will die of the disease. The incidence of pancreatic cancer is highest between ages 50 and 70, men are more likely to develop it than women, and patients from disadvantaged social classes are more frequently affected. The etiology of pancreatic cancer is unclear, but some risk factors have been well known for a long time. Probably the most important risk factor is smoking; the risk is proportional to the amount of tobacco smoked. The majority of pancreatic cancers arise in the exocrine glandular areas of the pancreas. Eighty percent of these carcinomas correspond histologically to an adenocarcinoma. These carcinomas are generally ductal in origin and are mostly localized in the head of the pancreas. FDG-PET should be performed when the conventional work-up produces indeterminate results concerning the nature of the lesion or the presence of metastases, or if the different morphologic imaging modalities produce contradictory results [1]. Any focal uptake with an SUV >3 is suspicious for malignancy. Sensitivity and specificity for FDG-PET are reported at between 80% and 90%. Rarely, a lesion with a higher SUV is a pancreatic abscess. This is a rare late complication of chronic pancreatitis. Lesions with SUVs between 2 and 3 may also be malignant. However, there is some overlap with inflammatory pseudotumors. The detection rate for lymph node metastasis is similar compared to CT and endosonography and ranges around 60% [2]. Specificity is about 85%. T1 and T-in-situ tumors will be detected with a rate of 50–70%. Sensitivity is lower for small lesions compared to larger tumors that are detected with 90% sensitivity (unpublished data).

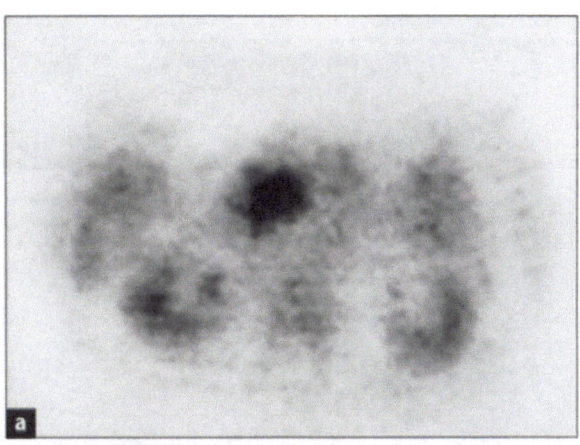

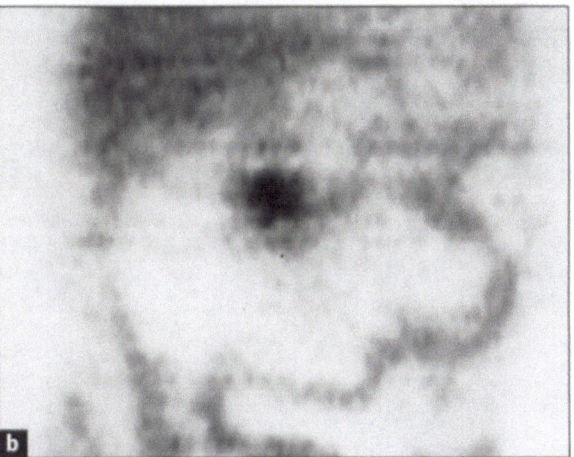

Figure 1 a, b

Patient and History: 69-year-old patient with a suspicious pancreatic mass on CT and a high grade stenosis of the pancreatic duct in ERCP.

Technique: 360 MBq FDG i.v. 45 min prior to start of emission. ECAT 931 scanner. 10'/BP with attenuation correction. Iterative reconstruction.

PET Results: The large intensive focal uptake in pancreatic head is typical for malignancy. The SUV was 4.6.

Histology: Ductal adenocarcinoma, pT3pN0.

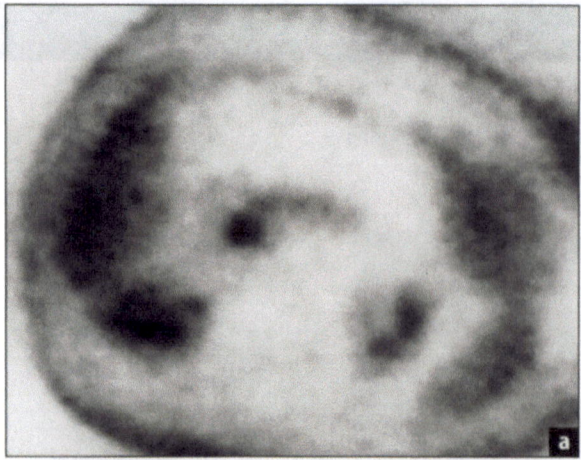

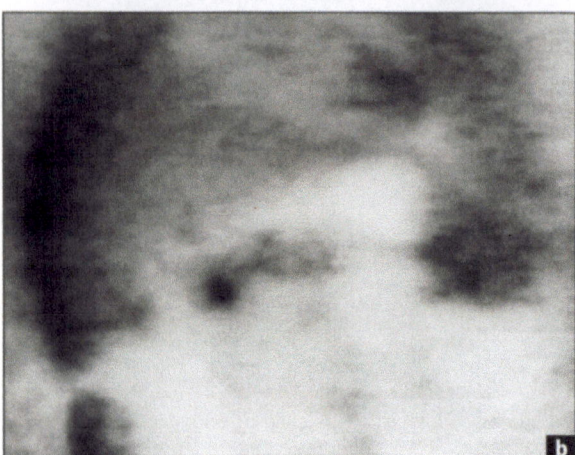

Figure 2 a, b

Patient and History: 63-year-old patient with a suspicious pancreatic mass on CT and MRI.

Technique: Hydro-PET technique: well-hydrated patient examined in right lateral position immediately following oral application of 400 ml water and 40 mg Buscopan i.v. and 470 MBq FDG i.v. 1 h prior to start of emission. ECAT HR+ scanner. 12'/BP without attenuation correction. Iterative reconstruction. Postprocessing with clockwise 90° rotation of transverse images so the patient appears to be supine on images.

PET Results: There is a large intensive focal uptake in pancreatic head strongly suggestive of malignancy. In addition, the pancreatic body and tail show moderate diffuse uptake indicative of poststenotic pancreatitis. Lymph node metastases are not seen.

Histology: Ductal adenocarcinoma, pT3pN1.

Cave! With non-attenuation corrected images, any focal uptake of the pancreas is suspicious for malignancy that is more intense than the liver in a segment that is found on the coronal image along a line-sight drawn vertically through the lesion. Also of note: the hydro-PET technique is easily identified by a fluid filled stomach with a vertical fluid-air interface and partial or complete duodenal hypotony (coronal image).

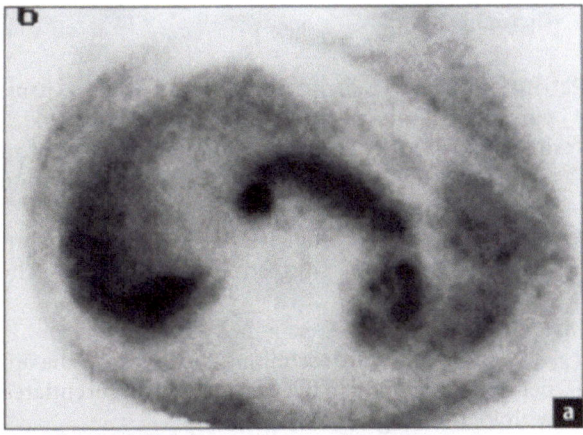

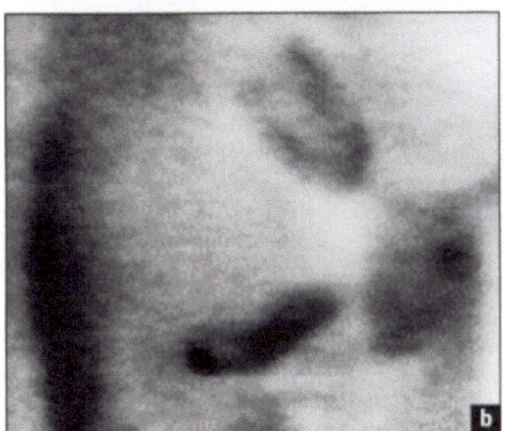

Figure 3 a, b

Patient and History: 43-year-old woman with a history of pancreatitis and a suspicious pancreatic mass on CT.

Technique: Hydro-PET technique (see Figure 2). 347 MBq FDG i.v. 1 h prior to start of emission. ECAT HR+ scanner. 12'/BP without attenuation correction. Iterative reconstruction.

PET Results: There is a relatively small intensive focal uptake in the pancreatic head strongly suggestive of malignancy. In addition, the pancreatic body and tail show intensive diffuse uptake indicative of active poststenotic pancreatitis.

Histology: Ductal adenocarcinoma, pT3.

Cave! The fluid filled slightly distended stomach with a vertical fluid-air interface is nicely seen on the coronal image for better anatomic appreciation.

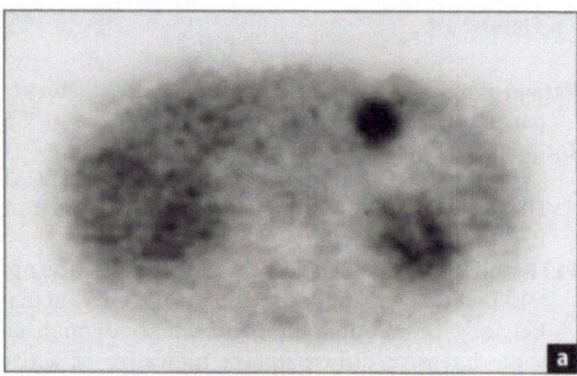

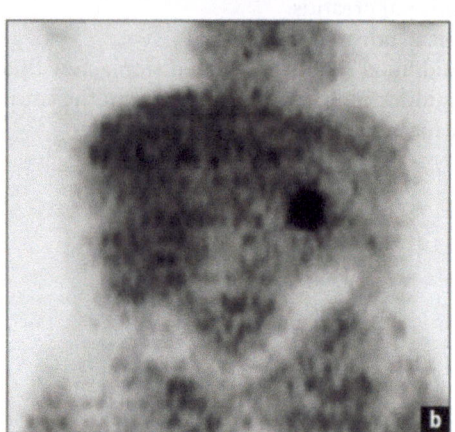

Figure 4 a, b

Patient and History: 48-year-old woman with a suspicious mass in the pancreatic tail on CT.

Technique: 235 MBq FDG i.v. 45 min prior to start of emission. ECAT 931 scanner. 10'/BP with attenuation correction. Iterative reconstruction.

PET Results: There is an intensive focal uptake in the pancreatic tail strongly suggestive of malignancy. The SUV is 3.7.

Histology: Ductal adenocarcinoma, pT2pN0.

Cave! Without the hydro technique, the organs of the upper abdomen and the liver may not be differentiated with PET (cf. Fig. 2).

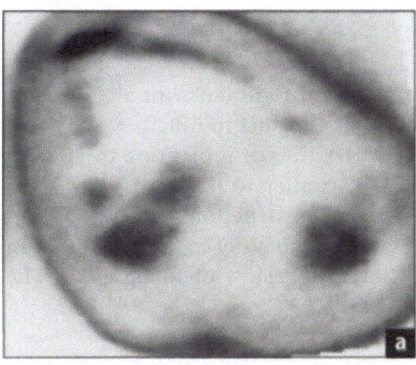

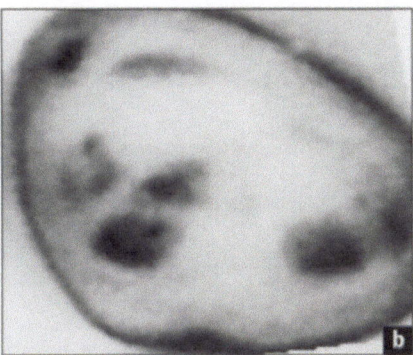

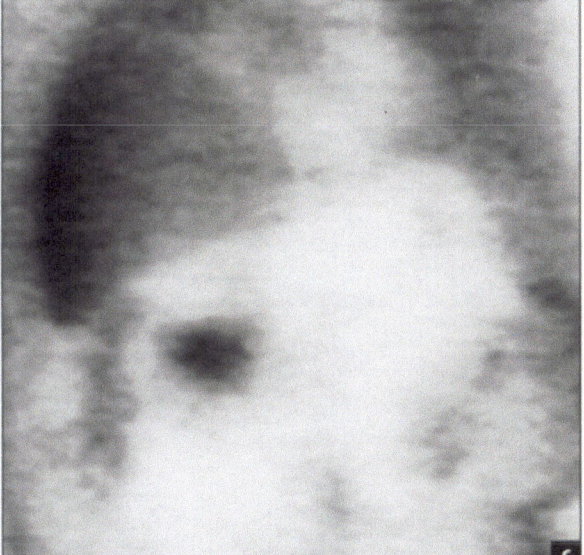

Figure 5 a–c

Patient and History: 71-year-old man with a diffusely enlarged pancreatic head on CT.

Technique: Hydro-PET technique (see Fig. 2). 540 MBq FDG i. v. 1 h prior to start of emission. ECAT HR+ scanner. 12'/BP without attenuation correction. Iterative reconstruction.

PET Results: There is an intensive diffusely increased uptake in the pancreatic head strongly suggestive of malignancy. Best seen in the transverse views (**a, b**), the lesion is surrounded by small adjacent separate lesions suggestive of lymph node metastasis.

Histology: Ductal adenocarcinoma, pT2pN1.

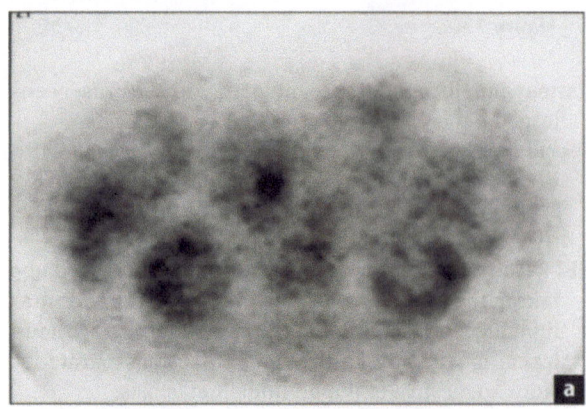

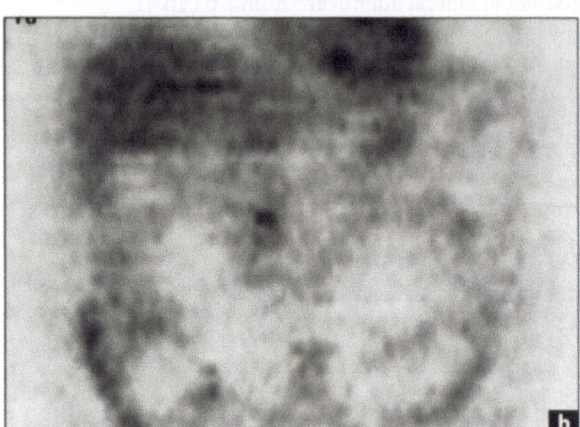

Figure 6 a, b

Patient and History: 68-year-old man with a suspicious stenosis of the pancreatic duct in ERCP.

Technique: 235 MBq FDG i.v. 45 min prior to start of emission. ECAT 931 scanner. 10'/BP with attenuation correction. Iterative reconstruction.

PET Results: There is a small focus of increased uptake in the pancreatic head suggestive of malignancy. The SUV is 2.8.

Histology: Ductal adenocarcinoma, pT1a pN0.

12.2 Other Malignant Tumors

Ampullary carcinoma, which originates in the papilla of Vater, appears less frequently, more often affecting young women, and has a better prognosis. The detection rate with FDG-PET for ampullary carcinoma is around 70–80% and is therefore somewhat lower than for ductal adenocarcinoma. This may be due to a smaller size compared to ductal adenocarcinoma. Bile-duct carcinoma is often localized within the head of the pancreas. Like ampullary carcinoma, it is usually smaller than pancreatic carcinoma due to early occlusion of the bile duct and therefore earlier clinical presentation. The detection rate is 50–60% (own unpublished data). This may also be due to a smaller size compared to ductal adenocarcinoma. Cystadenocarcinomata arise from acinar cells and present macroscopically with large cysts of varying sizes. The detection rate for cystic malignancies in the pancreas may be only around 50%. However, only a small number of patients have been studied so far. Tumors with large cysts and thin septa may not be detectable.

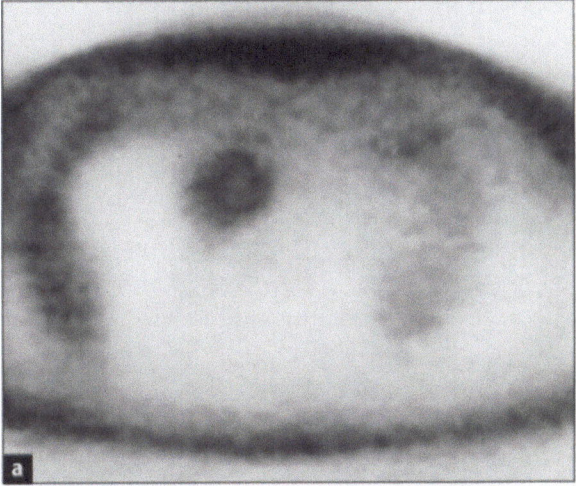

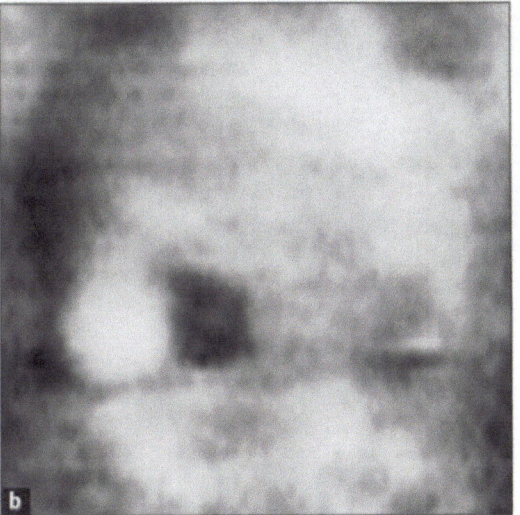

Figure 7 a, b

Patient and History: 62-year-old woman with a high grade stenosis of the proximal pancreatic duct in ERCP.

Technique: 361 MBq FDG i.v. 45 min prior to start of emission. ECAT 931 scanner. 12'/BP without attenuation correction. Iterative reconstruction.

PET Results: There is a relatively large focus of increased uptake in the pancreatic head suggestive of malignancy. The margins of the lesion show some focal bulging on the coronal view (**b**) consistent with metastases of adjacent lymph nodes.

Histology: Ampullary carcinoma, pT2pN1.

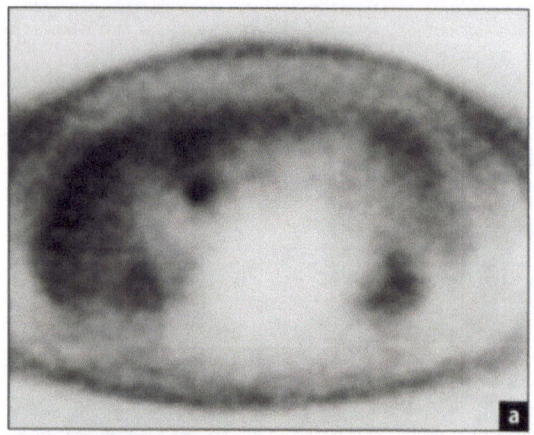

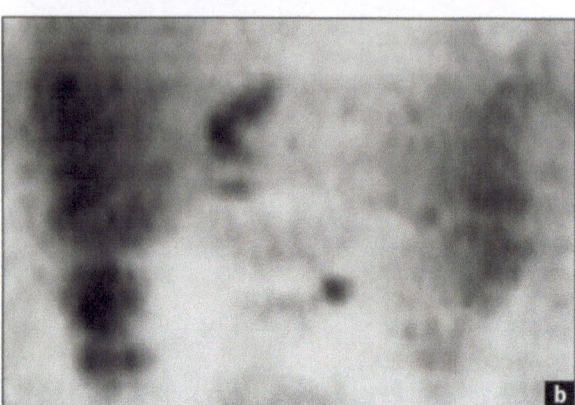

Figure 8 a, b

Patient and History: 63-year-old woman with painless jaundice.

Technique: 209 MBq FDG i.v. 45 min prior to start of emission. ECAT 931 scanner. 12'/BP without attenuation correction. Iterative reconstruction.

PET Results: Images show a small lesion with increased uptake in the pancreatic head suggestive of malignancy (**a, b**). On the coronal image, the lesion extends into the left lobe of the liver (**b**). Also, there are small focal uptakes inferior to the lesion and in the retroperitoneal area (**b**) consistent with lymph node metastases.

Histology: Bile duct carcinoma, pT3pN1.

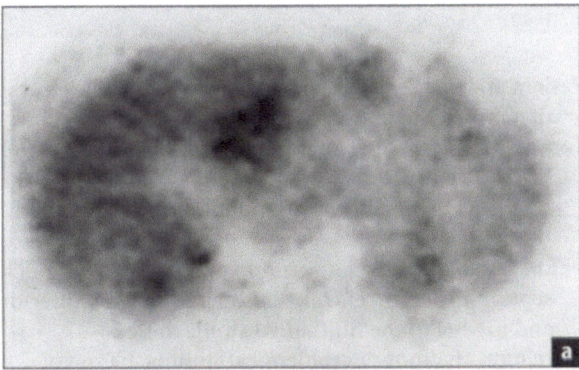

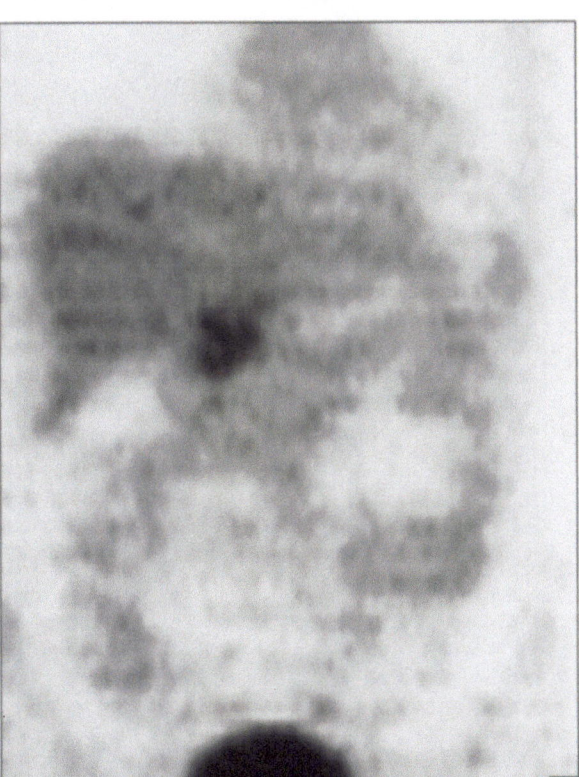

Figure 9 a, b

Patient and History: 57-year-old woman with a cystic mass in the pancreatic head in CT.

Technique: 287 MBq FDG i.v. 45 min prior to start of emission. ECAT 931 scanner. 10'/BP with attenuation correction. Iterative reconstruction.

PET Results: There is an irregularly shaped moderately increased FDG uptake in the pancreatic head (**a, b**).

Histology: Mucinous cystadenocarcinoma, pT3pN1.

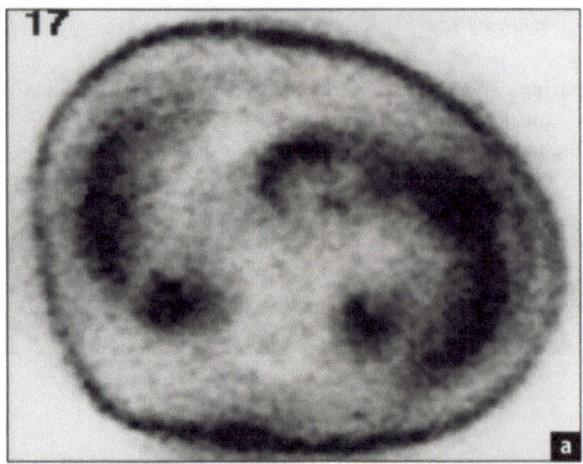

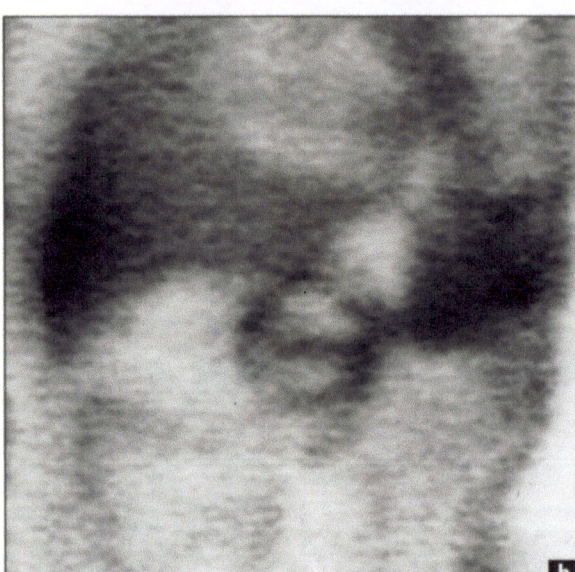

Figure 10 a, b

Patient and History: 67-year-old woman with a large cystic mass in the pancreatic body in CT.

Technique: Hydro-PET technique (see Fig. 2). 410 MBq FDG i.v. 1 h prior to start of emission. ECAT HR+ scanner. 12'/BP without attenuation correction. Iterative reconstruction.

PET Results: There is a large round cystic mass with thick septa and large central photopenic defects inferior and medial to the fluid filled stomach (**a, b**).

Histology: Mucinous cystadenocarcinoma, pT3pN0.

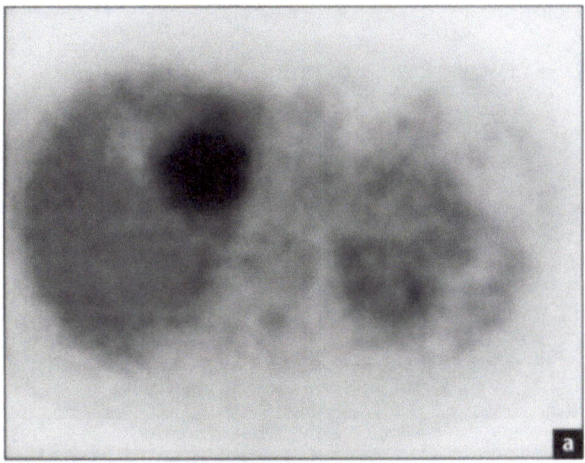

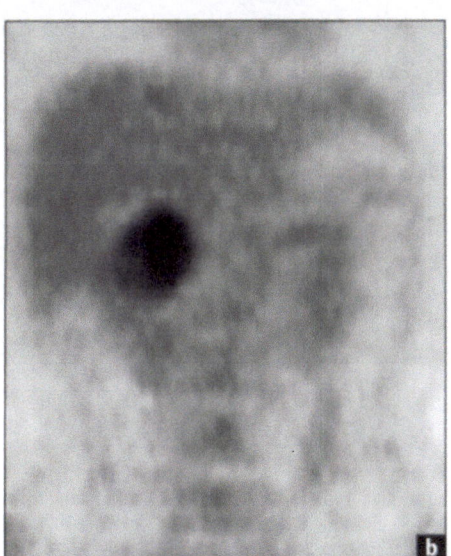

Figure 11 a, b

Patient and History: 30-year-old woman with a large round well demarcated mass in the pancreatic head in CT.

Technique: 330 MBq FDG i.v. 45 min prior to start of emission. ECAT 931 scanner. 10'/BP with attenuation correction. Iterative reconstruction.

PET Results: There is a well delineated round mass in the pancreatic head that has a highly increased FDG uptake. The SUV is 8.3.

Histology: Papillary cystic pseudotumor.

Cave! This is not a truly malignant tumor. However, this tumor has a >10% risk of becoming malignant in subsequent years.

12.3 Metastases

Metastases to the pancreas are occasionally found at surgery and are indistinguishable from pancreatic malignancies, if singular. In the liver, all untreated metastases >1 cm are usually detected with PET. About half of the metastases smaller than 1 cm that can be retrospectively identified with CT are prospectively seen with PET [3]. Lymph node metastases can be detected frequently (see Sect. 12.1); however, microscopic spread to lymph nodes is invisible. Peritoneal spread is difficult to detect if the spread is thin on the peritoneum and not well localized. PET may identify as many as 30% of patients [1] with peritoneal metastases.

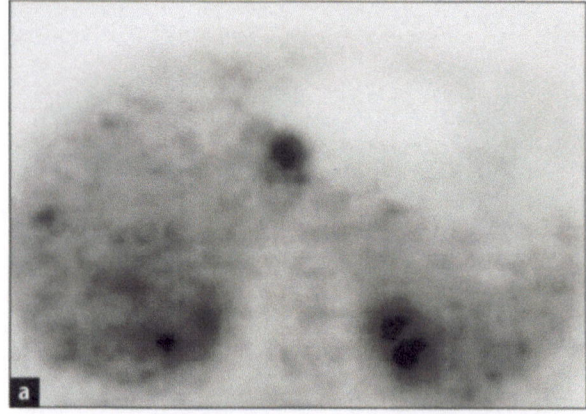

Figure 12 a, b

Patient and History: 50-year-old man with a pancreatic carcinoma and a few indeterminate 5-mm hypo-attenuating lesions in the liver.

Technique: 360 MBq FDG i.v. 45 min prior to start of emission. ECAT 931 scanner. 10'/BP with attenuation correction. Iterative reconstruction.

PET Results: There is a small round lesion in the pancreatic head that has a highly increased FDG uptake (**a**). This is the pancreatic tumor. In addition, all three hepatic lesions seen with CT (**b**) have an increased FDG uptake.

Histology: Multiple hepatic metastases.

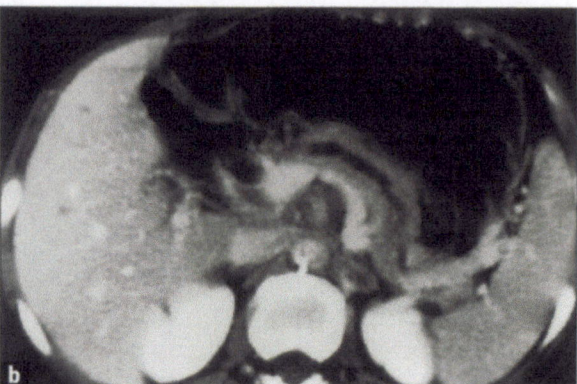

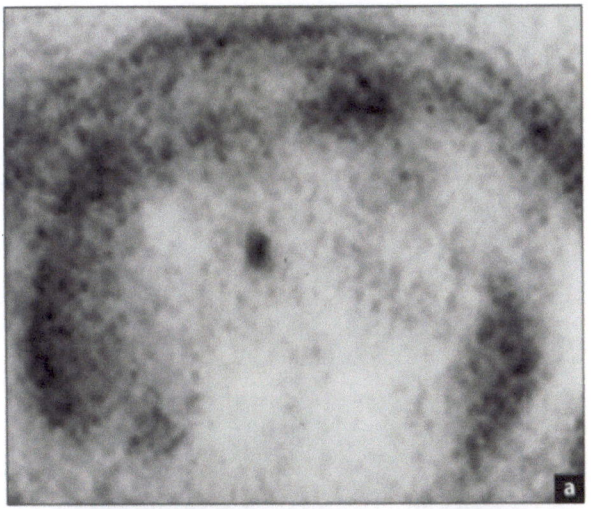

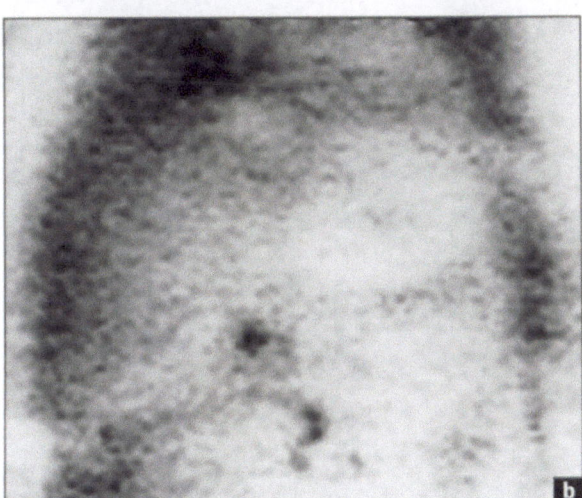

Figure 13 a, b

Patient and History: 68-year-old man with a suspicious mass in the pancreatic head. No metastases were detected with sonography, CT, MRI, endosonography, ERCP and angiography.

Technique: Hydro-PET technique (see Fig. 2). 358 MBq FDG i.v. 1 h prior to start of emission. ECAT HR+ scanner. 12'/BP without attenuation correction. Iterative reconstruction.

PET Results: There is a small lesion in the pancreatic head with focally increased FDG uptake (**a**). In addition, there are multiple small focal lesions in the abdomen indicative of peritoneal spread (**b**).

Histology: Bile duct carcinoma, pT3pN1, with peritoneal metastases.

Cave! Unspecific bowel uptake must be differentiated from peritoneal metastases. Unspecific bowel uptake usually has a longitudinal pattern while peritoneal lesions are round.

12.4 Chronic Pancreatitis

Most patients with chronic pancreatitis and mass forming pseudotumor exhibit no or only diffuse FDG uptake. This makes chronic mass forming pancreatitis distinguishable from pancreatic malignancy with an accuracy of 80–90 % [1, 2]. On the contrary, with conventional imaging, mass forming chronic pancreatitis often mimics pancreatic carcinoma, and the two conditions are indistinguishable [4].

Figure 14 a, b

Patient and History: 58-year-old man with an indeterminate mass in the pancreatic head with CT and a history of chronic pancreatitis.

Technique: Hydro-PET technique (see Fig. 2). 418 MBq FDG i.v. 1 h prior to start of emission. ECAT HR+ scanner. 12'/BP without attenuation correction. Iterative reconstruction.

PET Results: Normal abdominal study with minimal FDG uptake in the pancreatic region. No sign of acute on chronic pancreatitis or malignancy.

Histology: Chronic sklerosing pancreatitis.

Cave! The pancreas is located dorsal and inferior to the fluid filled stomach. The fluid-air interface in the stomach should always be seen with a properly performed hydro technique.

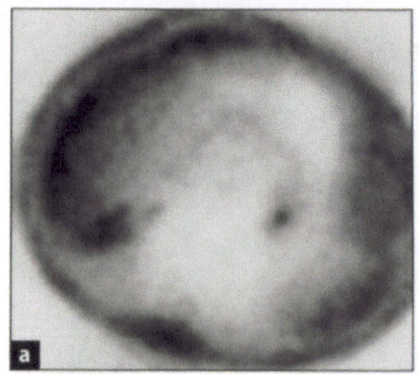

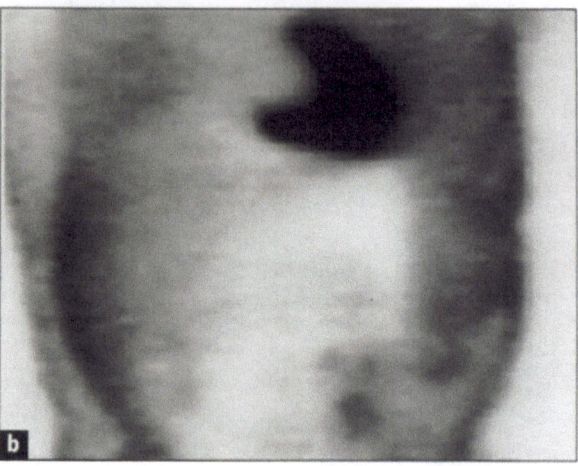

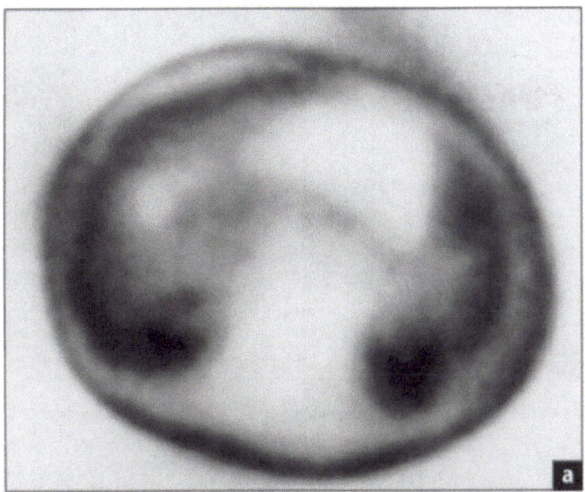

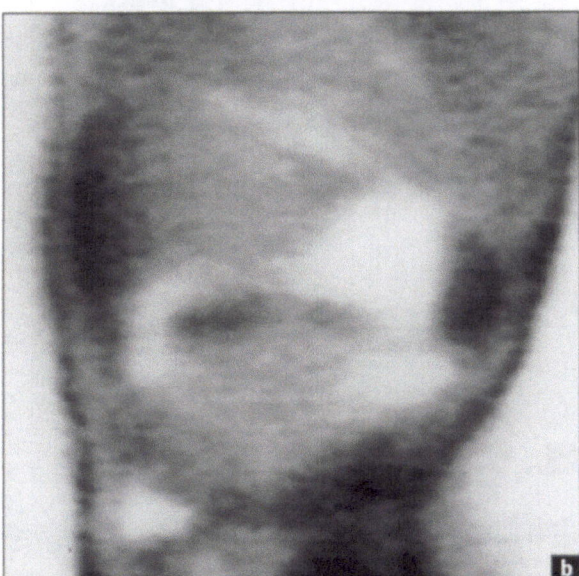

Figure 15 a, b

Patient and History: 40-year-old woman with a mass in the pancreatic head on CT and a history of chronic pancreatitis.

Technique: Hydro-PET technique (see Fig. 2). 448 MBq FDG i.v. 1 h prior to start of emission. ECAT HR+ scanner. 12'/BP without attenuation correction. Iterative reconstruction.

PET Results: The pancreas shows a diffusely slightly inhomogeneous increased FDG uptake.

Histology: Active diffuse pancreatitis.

Cave! In this example of the hydro technique, there is complete hypotony of both stomach and duodenum. This allows a clear delineation of the pancreas versus both liver and stomach.

12.5 Pitfalls

The most commonly recognized false positive findings are acute abdominal conditions including acute bouts of chronic pancreatitis [5–7]. Positive PET findings of patients that have signs of acute disease like abdominal pain, elevated WBC or C-reactive protein should therefore be interpreted with care. False positive liver findings can appear in patients that have markedly dilated bile ducts and have subsequent small cholangitic abscesses [3]. Peritoneal metastasis can be erroneously diagnosed if there is infrequent, atypically patchy, non-specific intestinal accumulation of FDG. Also of note is the possibility of mistakenly calling extrapancreatic unspecific foci. Sometimes, a collapsed stomach, a spastic transverse colon or even an abnormal and deformed right kidney may simulate pathologic uptake in the "pancreatic region." For most findings, a simultaneous reading of a CT and/or MRI is therefore mandatory.

Small size limits detection. With a full ring scanner, detectability of pancreatic metastasis in the liver decreases with lesions <1 cm [3]. The same is true for pancreatic lesions: About half of the smaller T1 and T-in-situ lesions and most of the highly differentiated tumors may be missed by FDG-PET. Also, the detection of cystic tumors, bile duct carcinomas and ampullary carcinomas is more difficult than the detection of ductal adenocarcinoma (unpublished data). Another variable to be kept in mind is plasma glucose. Plasma glucose levels at the time of FDG application is negatively correlated with the tumor SUV [8]. Care with interpretation should be taken when the scan is negative and the glucose value exeeds 130 mg/dl. As with false positive findings, misinterpretation may be a problem. A supposed "atypical" uptake in the "pancreatic region" may be mistaken to be unspecific uptake of adjacent bowel. Co-reading with existing CT and/or MRI is essential to avoid this kind of error.

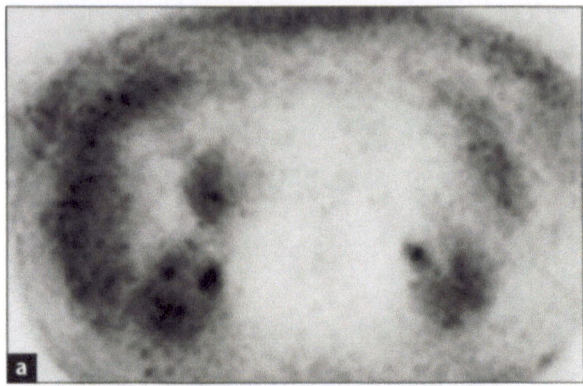

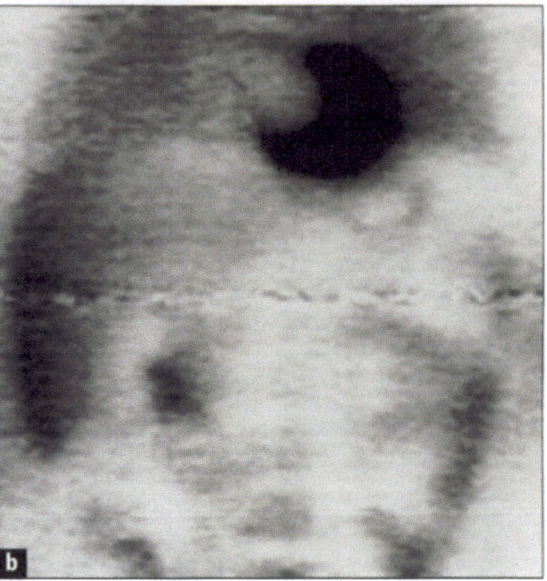

Figure 16 a, b

Patient and History: 27-year-old man with abdominal pain and a suspicious mass in the pancreatic head on CT.

Technique: Hydro-PET technique (see Fig. 2). 322 MBq FDG i.v. 1 h prior to start of emission. ECAT HR+ scanner. 12'/BP without attenuation correction. Iterative reconstruction.

PET Results: There is an intensive, diffusely increased uptake in the pancreatic head suggestive of malignancy (**a, b**). The lesion is surrounded by small adjacent separate lesions that look like lymph node metastasis. However, in the face of acute abdominal pain the differential diagnosis is acute or chronic mass forming pancreatitis with adjacent active inflammatory lymph nodes.

Histology: Acute or chronic pancreatitis.

Cave! Please note the similarity with Fig. 5. Patient history and blood chemistry values (white blood count, C-reactive protein) are useful information.

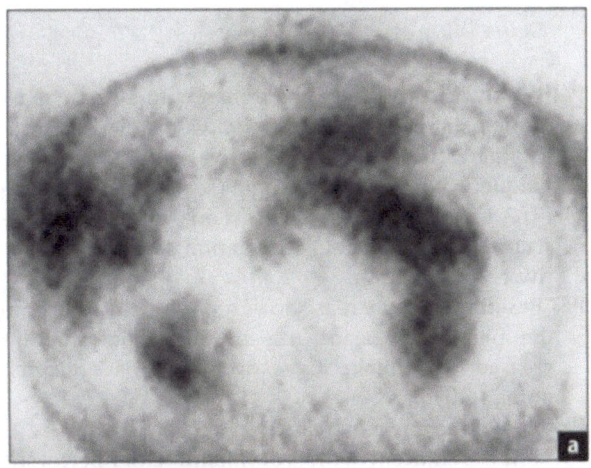

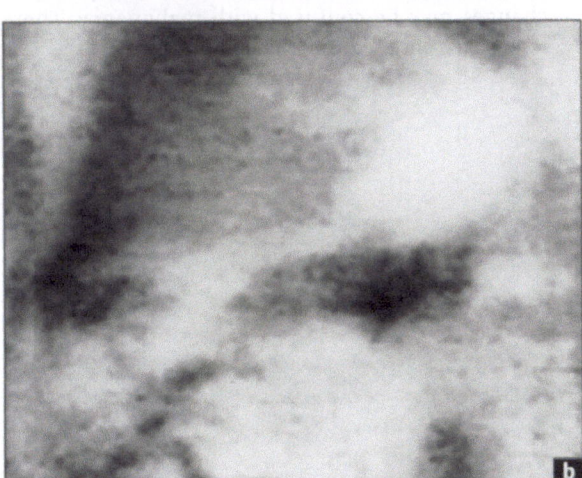

Figure 17 a, b

Patient and History: 68-year-old man with a suspicious mass in the pancreatic head on CT and a history of chronic pancreatitis.

Technique: Hydro-PET technique (see Fig. 2). 356 MBq FDG i.v. 1 h prior to start of emission. ECAT HR+ scanner. 12'/BP without attenuation correction. Iterative reconstruction.

PET Results: The pancreas shows a diffusely increased FDG uptake due to of active pancreatitis (**a, b**). A tumor is not seen.

Histology: 2-cm bile duct carcinoma and poststenotic pancreatitis.

Cave! The tumorous FDG uptake is obscured by poststenotic pancreatitis. Compare with Figs. 2 and 3.

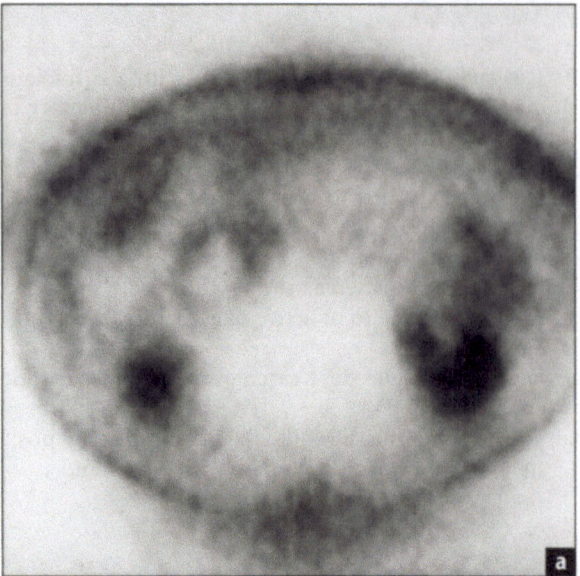

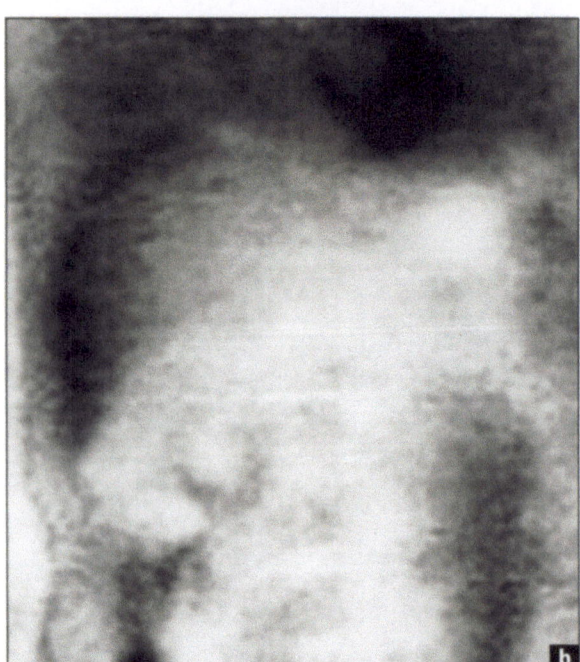

Figure 18 a, b

Patient and History: 41-year-old man with a cystic mass in the pancreatic head on CT and a history of chronic pancreatitis. Normal C-reactive protein.

Technique: Hydro-PET technique (see Fig. 2). 496 MBq FDG i.v. 1 h prior to start of emission. ECAT HR+ scanner. 12'/BP without attenuation correction. Iterative reconstruction.

PET Results: The pancreas shows a photopenic defect in the pancreatic head with irregular marginal increased FDG uptake suggestive of a cystadenocarcinoma (**a, b**).

Histology: Chronic pancreatitis with pseudocyst.

Cave! Bowel adjacent to cysts or inflammatory pericystic changes may be confused with malignancy. Therefore, scans should be co-read with CT and/or MRI.

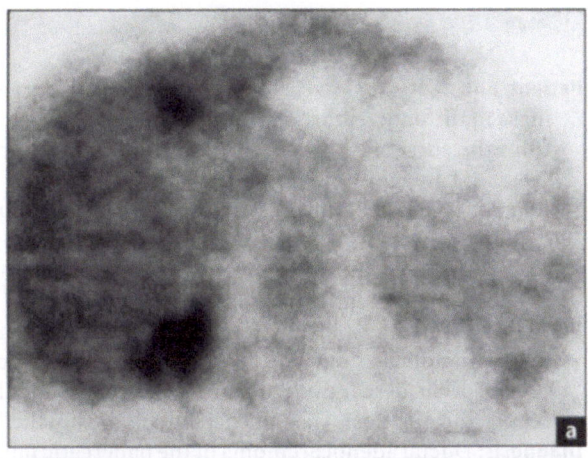

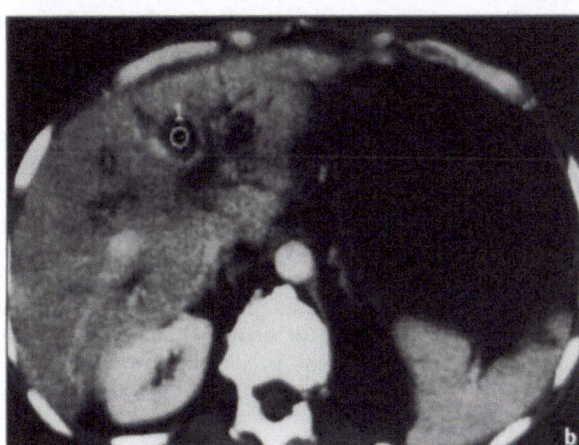

Figure 19 a, b

Patient and History: 60-year-old man with a suspicious mass in the pancreatic head and dilated intrahepatic bile ducts.

Technique: 360 MBq FDG i.v. 45 min prior to start of emission. ECAT 931 scanner. 10'/BP with attenuation correction. Iterative reconstruction.

PET Results: There is a focally increased FDG uptake in segment IV of the liver (**a**) corresponding to a hypo-attenuating mass in CT. In the presence of dilated bile ducts (see CT, **b**), this finding may be either metastasis or inflammatory granuloma.

Follow-up Diagnosis: Cholangitic granuloma. No hepatic metastases.

Cave! Without the knowledge of dilated bile ducts the PET result may be false positive.

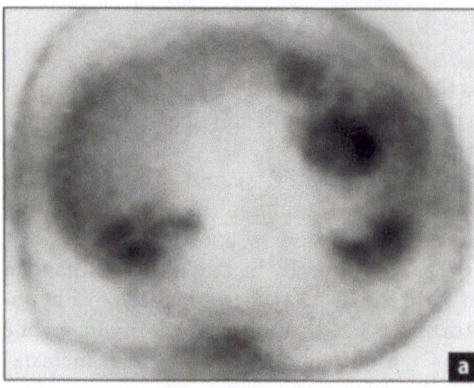

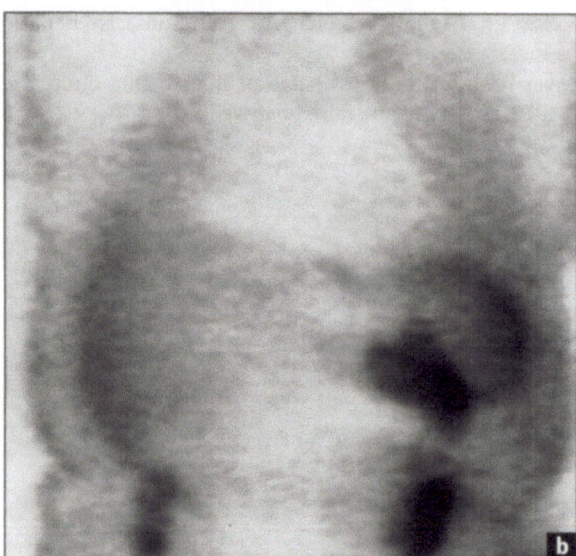

Figure 20 a, b

Patient and History: 71-year-old woman with a large mass in the pancreatic tail. However, the referral note from the surgeon was simply "suspicious pancreatic mass." CT images were not provided.

Technique: Hydro-PET technique (see Fig. 2). 507 MBq FDG i.v. 1 h prior to start of emission. ECAT HR+ scanner. 12'/BP without attenuation correction. Iterative reconstruction.

PET Results: There is a focally increased FDG uptake in the region of the pancreatic tail and also unspecific uptake of the descending colon (**a, b**). On the original report, the diagnosis was "unspecific colonic uptake."

Diagnosis: Ductal adenocarcinoma of the pancreatic tail.

Cave! Precise history and co-reading with morphologic imaging is necessary for proper interpretation of PET.

References

1. Diederichs CG, Staib L, Vogel J, Glatting G, Glasbrenner B, Brambs H-J, Beger HG, Reske SN (2000) Values and limitations of FDG-PET in pancreatic masses. Pancreas (in press)
2. Diederichs CG, Sokiranksi R, Pauls S, Schwarz M, Guhlmann C, Glatting G, Glasbrenner B, Moller P, Beger HG, Brambs H-G, Reske SN (1999) Preoperative diagnosis of pancreatic tumors: what is the role of FDG-PET following endosonography (ES), ERCP, Spiral-CT (CT), and MRI? J Nucl Med 40/5 Suppl:104P
3. Fröhlich A, Diederichs CG, Staib L, Vogel J, Beger HG, Reske SN (1999) Detection of liver metastases from pancreatic cancer using FDG-PET. J Nucl Med 40:250–255
4. Neff CC, Simeone JF, Wittenberg J, Mueller PR, Ferrucci JT Jr. (1984) Inflammatory pancreatic masses: problems in differentiating focal pancreatitis from carcinoma. Radiology 150:35–38
5. Shreve PD (1998) Focal fluorine-18 fluorodeoxyglucose accumulation in inflammatory pancreatic disease. Eur J Nucl Med 25:259–264
6. Zimny M, Buell U, Diederichs CG, Reske SN (1998) False-positive FDG-PET in patients with pancreatic masses: an issue of proper patient selection? Eur J Nucl Med 25:1352
7. Diederichs CG, Staib L, Glasbrenner B, Guhlmann A, Glatting G, Pauls S, Beger HG, Reske SN (1999) F-18 fluorodeoxyglucose (FDG) and C-reactive protein (CRP). Clin Pos Imaging Vol. 2(3): 131–136
8. Diederichs CG, Staib L, Glatting G, Beger HG, Reske SN (1998) FDG-PET: elevated plasma glucose reduces both uptake and detection rate of pancreatic malignancies. J Nucl Med 39:1030–1033

Brain Tumors

13.1 PET Imaging Protocol Used in This Chapter

- PET scanner:
  GE Advance (Milwaukee, WI, USA)
- Patient preparation:
  Patient fasts for 4–6 h prior to the study.
- Radiopharmaceutical:
  F-18 Fluorodeoxyglucose (FDG), 10 mCi (adult dose), intravenously.
- Uptake phase:
  The patient remains in a quiet, dimly lit room for 30 min following injection of FDG and prior to imaging.
- Image acquisition:
  1. Positioning: 2D emission scan (1–2 min) for the purpose of localization.
  2. Imaging: 3D emission scan (approximately 6 min), single bed position.
- Image reconstruction:
  1. 3D filtered backprojection
     Transaxial filter: Hanning, 4.5 mm cutoff
     Axial filter: ramp, 8.5 mm cutoff
     25.6-mm field-of-view, 128 × 128-pixel matrix
     4.25-mm transaxial slice thickness
  2. Calculated attenuation-correction applied
  3. Co-registration with MRI using surface fit technique (Pelizzari et al. 1989)
- Image display:
  Software allows the axial MRI images to be displayed along with the co-registered PET images. Interactive features include:
  1. Ability to rapidly alternate between the co-registered images, or to fade from one modality to the other along a continuum.
  2. Reconstruction in axial, coronal, or sagittal planes, and
  3. Adjustment of image grayscale.

13.2 Primary Tumor: High Grade

The majority of primary intracranial tumors are glial in origin. The most common glial tumors are astrocytic tumors, which include low grade astrocytoma, anaplastic astrocytoma, and glioblastoma multiforme. The latter two forms are aggressive, high-grade tumors. FDG PET has a well-established role for distinguishing low grade from high grade tumors, and there appears to be a relationship between the degree of FDG uptake and prognosis in these patients (Alavi et al. 1988). Furthermore, these tumors are often heterogeneous, and PET can identify focal regions within the tumor which likely contain high grade elements. Finally, FDG PET can be used to follow patients for evidence of recurrence following therapy (Barker et al. 1997).

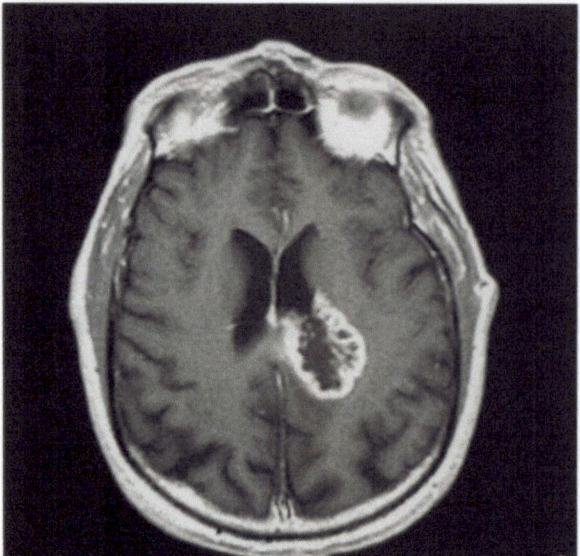

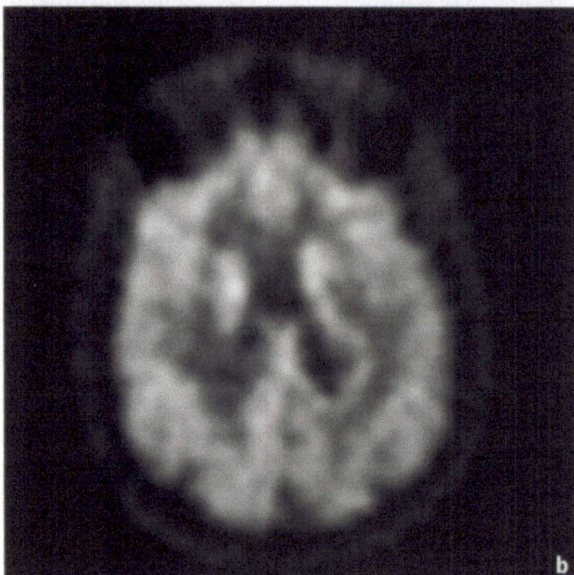

Figure 1 a, b

Patient and History: 76-year-old male with 2-week history of gait difficulties and dragging of his right lower extremity.

PET Results: Contrast-enhanced T1-weighted MRI (**a**) demonstrates enhancing mass in the left parietal lobe. Co-registered PET image (**b**) reveals corresponding rim-like hypermetabolic activity, equal or exceeding that of gray matter, consistent with high-grade tumor.

Histology: Stereotactic biopsy diagnostic of glioblastoma multiforme.

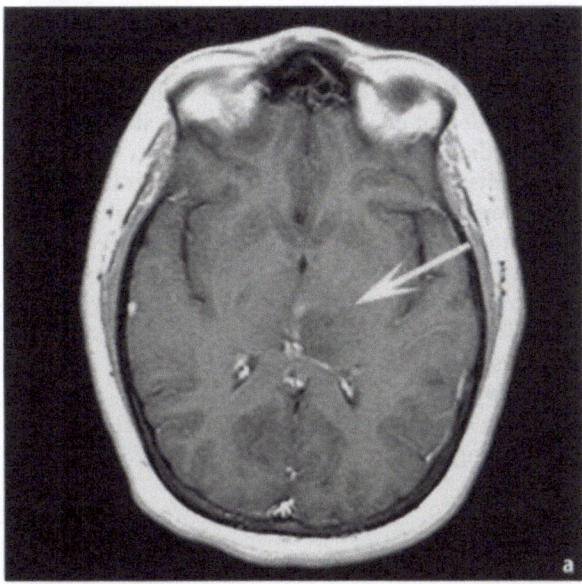

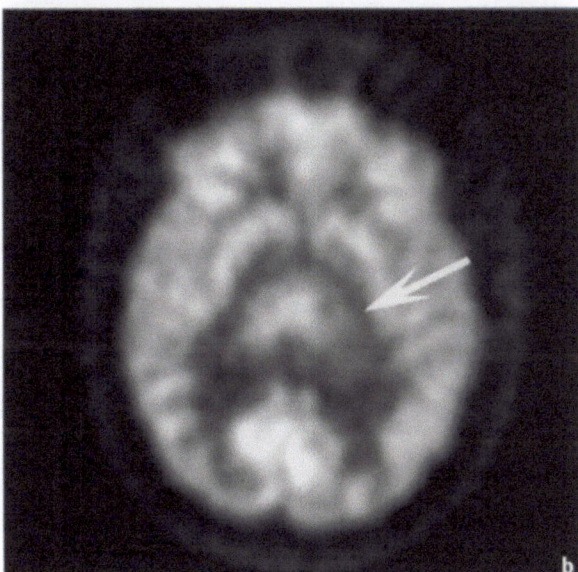

Figure 2 a, b

Patient and History: 33-year-old female with no neurological symptoms and a 5-year history of thyroid disease. She had an MRI to evaluate her pituitary and was found to have a thalamic lesion.

PET Results: MRI demonstrated abnormal T2 signal in the left thalamus (T2-weighted images not shown) with low signal and only minimal, wispy enhancement on post-gadolinium T1-weighted images (**a**). Co-registered FDG image (**b**) shows corresponding FDG accumulation within the thalamic abnormality (*arrow*) which is similar to that of the normal contralateral thalamus, suggesting a high-grade tumor.

Histology: Stereotactic biopsy revealed anaplastic astrocytoma.

Cave! In evaluating lesions within white matter structures, such as basal ganglia or thalamus, FDG accumulation equaling that of the normal structure represents hypermetabolic activity, and suggests high-grade tumor.

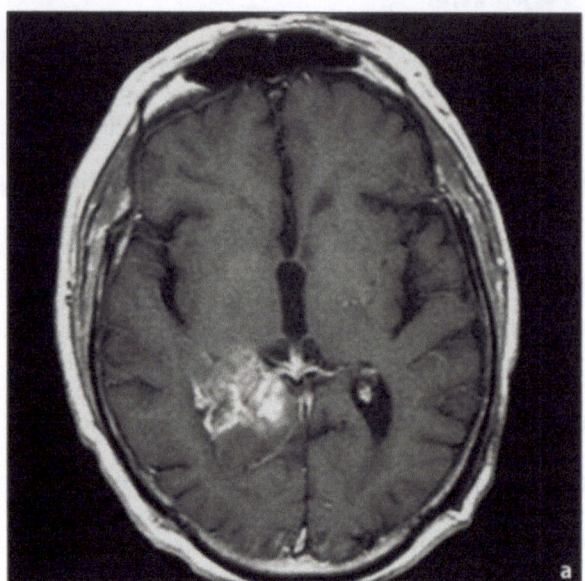

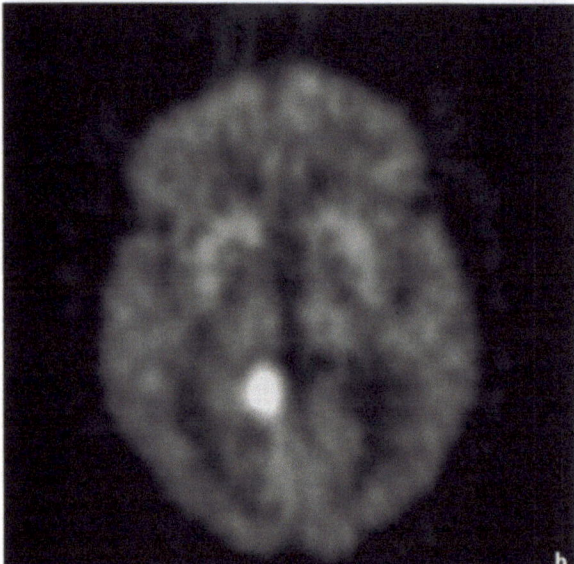

Figure 3 a, b

Patient and History: 65-year-old male who presents for evaluation of anaplastic astrocytoma after undergoing radiation therapy.

PET Results: T1-weighted MRI (**a**) demonstrates heterogeneously enhancing lesion in the posteromedial right temporal lobe. Co-registered PET image (**b**) reveals focal intense hypermetabolic activity (much greater than normal cortical gray matter) within the medial aspect of the enhancing mass, consistent with persistent high-grade tumor following radiation therapy.

Histology: Residual high-grade anaplastic astrocytoma following therapy.

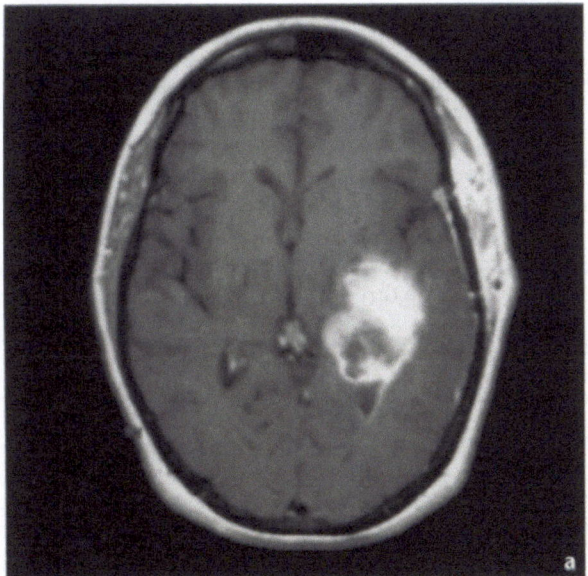

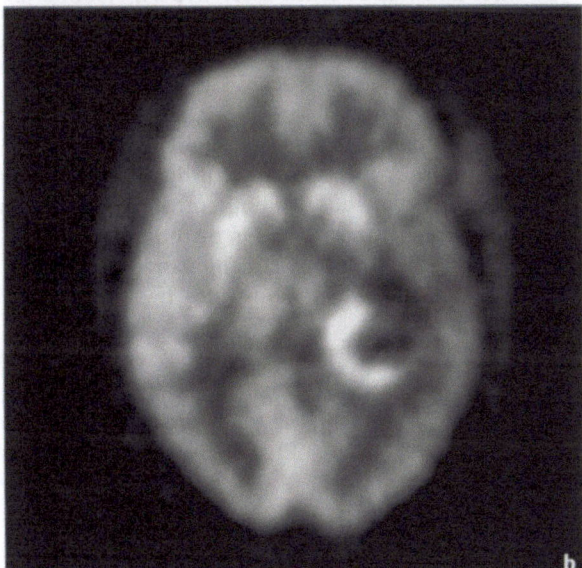

Figure 4a, b

Patient and History: 47-year-old female with left temporal lobe tumor. A subtotal resection was done 1 month prior to obtaining these images.

PET Results: Contrast-enhanced T1-weighted MRI (**a**) and co-registered PET image (**b**) reveal a surgical defect in the left temporal lobe with adjacent intense hypermetabolic activity, greater than normal gray matter, along the medial aspect of the surgical site, compatible with residual high grade tumor.

Histology: Surgical pathology at resection was diagnostic for glioblastoma multiforme. Following these imaging studies, the patient received external radiation therapy, but continued progression was noted on MRI 2 months later. She then underwent 11 cycles of chemotherapy, but MRI continues to show progressive disease 6 months following resection.

Cave! Postoperative changes do not influence the evaluation of the surgical resection bed.

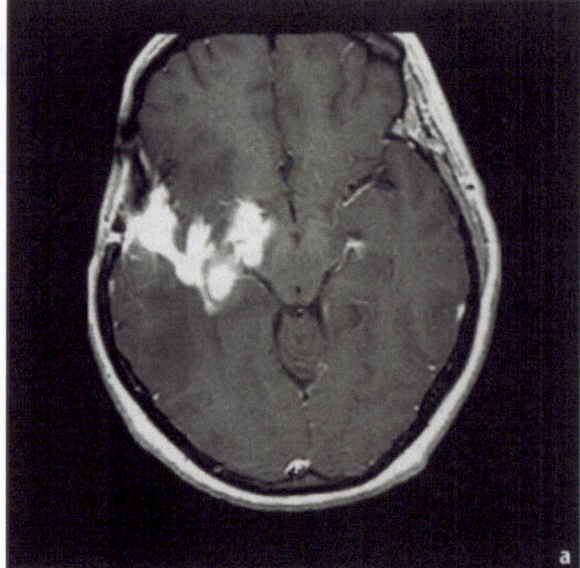

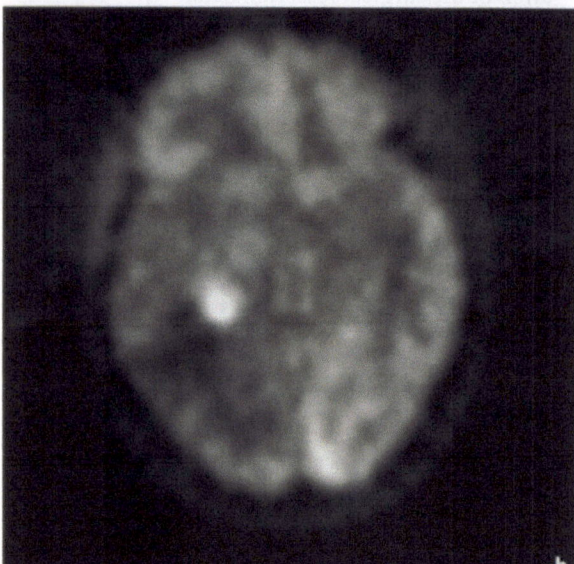

Figure 5 a, b

Patient and History: 44-year-old female diagnosed with right temporal lobe glioblastoma multiforme 13 months ago. Treatment has included surgical resection followed by radiation therapy. Subsequently, patient had re-resection and high dose therapy using radiolabeled (I-131) monoclonal antibodies injected into the surgical resection cavity. More recently, she has undergone three cycles of BCNU/CPT-11 chemotherapy.

PET Results: Surgical resection cavity is demonstrated on contrast-enhanced T1-weighted MRI study (**a**) in the right temporal lobe. There is a rim of gadolinium enhancement surrounding the surgical resection cavity on the MR scan, with corresponding FDG uptake (**b**). This has been largely stable, and felt to represent radiation necrosis. However, a focus of nodular enhancement is also noted which has increased in size on MRI and has become more hypermetabolic on PET study over 6 weeks. This site was suspected for focal tumor recurrence, and was biopsied stereotactically.

Histology: Prominent reactive gliosis and necrosis. No evidence of malignancy or granulomatous infection, and no microorganisms were identified.

Cave! Following high dose radiotherapy, radiation necrosis and recurrent tumor can be indistinguishable on MRI and FDG PET. MRI demonstrates enhancement and FDG PET demonstrates hypermetabolic activity.

13.3 Primary Tumor: Low Grade

Primary low-grade glial tumors include juvenile pilo-cytic astrocytoma, oligodendroglioma, and low-grade astrocytoma. These tumors generally demonstrate hypometabolic activity relative to normal brain. In low grade astrocytomas, the appearance of hypermetabolic activity portends more malignant transformation and poorer prognosis (DeWitte et al. 1996). In other low-grade tumors, particularly pilocytic astrocytoma, hypermetabolic activity can be observed in the absence of aggressive behavior, and the significance of this finding has yet to be established.

Figure 6 a, b

Patient and History: 43-year-old male presented with progressive headaches.

PET Results: A mass in the left posterior frontal lobe has low signal on T1-weighted images, and only mild contrast enhancement (**a**). Co-registered PET image (**b**) demonstrates hypometabolism within this mass, similar to adjacent white matter, that is compatible with a low-grade tumor.

Histology: Stereotactic biopsy revealed well-differentiated astrocytoma.

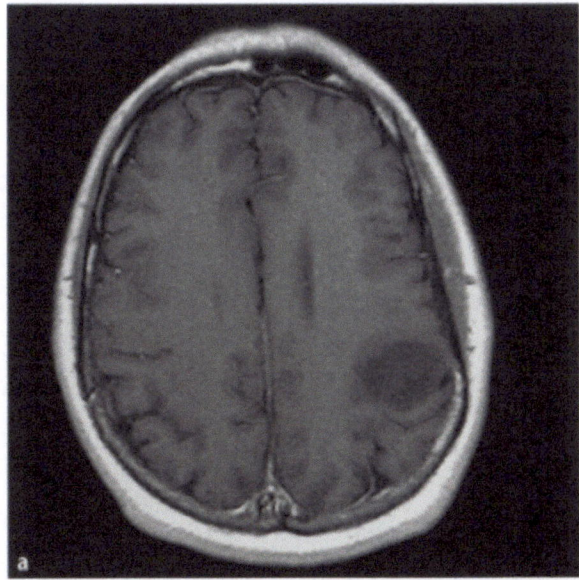

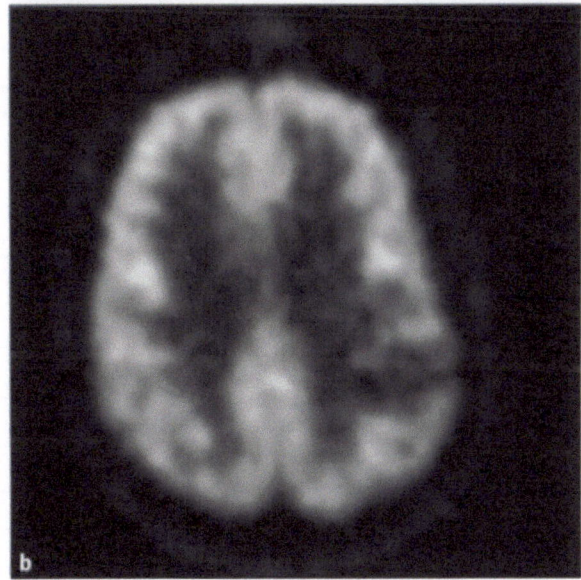

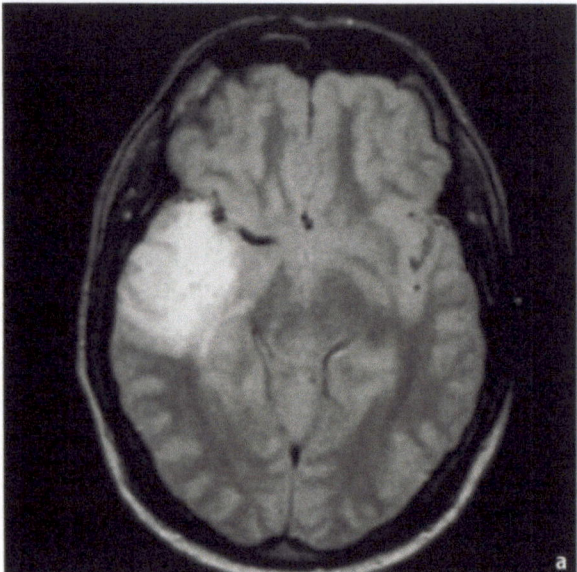

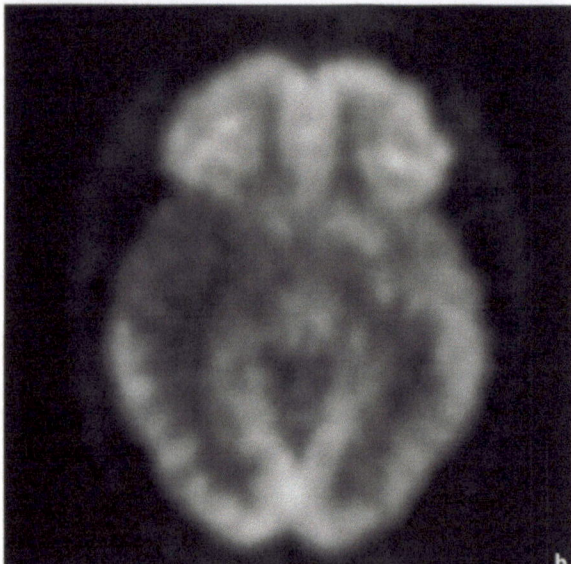

Figure 7 a, b

Patient and History: 28-year-old male with head injury 9 months ago. CT was done to evaluate this injury, and right temporal lobe lesion was discovered. Subsequently, the patient has had several seizures.

PET Results: Proton-density-weighted MR images (**a**) demonstrates a high-signal abnormality in the right temporal lobe, consistent with an infiltrating tumor. The co-registered PET image (**b**) reveals corresponding abnormality which is intermediate between white matter and gray matter, but closer to white matter, suggesting low-grade neoplasm.

Histology: This mass was surgically resected, with pathologic diagnosis of well-differentiated oligodendroglioma.

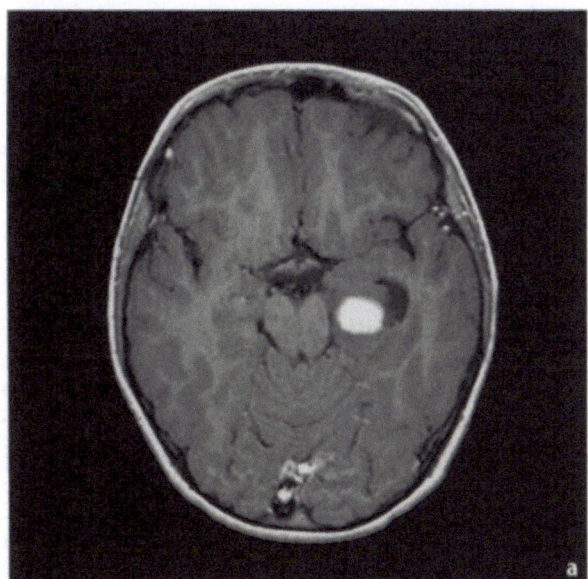

Figure 8 a, b

Patient and History: 9-year-old male presented with several episodes of staring spells followed by aphasia lasting about 1 min.

PET Results: T1-weighted MRI reveals a well-circumscribed left mesiotemporal lesion which densely and homogeneously enhances following gadolinium administration (**a**). The mass measures approximately 1.7 × 1.8 × 1.7 cm and primarily involves the left parahippocampal gyrus. Co-registered FDG PET images (**b**) demonstrate metabolic activity within the enhancing lesion to be intermediate between white and gray matter, but closer to that of white matter, suggesting a low-grade neoplasm.

Histology: Surgical resection was performed, revealing pilocytic astrocytoma, WHO grade I.

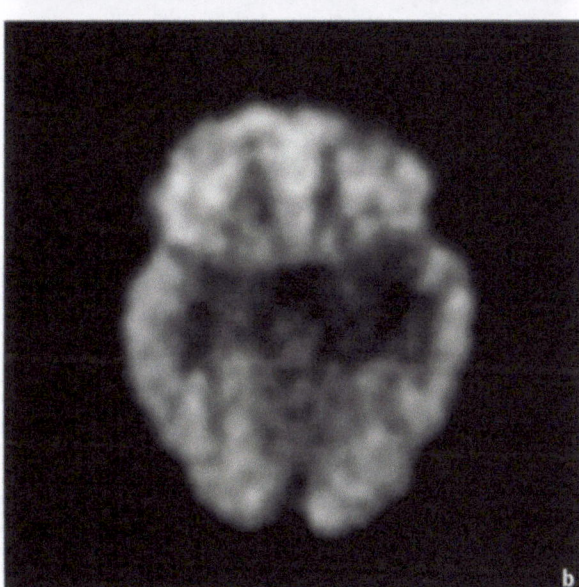

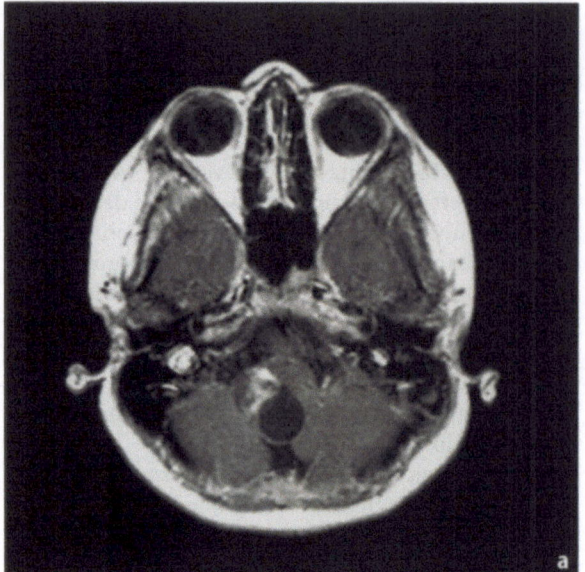

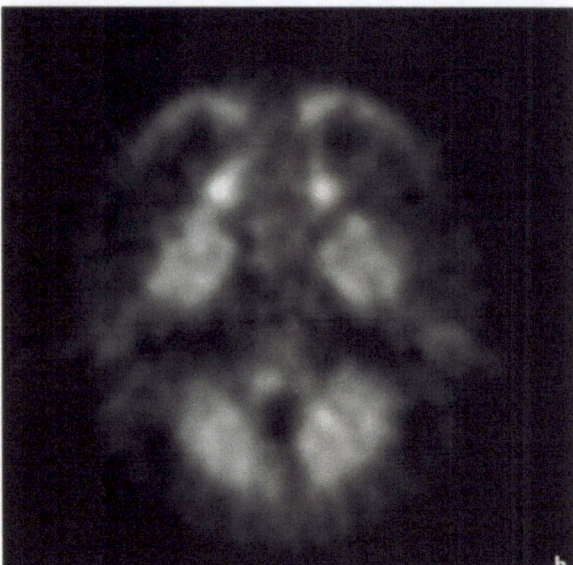

Figure 9 a, b

Patient and History: 12-year-old female with history of juvenile pilocytic astrocytoma.

PET Results: T1-weighted MR image (**a**) demonstrates a mass in the right medulla with a large cystic component and a peripheral enhancing nodule. Co-registered PET image (**b**) shows hypermetabolic activity (closer to gray matter) corresponding to nodular enhancing focus.

Histology: Juvenile pilocytic astrocytoma.

Cave! Juvenile pilocytic astrocytomas may demonstrate hypermetabolic features, even though they tend to be sharply delineated, resectable, and carry a favorable prognosis. One explanation is that, unlike malignant gliomas, these tumors contain a high number of fenestrated epithelial cells, which may be hyperplastic and thus preferentially accumulate FDG (Roelcke et al. 1998).

13.4 Primary Tumor: Others

Non-glial primary tumors of the brain are relatively un-common. As with most glial tumors, high-grade tumors would be expected to exhibit avid FDG accumulation. However, the PET appearance of these tumors is less well characterized.

Figure 10 a, b

Patient and History: 36-year-old male with HIV infection. The patient had a recent history of aseptic meningitis, presenting with headache, vomiting, photophobia, and neck stiffness.

PET Results: T1-weighted MR image following gadolinium administration (**a**) demonstrates multiple ring-enhancing lesions within the cerebellum, suggesting either infection (e.g., toxoplasmosis) or neoplasm (e.g., lymphoma). The co-registered PET image (**b**) shows hypermetabolic activity within these lesions exceeding that of normal gray matter, and is consistent with CNS lymphoma.

Histology: Biopsy was performed, revealing large B-cell lymphoma, with positive staining for EBV-associated antigens EBNA-2 and LMP-1.

Cave! CNS lymphoma demonstrates high metabolic activity compared with inflammatory lesions, and this distinction can be particularly helpful in evaluating immunocompromised patients who present with multiple intracranial lesions.

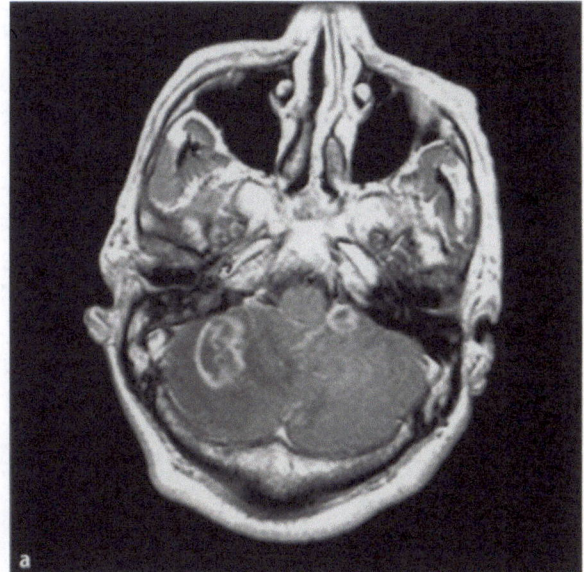

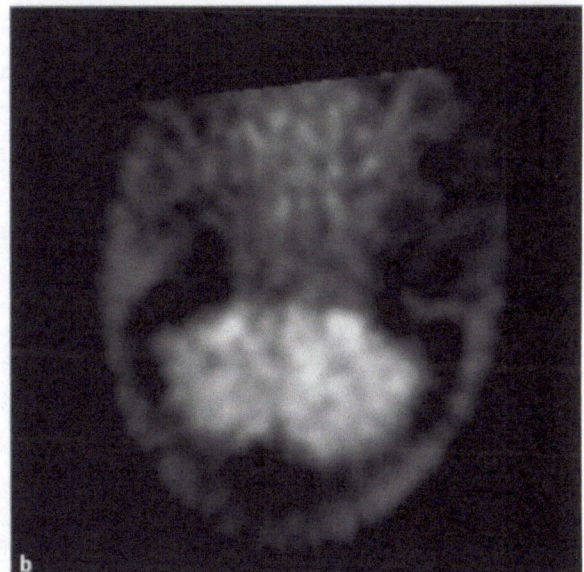

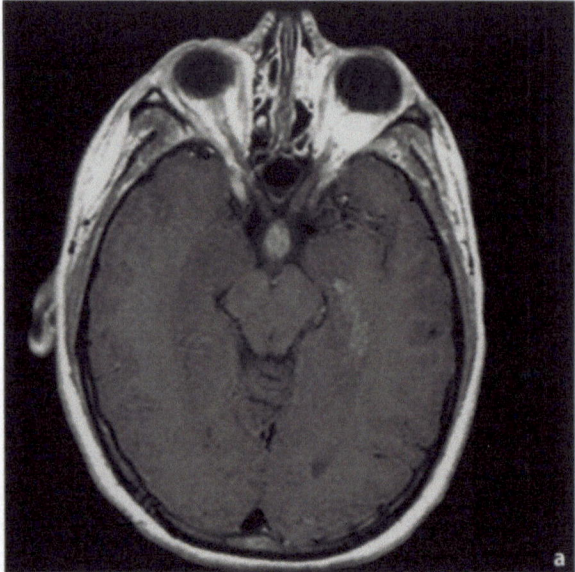

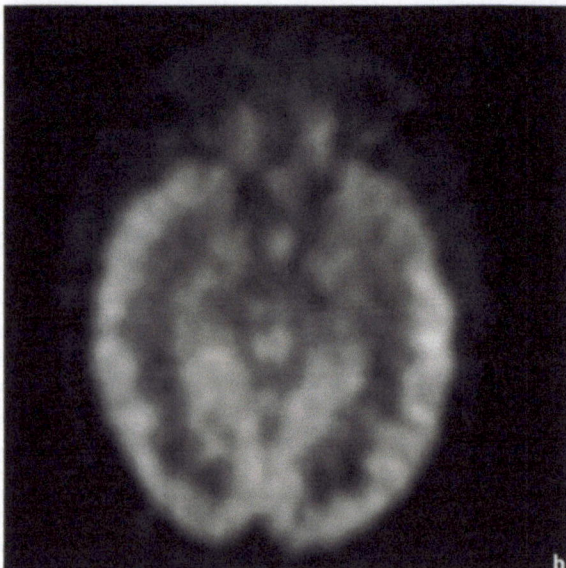

Figure 11 a, b

Patient and History: 28-year-old male admitted following a motor vehicle accident. He was noted to produce 6 l urine over 24 h, with an increase in serum sodium to 150 mmol/l (normal 135–145 mmol/l). Patient had symptoms of panhypopituitarism over several months, including erectile dysfunction, cold intolerance, and tachycardia.

PET Results: Enhancing mass involving the infundibulum is identified on postcontrast T1-weighted MRI (**a**). Diagnostic considerations for an infundibular stalk mass include neurosarcoid, germinoma, and metastatic disease. Co-registered PET image (**b**) reveals corresponding hypermetabolic activity, similar to that of cortical gray matter.

Histology: Microscopic examination of the surgical specimen revealed lymphocytes and sheets of large anaplastic cells having prominent nucleoli. Pathologic diagnosis was germinoma.

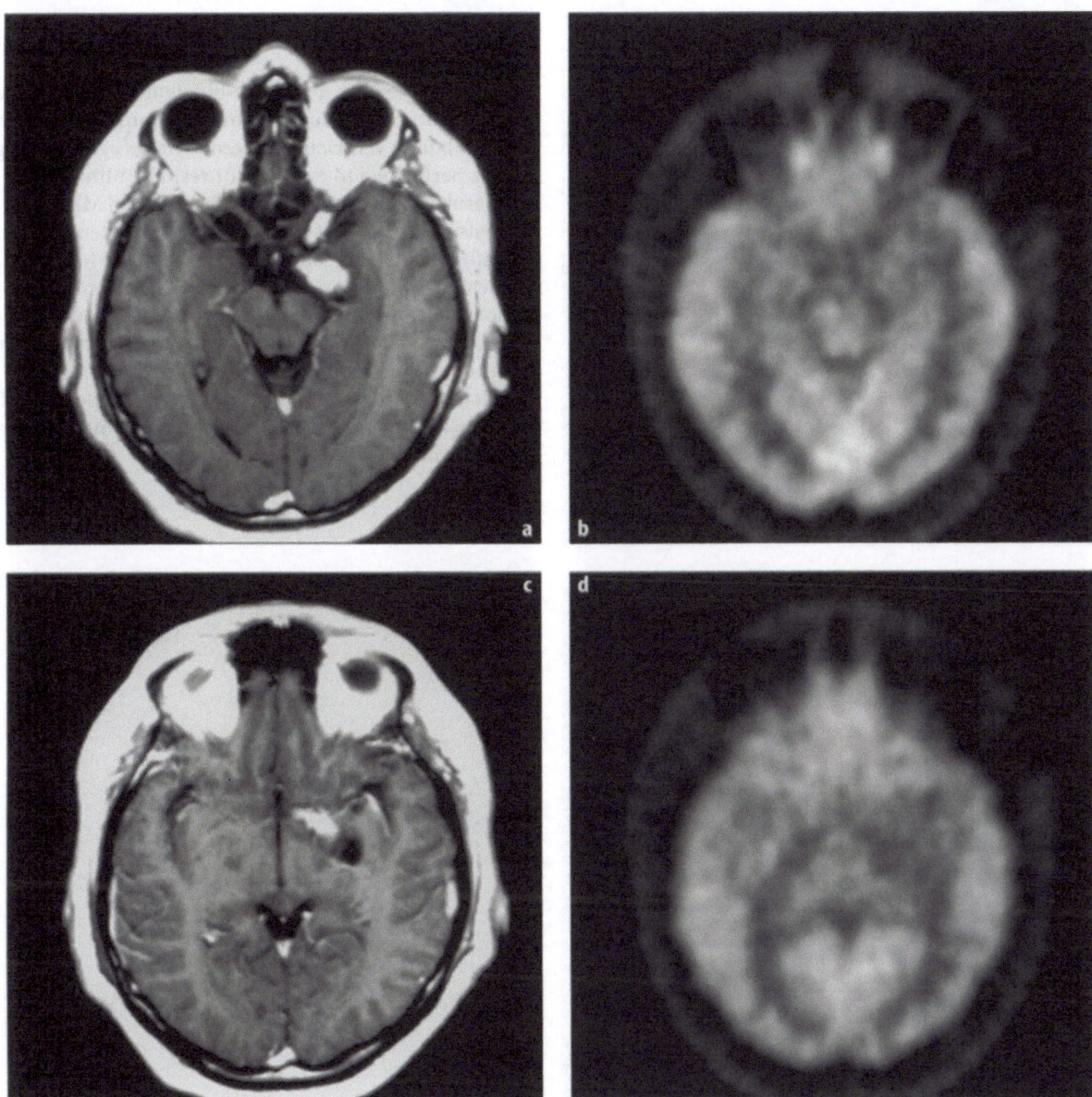

Figure 12 a–c

Patient and History: 46-year-old male with a 14-year history of seizures. Currently, seizures involve staring, aphasia, tinnitus, and head movement to the right.

PET Results: T1-weighted MRI (**a, c**) demonstrates a densely enhancing 1.9×1.3-cm mass involving the hippocampal head, posterior amygdala, and para-hippocampal gyrus in the left temporal lobe. Co-registered PET images (**b, d**) demonstrate corresponding hypermetabolic activity, intermediate between white and gray matter, and suggestive of a high grade glioma or pilocytic astrocytoma. The appearance is also not typical for a seizure focus.

Histology: Ganglioglioma, WHO grade I.

Cave! It has been previously suggested that gangliogliomas are hypometabolic (Kincaid et al. 1998). However, in a series of six patients with gangliogliomas at our institution (Provenzale et al. 1999), all gangliogliomas were found to have regions of hypermetabolic activity when evaluated using co-registered PET and MR images. The image co-registration allowed the hypermetabolic activity within the tumor to be accurately distinguished from what otherwise might be presumed to be adjacent normal gray matter. More studies with co-registered images need to be done to further characterize the metabolic patterns of these tumors.

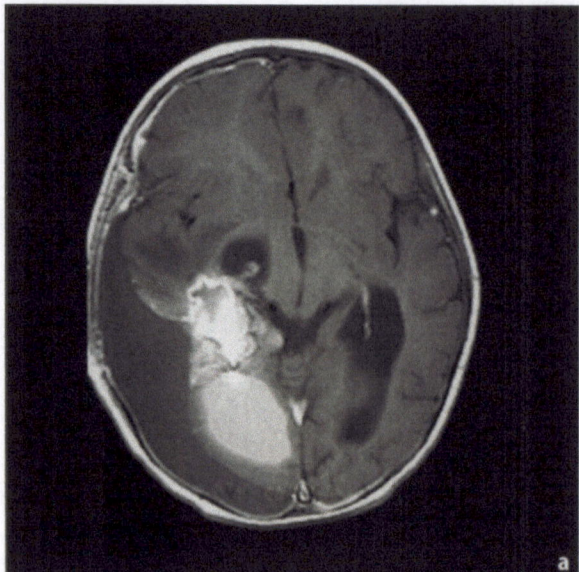

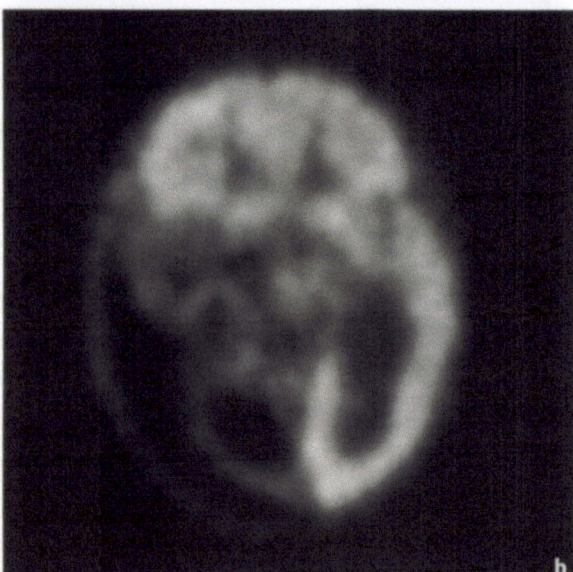

Figure 13 a, b

Patient and History: 15-month-old female who had a large choroid plexus carcinoma removed from the right lateral ventricular system 5 weeks ago. Imaging was performed to evaluate for residual tumor.

PET Results: Contrast-enhanced T1-weighted MRI (**a**) reveals postsurgical changes in the right hemisphere, with residual ring enhancement adjacent to the surgical resection site. Co-registered PET (**b**) reveals associated intermediate metabolic activity approaching that of normal gray matter. This is compatible with residual tumor.

Histology: Additional surgical resection was performed prior to chemotherapy. Pathology confirmed residual choroid plexus carcinoma.

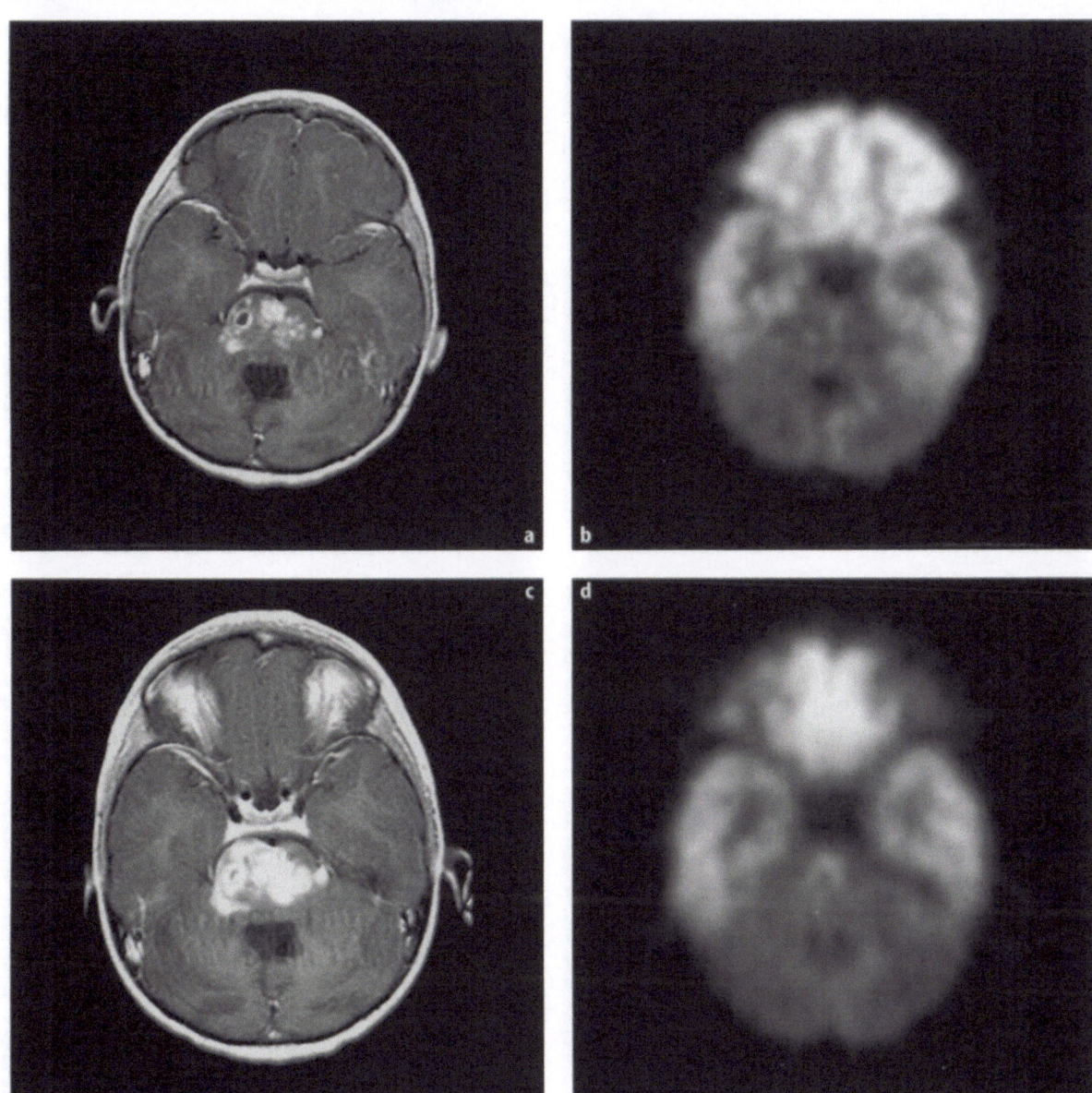

Figure 14 a–d

Patient and History: 8-year-old male initially presented with posterior fossa tumor at age 2, and underwent multiple resections. Treatments have included chemoradiation therapy and bone marrow transplantation. He now presents with progressive symptoms of dysarthria, gait ataxia, and diplopia.

PET Results: Contrast-enhanced T1-weighted MRI (**a, c**) demonstrates enhancing brainstem tumor involving the pons, midbrain, and medulla. Co-registered PET images (**b, d**) demonstrate heterogeneous FDG accumulation within the region of enhancement, with focal areas of hypermetabolic activity approaching that of normal gray matter. This suggests persistent or recurrent neoplasm, with focal areas of high grade tumor.

Histology: Malignant embryonal neoplasm. Previous pathology had revealed this tumor to have neuroblastic differentiation without evidence for glial or ependymal differentiation. Retromastoid craniectomy following these studies revealed recurrent tumor.

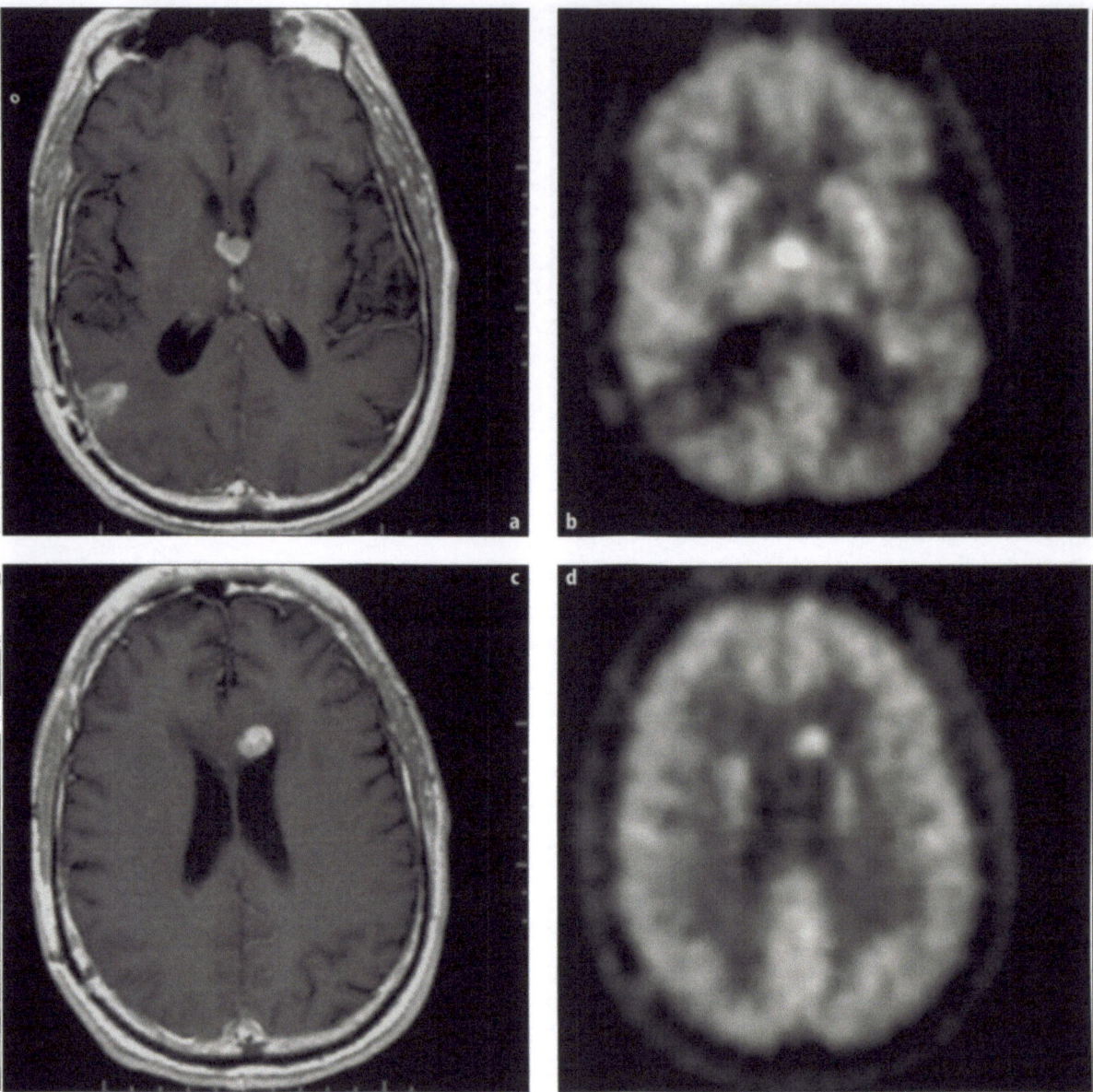

13.5 Intracranial Metastases

Figure 15 a–d

Brain metastases are frequently small in size and may range from hypermetabolic or hypometabolic in relative FDG uptake. For these reasons, the sensitivity for PET is relatively low (68 % in a study by Griffeth et al. 1993). Another study (Palm et al. 1999) reported a higher sensitivity for detecting brain metastases from lung cancer (82 %), but at the expense of low specificity (38 %). In a series of 273 patients with suspected malignancy, cerebral metastases were found in 1.5 %, and first diagnosed by PET in only 0.7 % of cases (Larcos and Maisey 1996). Contrast-enhanced MRI remains the most sensitive technique for detecting intracranial metastases.

Patient and History: 54-year-old male diagnosed with melanoma, unknown primary site, now presenting with gait disturbance, feeling off balance, and drifting while walking. At an outside hospital, a brain lesion was noted on MRI and a lesion in the right parietal lobe was resected. More recent MRI showed progression, and he was referred for consideration of further therapy.

PET Results: Contrast-enhanced T1-weighted MRI images (**a, c**) demonstrate that a new enhancing left parieto-occipital lesion has appeared, and other smaller lesions in the corpus callosum and third ventricle have progressed. Co-registered PET images (**b , d**) demon-

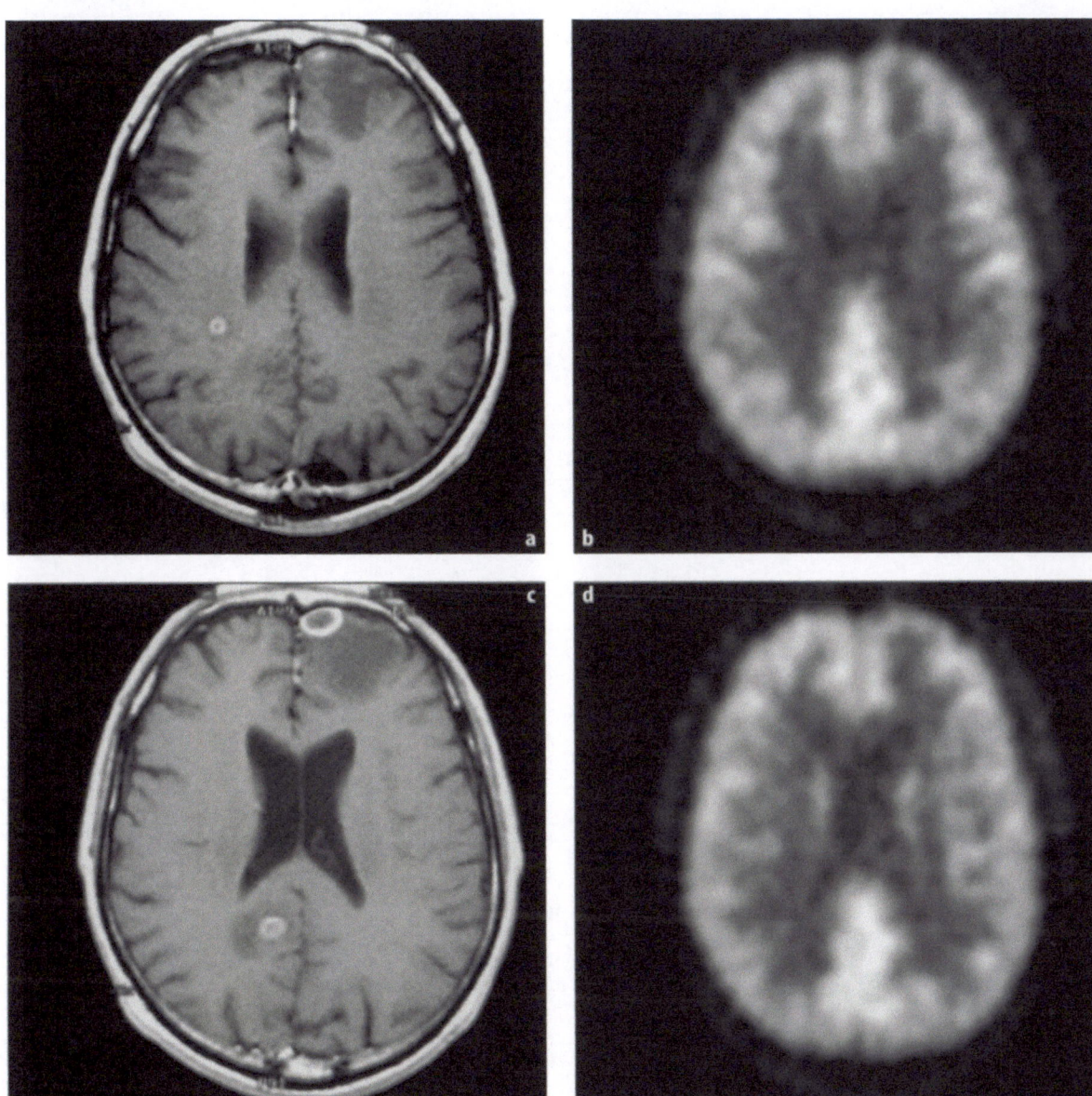

Figure 16 a–c

strate corresponding intense hypermetabolism (greater than gray matter) in these lesions, consistent with aggressive metastatic disease. There appears to be less hypermetabolism associated with the previously resected right parieto-occipital lesion.

Histology: Metastatic melanoma.

Cave! Whole-body PET imaging is proving to be valuable for the evaluation of primary and metastatic melanoma, which typically demonstrates intense FDG accumulation.

Patient and History: 61-year-old male diagnosed with stage IIIA non-small cell lung cancer 1 year ago, which presented as a 3×3×2-cm mass in the right upper lobe on CT with possible mediastinal adenopathy. At the time of diagnosis, head CT and bone scans were negative. More recently, MRI showed multiple enhancing lesions consistent with metastatic disease.

PET Results: Multiple enhancing nodules with surrounding edema typical of metastases are identified on T1-weighted MR images (**a, c**). Co-registered PET images demonstrate no corresponding focal hypometabolic or hypermetabolic activity.

Histology: Brain metastases from lung carcinoma (biopsy not performed).

Cave! This case demonstrates how inconspicuous intracranial metastases can be on PET scan alone.

References

Alavi et al. (1988) Cancer 62:1074
Barker et al. (1997) Cancer 79:115
DeWitte et al. (1996) Neurosurgery 39:470
Griffeth et al. (1993) Radiology 186:37
Palm et al. (1999) Med Klin 94:224
Kincaid et al. (1998) AJNR 19:801
Larcos and Maisey (1996) Nucl Med Commun 17:197
Pelizzari et al. (1989) J Comput Assist Tomogr 13:20
Provenzale et al. (1999) AJR 172:1103
Roelcke U et al. (1998) J Neuro Oncol 36:279–283

Chapter 14

Gynecological Tumors (Except Breast Cancer)

H. Bender and H. Palmedo

Ovarian cancer is the fourth most frequent cause of cancer death in women and the leading cause of gynecological cancer deaths. More women die of ovarian cancer than from cervical and endometrial carcinoma combined. Roughly 20,000 new ovarian cancer cases are diagnosed every year in the United States and 12,000 women will die. Approximately 1 woman in 70 will develop the disease and about 1 % of all female deaths are due to ovarian cancer. A steady increase in age-adjusted ovarian cancer death rates has been observed over the last 4 decades.

Histologically, epithelial carcinoma accounts for 80–90 % of ovarian malignancies. Epithelial tumors disseminate primarily by surface shedding, lymphatic spread, or, rarely, hematogenously.

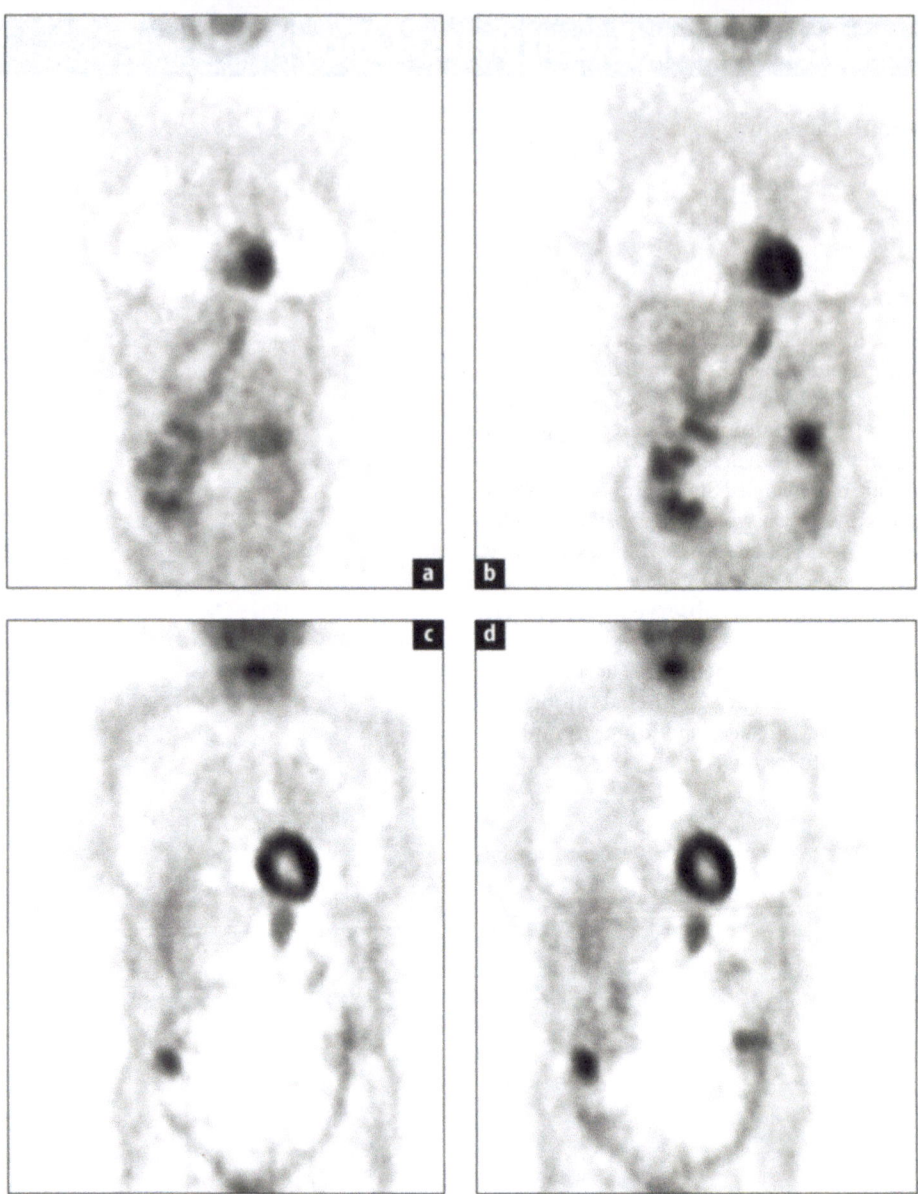

Figure 1 a–d

Diagnosis: Ovarian carcinoma with multifocal perito-neal spread/recurrence.

Patient and History: 75-year-old patient with ovarian carcinoma detected in 1982; the patient had received standard surgery, chemotherapy and radiation therapy. In 1991, she suffered a tumor recurrence which could be surgically removed. In 1995, increasing CA 125 levels were observed, but conventional imaging did not detect a tumor site.

Technique: Emission scans with a slice thickness of 4 mm, image reconstruction by filtered backprojection.

PET Results: The series of coronal images (**a–d**) show slightly enhanced tracer uptake in projection on parts of the small and large intestine. Focally enhanced uptake can be seen in the lower right abdomen as well as two hot spots, (**a**) right lateral abdomen and (**b**) left lateral abdomen. No extraabdominal tracer accumulation was observed. In addition, high tracer uptake is found in the myocardium and in the larynx (normal variants).

Histology: Ovarian carcinoma with peritoneal spread.

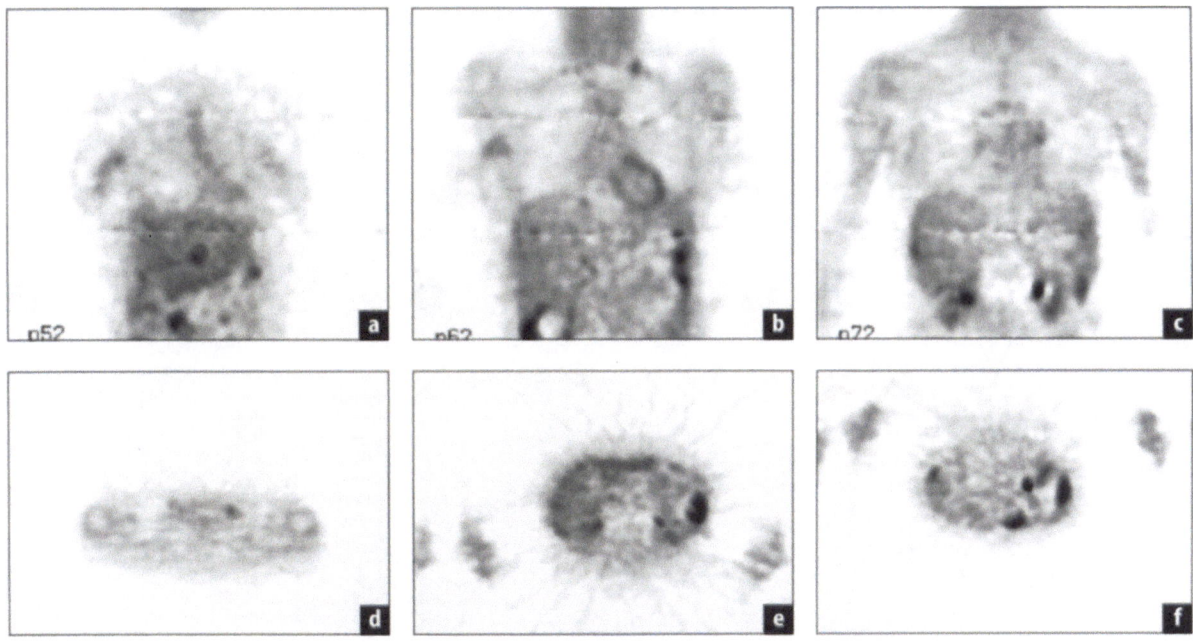

Figure 2 a–f

Diagnosis: Ovarian carcinoma with peritoneal spread and lymph node metastases.

Patient and History: 47-year-old patient with ovarian cancer in 1993. Patient received standard surgery, chemotherapy and radiation therapy. In 1995 increasing tumor markers were observed.

Technique: Transmission-corrected scans with a slice thickness of 4 mm, image reconstruction by filtered backprojection.

PET Results: The series of coronal (**a–c**) and transaxial (**d–f**) views show multiple hot spots within the abdomen, in the liver and one in the left supraclavicular region. Faint uptake in mediastinal lymph nodes.

Histology: Ovarian carcinoma, FIGO III.

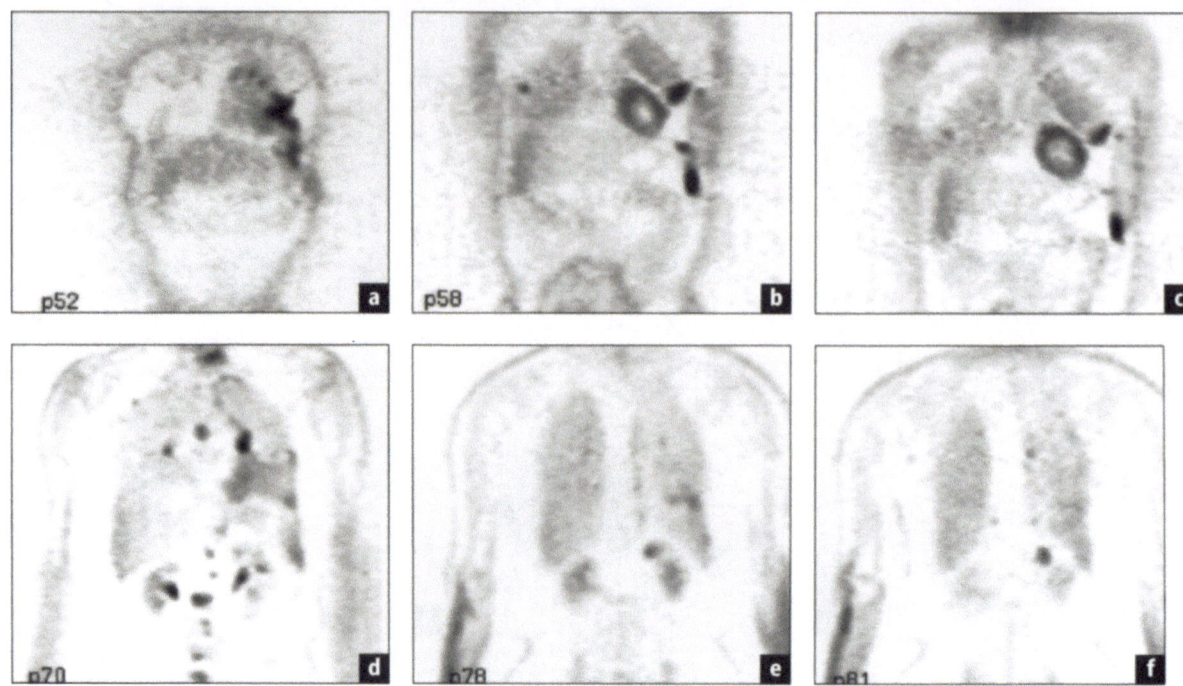

Figure 3 a–f

Diagnosis: Ovarian carcinoma with lung/pleural metastases.

Patient and History: 43-year-old patient with ovarian carcinoma (1990). Patient received standard surgery and chemotherapy. In 1993 increasing tumor markers (CA 125) were observed.

Technique: Emission scans with a slice thickness of 4 mm from ventral to dorsal, image reconstruction by filtered backprojection.

PET Results: The series of coronal views (**a–f**) show multiple foci in projection on the left lung/pleura (extensive), right lung/thorax wall, mediastinum, and left lateral upper abdomen.

Histology: Ovarian carcinoma with distant metastases.

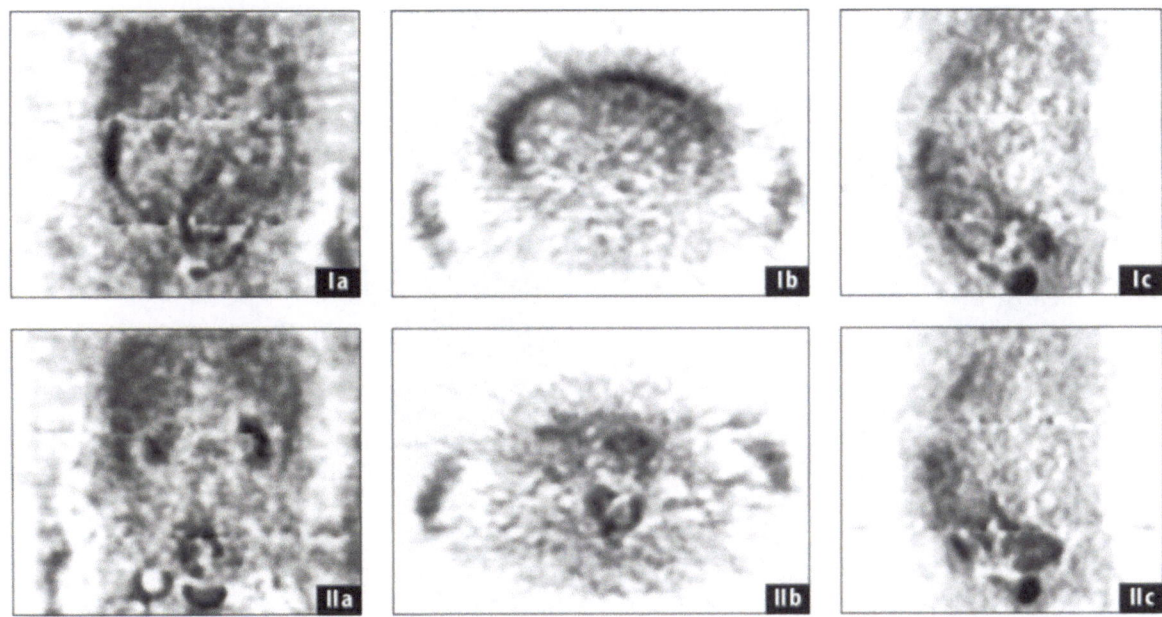

Figure 4/I a–c/II a–c

Diagnosis: Ovarian cancer with peritoneal effusion (malignant ascites).

Patient and History: 75-year-old patient with newly developed massive ascites.

Technique: Transmission-corrected scans with a slice thickness of 4 mm, image reconstruction by filtered backprojection.

PET Results: The series (**I–II**) of coronal (**a**), transaxial (**b**) and sagittal (**c**) views show intense tracer uptake in projection along some parts of the small and large bowel. In addition, the abdomen shows a diffuse tracer uptake in the range of the liver activity, which can be barely seen.

Histology: Ovarian carcinoma with malignant ascites

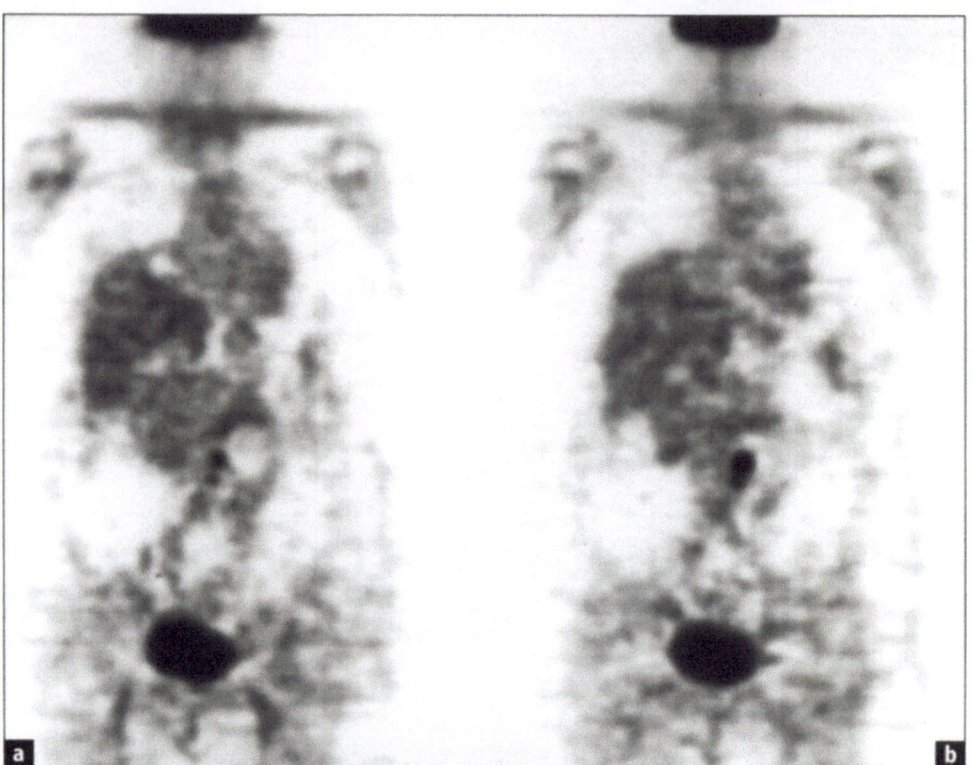

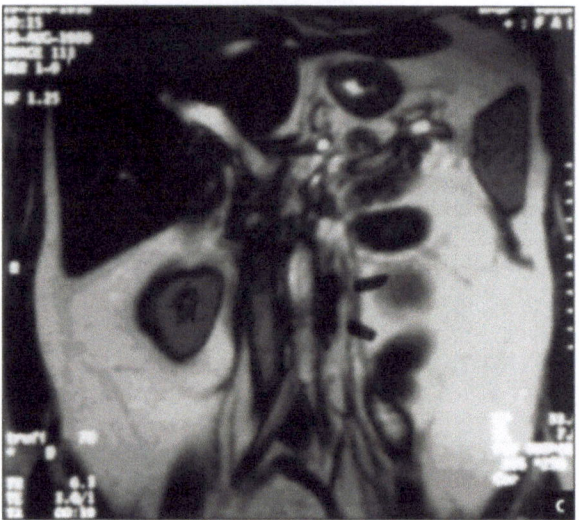

Figure 5 a–c

Diagnosis: Lymph node metastases of a corpus carcinoma.

Patient and History: 61-year-old patient with corpus carcinoma (November 1997). Patient received conventional surgery, radiation therapy and local brachytherapy. Two CT scans within 3 months detected two paraaortic lymph nodes (around 1 cm) which were suspicious and showed questionable increasing size.

Technique: Transmission-corrected scans with a slice thickness of 4 mm, image reconstruction by filtered backprojection.

PET Results: The coronal (**a, b**) views show two confluent foci, localized paravertebrally in the left abdomen corresponding with the lesions described in the MRI scan (**c**) 2 days before.

Histology: Adenocarcinoma of the corpus uteri.

Subject Index